FRCPath P1 Histopathology

Volume 1

Foundations and Visceral Pathology

The Vayden Academic Press

FRCPath Companion Series

❖

Other titles in the series

FRCPath Part 1 — Haematology, Volume 1
General Haematology, Haemostasis and Thrombosis

FRCPath Part 1 — Haematology, Volume 2
Transfusion, Malignant Haematology

FRCPath Part 1 — Histopathology, Volume 2
Surgical Subspecialties

❖

Companion volumes

Integrated Pathology: From Concepts to Diagnosis
Volumes 2A and 2B

Algorithmic Diagnostic Immunohistochemistry
A bench-side companion for surgical pathology

Pathology in Patterns
USMLE companion

Pathway to USMLE
Volumes 1, 2, and 3

All titles available from Amazon worldwide and direct from www.vaydenpress.com.

FRCPath P1 Histopathology

Volume 1

Foundations and

Visceral Pathology

Vishal Tayade

MD Pathology, FRCPath Part 1

Assistant Professor of Pathology

Grant Government Medical College and Sir J.J. Group of Hospitals, Mumbai

VAYDEN ACADEMIC PRESS

Mumbai

Vayden Academic Press

Mumbai 400012, Maharashtra, India

publishing@vaydenpress.com | www.vaydenpress.com

FRCPath Part 1 — Histopathology, Volume 1: Foundations and Visceral Pathology

First edition, 2026

ISBN: 978-81-686730-2-1

Disclaimer

This book has been prepared as a postgraduate revision aid for candidates preparing for the Royal College of Pathologists' Part 1 examination in Histopathology and for qualified medical professionals seeking a structured review of the syllabus content. The text draws on authoritative primary sources (the WHO Classification of Tumours fifth edition, the AJCC Cancer Staging Manual eighth edition, the Royal College of Pathologists' cancer datasets, the International Collaboration on Cancer Reporting datasets, the British Society for Haematology guidelines where overlap with histopathology obtains, and NICE clinical pathways) but is not a substitute for those documents. Examination candidates should consult the current versions of the cited primary sources before the date of their sitting. Diagnostic decisions and reporting practice in routine clinical work should always rest on individual clinical judgement, departmental protocol, and the most recent editions of the authoritative texts named above.

Trademark notice

Distributed internationally via Amazon. Indian direct distribution via www.vaydenpress.com and partnered medical bookstores.

To my parents, with gratitude.

To my teachers, who taught me to look first.

To my students, who taught me what to teach.

⁂

Preface

The Royal College of Pathologists' Part 1 examination in Histopathology, colloquially the FRCPath P1, operates as the principal gatekeeping assessment for higher histopathology training in the United Kingdom and in several Commonwealth pathways modelled upon it. The written paper combines best-of-five single best answer items with extended matching questions drawn from across the discipline, and demands not only factual recall but pattern recognition, classification fluency, and the ability to translate a microscopic observation into the appropriate downstream investigation.

This volume — the first of a two-part companion series under the Vayden Academic Press FRCPath imprint — covers the foundational laboratory sciences, cytopathology, and the medical organ systems most heavily examined in the first sitting: gastrointestinal, hepatobiliary, pulmonary and pleural, cardiovascular, endocrine, renal, and dermatopathological (medical). Volume 2 extends coverage to gynaecological, breast, soft tissue, bone, lymphoreticular, central nervous system, ophthalmic, head and neck, urological, and male genitourinary subspecialties, together with the supplementary paediatric and forensic remits expected at this level.

The pedagogical architecture is uniform across both volumes: mechanism-first stems, two-paragraph rationales, three single best answer questions and one themed extended matching question per chapter, and a citation policy restricted to authoritative sources — the WHO Classification of Tumours fifth edition, the AJCC TNM staging eighth edition, the Royal College of Pathologists' cancer datasets, the International Collaboration on Cancer Reporting datasets, the British Society for Haematology guidelines where overlap with histopathology obtains, and NICE clinical pathways. Secondary textbooks and uncurated online compendia are deliberately excluded from citation, on the principle that examination preparation profits more from primary literacy in the few documents the examiners themselves consult than from breadth across many.

Errata and addenda are published on the Vayden Academic Press website. Correspondence regarding factual content — and especially regarding any deviation from the most recent dataset revision — is welcomed via the publisher and will be acknowledged in subsequent editions.

Vishal Tayade

Mumbai, May 2026

How to Use This Book

Each chapter follows a fixed structure — a brief contextual introduction, anatomical or syndromic orientation where relevant, a systematic walk through the entities encountered at FRCPath P1 level, embedded reporting and grossing notes where directly examined, three single best answer questions with two-paragraph rationales, and a themed extended matching question with ten options and five stems. The rationales serve not as marking schemes but as teaching paragraphs, and frequently extend beyond the immediate stem to flag adjacent traps, recent classification updates, and immunohistochemistry pitfalls.

Visual grammar

The cream box flags worked examples, reporting pearls, and explicit pitfalls. The gold horizontal rule separates major substantive sections. Navy headings denote chapter-level and major divisions; teal headings demarcate finer-grained subdivisions. Figures are numbered by chapter and embedded close to the text they illustrate.

Recommendations for study

Three practical recommendations attend the use of this volume. First, the SBAs should be attempted under timed conditions before the rationale is read — sixty to ninety seconds per stem approximates the examination pace. Second, the EMQ option list at the head of each themed set should be read in full before any stem is attempted, since the examiners construct option lists to discriminate near-miss diagnoses; cursory reading defeats the testing principle. Third, the recommended primary sources at the end of each chapter, drawn exclusively from WHO 5, AJCC 8, RCPath cancer datasets, ICCR datasets, BSH guidelines, and NICE, should be downloaded in current form before any examination sitting; revisions occur frequently, and the dataset version current at the time of writing is annotated where ambiguity may otherwise arise.

Relationship to Volume 2

Volume 1 and Volume 2 are designed to be used in combination. Concepts foregrounded in Volume 1, notably the foundational laboratory sciences and the cytopathology overview, are referenced, not repeated, in Volume 2. The two volumes are available individually or as a paired set at a reduced cover price.

A note on abbreviations and citations

A conservative abbreviations list appears in the back matter. Abbreviations not on the list are spelled out at first use within each chapter. Citations are minimal and restricted to the authoritative source set named above; secondary textbooks and uncurated online resources are not cited. Where a clinical pathway document carries an authoring society other than those listed, the citation is annotated to indicate the consensus source. Errata corrections are published openly on the Vayden Academic Press website and incorporated in subsequent printings.

About the Author

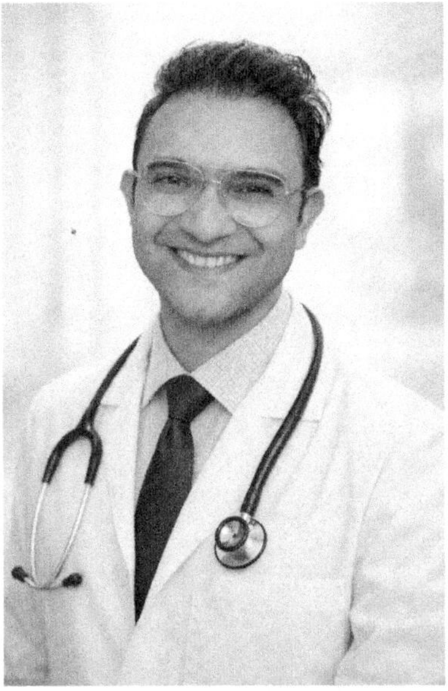

Vishal Tayade

MD Pathology · FRCPath Part 1

Vishal Tayade is Assistant Professor of Pathology at Grant Government Medical College and Sir J.J. Group of Hospitals, Mumbai, where he trains residents in surgical pathology, haematopathology, and cytopathology. He completed his MD in Pathology and training in oncopathology at Tata Memorial Centre, Mumbai. He holds Part 1 of the FRCPath, Royal College of Pathologists, London.

His academic interests sit at the intersection of pattern recognition, integrated diagnostics, and pathology education. He has published in peer-reviewed journals on haematopathology, cytology artefacts, and laboratory diagnostics, and contributes images to the ASH Image Bank.

He is the founder of Vayden Academic Press, dedicated to writing focused, examination-grade textbooks for postgraduate pathology and laboratory medicine. Pathology in Patterns is the USMLE rapid-revision companion to his Pathway to USMLE series, alongside his FRCPath First Paper preparation volumes and the two-volume Integrated Pathology textbook.

Outside the laboratory, he writes literary fiction. His published novels include Love in Chaos, Resonance, the Dr Vishal Sarkar Mystery trilogy, and the literary novels The Chalk Line and No One Was Responsible.

He lives in Mumbai.

Contents

Preface......ix
How to Use This Book......xi
About the Author......xiii

Part I Foundations of Histopathology Practice
Chapter 1. Pre-analytical handling, fixation, processing, and staining......1
Chapter 2. Immunohistochemistry: principles, antibody panels, and controls......20
Chapter 3. Molecular pathology: extraction, PCR, NGS, and variant interpretation......37
Chapter 4. Frozen sections and intraoperative diagnosis......53
Chapter 5. Reporting standards, quality assurance, and error management......67
Chapter 6. Autopsy practice......80

Part II Cytopathology
Chapter 7. Cytopathology principles......91

Part III Gastrointestinal Tract
Chapter 8. Oesophagus......102
Chapter 9. Stomach......115
Chapter 10. Small bowel and appendix......125
Chapter 11. Colon, rectum, and anus......134

Part IV Hepatobiliary and Pancreatic Pathology
Chapter 12. Liver......142
Chapter 13. Biliary tree and gallbladder......151
Chapter 14. Pancreas......158

Part V Pulmonary and Pleural Pathology
Chapter 15. Lung......166
Chapter 16. Pleura......174

Part VI Cardiovascular Pathology
Chapter 17. Cardiac pathology......181
Chapter 18. Vascular pathology......188

Part VII Endocrine Pathology
Chapter 19. Thyroid and parathyroid......195
Chapter 20. Adrenal, pituitary, paraganglioma......202

Part VIII Renal Pathology

Chapter 21. Medical renal disease 209

Chapter 22. Renal tumours 217

Part IX Medical Dermatopathology

Chapter 23. Skin (medical dermatopathology) 224

Abbreviations **231**

Key Sources and Further Reading **233**

Examination Preparation Notes **235**

Index **237**

Chapter 1 — Pre-analytical handling, fixation, processing, and staining

Every histopathological diagnosis rests on a chain of pre-analytical steps that are largely invisible in the final report. A specimen that is malfixed, processed in a tired schedule, or sectioned through a chattered ribbon will yield interpretive errors that no immunohistochemistry or molecular addendum can fully retrieve. The FRCPath Part 1 examiners regard this chain, from theatre handover to the stained slide, as core knowledge, and image-SBA stems frequently embed an artefact that the candidate is expected to recognise as a processing failure rather than a pathological pattern. This chapter sets out the chemistry, mechanics, and quality framework of the routine laboratory workflow.

1.1 Pre-analytical handling

Biopsy and specimen types

Surgical specimens reaching the laboratory range from microscopic shavings to complete organs, and the diagnostic strategy depends on what arrives at cut-up. A needle core biopsy (TruCut) yields a cylindrical fragment two to three centimetres long and one to two millimetres in diameter, sampled blind or under image guidance, and represents a tiny but architecturally intact portion of the lesion. A punch biopsy of skin removes a small cylinder of full-thickness skin and is the workhorse of inflammatory dermatopathology. A shave biopsy removes only the superficial epidermis and papillary dermis; depth of sampling is correspondingly limited and a deep melanoma can be missed if the lesion was not flagged for excision. Incisional biopsy samples part of a lesion to confirm malignancy before definitive surgery, while excisional biopsy aims to remove the entire lesion with a margin and is at once diagnostic and therapeutic. The candidate should match biopsy modality to clinical question — a sentinel lymph node arrives for staging rather than histological subtyping, and a tru-cut breast core arrives for biomarker assessment rather than full architectural review.

Cytology specimens, treated in depth in Chapter 7, intersect the pre-analytical workflow at multiple points. Fine-needle aspiration (FNA) cytology samples cell-rich material from a focal lesion (thyroid nodule, salivary tumour, breast lump) and is processed either as a direct smear or, increasingly, by liquid-based methodology in which the aspirate is rinsed into a preservative fluid (CytoLyt, PreservCyt) and prepared as a monolayer slide. Exfoliative cytology samples spontaneously shed cells from a body fluid (urine, sputum, peritoneal washings, cerebrospinal fluid) and follows a similar liquid-based or cytospin pathway. Tissue arriving fresh for cytology — for example, a serous effusion — has to be processed promptly because cellular detail degrades within hours of collection.

Specimen reception and identification

The specimen journey begins in theatre or the clinic, and the laboratory has only partial control over what arrives at the cut-up bench. The three pillars of safe reception are unequivocal identification, fitness for purpose, and timely fixation. Identification failures — mismatched request forms, two-patient bottle swaps, illegible labels — are the single most-reported pre-analytical incident in RCPath audits. A rigorous two-identifier policy at booking-in, coupled with a positive specimen-tracking system, reduces but does not eliminate the risk. When discrepancy is found, the specimen is quarantined, the clinical team is contacted, and resolution is documented before any cut-up takes place.

Fitness for purpose covers specimen integrity, container appropriateness, and fixative volume. Small biopsies should arrive in a fixative volume ten-fold the tissue volume; large resections require pre-cut bread-loafing to allow penetration. A breast lumpectomy fixed intact will yield central autolysis and a falsely low Ki-67 fraction at the deep margin — a recurrent pitfall in oncology multidisciplinary review.

Fresh specimen routing

Selected specimens are received fresh rather than in fixative. The four classical indications are lymphoma work-up (for flow cytometry and cytogenetics), renal biopsy (for immunofluorescence and electron microscopy), muscle and nerve biopsy (for enzyme histochemistry and frozen-section preservation), and tissue intended for tumour banking. Each requires a pre-agreed handover protocol with the surgical team — a fresh lymph node arriving at the laboratory after the night porter has gone home will autolyse and lose the very antigens for which it was requested.

Grossing and dissection

Grossing — also called cut-up or specimen description — translates a three-dimensional surgical specimen into the two-dimensional sections that ultimately reach the microscope. Three principles govern good grossing: orientation, sampling, and inking. Orientation follows the surgeon's anchoring sutures or anatomical landmarks; loss of orientation in an unpinned colon segment is irreversible once formalin has set the mesentery. Sampling is dictated by ICCR and RCPath dataset guidance — for example, one block per centimetre of tumour diameter in colorectal cancer, with mandatory blocks of the closest radial margin. Inking with differential colours (black for circumferential, blue for proximal, yellow for distal) preserves margin orientation through processing.

Photography at cut-up has shifted from optional to expected. A photograph keyed to block numbers permits later correlation when a discrepant lymph-node count or an unexpected satellite nodule is queried at multidisciplinary meeting. Departmental digital archives — when stored to ISO 15189 retention standards — also support trainee teaching and medico-legal review.

Standardised cut-up datasets, published by the Royal College of Pathologists and harmonised internationally by the International Collaboration on Cancer Reporting (ICCR), define the minimum information that a resection report must contain. These datasets specify which margins are mandatory, what minimum block count is acceptable for each specimen category, and how individual data items (tumour grade, stage, lymph-node count, lymphovascular invasion, perineural invasion) are reported. ICCR datasets are aligned with AJCC TNM 8 staging and with WHO 5th edition classifications. Adherence is audited at peer review and at external accreditation visits, and a cut-up report that omits a mandatory data item is flagged as a minor non-conformity by UKAS assessors.

Specimen rejection criteria are written into every accredited laboratory standard operating procedure. Categories of mandatory rejection include unlabelled specimens, mismatched specimen and request form, specimens received in inappropriate fixative for the requested test (for example, formalin-fixed tissue submitted for flow cytometry), and specimens whose pre-analytical delay exceeds the locally defined limit. Borderline rejections — partial labelling, incomplete clinical details, ambiguous laterality — are escalated to the consultant on call and resolved with documented clinical contact before processing.

1.2 Fixation

Purpose and chemistry of fixation

Fixation arrests autolysis, stabilises tissue architecture, and renders proteins and nucleic acids resistant to the dehydration and clearing solvents used later. The ideal fixative — none exists in practice — would penetrate rapidly, preserve antigenic epitopes, leave nucleic acids intact, and impose minimal shrinkage. Real-world fixatives strike compromises across these axes, and the laboratory selects between them on the basis of tissue type, downstream test, and turnaround time.

Ten per cent neutral buffered formalin — abbreviated as 10% NBF, equivalent to four per cent formaldehyde — is the universal default. Formaldehyde acts by forming methylene bridges between basic amino acid residues (lysine, arginine, histidine) on adjacent proteins, producing cross-links that lock tertiary structure. The neutral phosphate buffer (pH 7.0–7.4) prevents the gradual oxidation of formaldehyde to formic acid, which would generate the brown granular formalin pigment classically seen in heavily haemorrhagic tissue. Penetration follows the Medawar equation — depth proportional to the square root of time — so a 4 cm-thick liver biopsy needs at least twenty-four hours, whereas a needle core fixes in one to two hours.

Under-fixation causes incomplete cross-linking, leaving the centre of a block soft and prone to chatter during microtomy. The hallmark is a pale, smudged, often holey central zone with a sharper outer rim — pathognomonic of formalin that has not reached the core. Over-fixation, by contrast, masks epitopes by excessive cross-linking; antigen retrieval can recover most antibodies but a small subset (notably some clones of oestrogen receptor and HER2) remain compromised. The ASCO/CAP breast biomarker guidance therefore caps formalin fixation of breast resections at seventy-two hours and sets a minimum of six hours.

Alternative fixatives

Bouin solution — picric acid, formaldehyde, and glacial acetic acid — is favoured for testicular and gastrointestinal biopsies because it accentuates nuclear detail and chromatin texture. The drawback is that picric acid degrades nucleic acids and renders the block unsuitable for downstream PCR or in-situ hybridisation. Bouin-fixed material is therefore avoided where molecular work is anticipated.

Zenker fluid and the related Helly fluid contain mercuric chloride and produce excellent nuclear preservation. They are now largely historical because mercury disposal is regulated and the residual mercury pigment — black, refractile, intracellular granules — must be removed from sections by iodine and thiosulphate treatment before staining. B5 fixative (a mercuric variant) was popular for bone marrow trephines but has been displaced by formalin-based protocols compatible with modern immunohistochemistry.

Alcohol-based fixatives — methanol, ethanol, and the proprietary alcohol formalin substitutes — preserve nucleic acids better than aldehyde fixatives, at the cost of greater tissue shrinkage and altered chromatin texture. They are used in cytology (CytoLyt, PreservCyt for liquid-based cervical cytology) and for selected molecular pathology protocols. Glutaraldehyde, a five-carbon dialdehyde, provides superior ultrastructural preservation and is the standard fixative for electron microscopy at concentrations of two to four per cent.

A summary of fixative trade-offs is set out in the next box.

Fixative selection — quick reference

10% NBF: default. Cross-links proteins; pH-buffered to suppress formalin pigment. Compatible with IHC, FISH, and most NGS assays after antigen and epitope retrieval.

Bouin: excellent nuclear detail; testis, GI biopsies. Avoid if PCR or ISH planned — picric acid degrades nucleic acids.

B5 / Zenker: mercury-based, sharp nuclear preservation. Largely historical; disposal-restricted. Watch for mercury pigment.

Alcohol fixatives: nucleic-acid sparing; favoured in cytology. Cause shrinkage and altered chromatin.

Glutaraldehyde 2–4%: electron microscopy. Penetrates slowly; tissue cubes have to be no more than 1 mm.

Formalin handling and safety

Formaldehyde is a category 1B carcinogen under the European CLP regulation, with an occupational exposure limit of 0.3 ppm (eight-hour TWA) and a short-term limit of 0.6 ppm. The laboratory therefore controls vapour through downdraught dissection benches, sealed transport containers, and pre-filled fixative cassettes that avoid open-bottle decanting. Spill response uses sodium bisulphite or a proprietary formalin neutraliser; waste formalin is collected for incineration rather than poured to drain.

Broader chemical and biological safety

Beyond formalin, the laboratory handles xylene (neurotoxic, hepatotoxic, sensitiser), ethanol (flammable; bulk storage demands fire-rated cabinets), strong acids (decalcification), and a range of dyes and silver-staining reagents. Each substance is documented under a COSHH (Control of Substances Hazardous to Health) risk assessment, with controls graded by exposure route, concentration, and duration of contact. Safety data sheets are kept readily accessible at every workstation, and trainees are introduced to the COSHH framework as part of induction. Eye protection, lab coats, and nitrile gloves are mandatory at cut-up; respirator-equipped helmets are used for autopsy work and for handling specimens of suspected high-pathogenicity disease.

Biological safety classifies infectious agents into containment levels (ACDP categorisation in the United Kingdom, BSL classification in the United States) that determine the laboratory engineering controls and personal protective equipment required for safe handling. Routine surgical specimens are managed at containment level 2, suitable for the majority of viral and bacterial agents encountered in everyday practice. Specimens from suspected or known cases of tuberculosis, hepatitis B and C, HIV, prion disease, and viral haemorrhagic fever attract level 3 handling, including the use of class II biological safety cabinets, double-bagged disposal, and dedicated waste streams. Prion disease (Creutzfeldt-Jakob disease and variants) is the highest-consequence pre-analytical risk because prions resist conventional formalin fixation and standard autoclave sterilisation; suspected cases follow a specific national protocol with dedicated single-use equipment.

Waste streams are segregated by hazard category. Yellow bags collect clinical waste destined for incineration; orange bags collect non-anatomical clinical waste for alternative treatment; sharps go into rigid yellow or purple containers depending on cytotoxic content; chemicals are collected in vendor-supplied bulk drums for licensed disposal. The laboratory keeps a waste log and reconciles vendor uplift against in-house generation.

Workforce roles and integration

Histopathology is a team service. Consultant pathologists hold ultimate diagnostic responsibility and lead multidisciplinary review. Specialty registrars rotate through subspecialty firms during training. Biomedical scientists (BMS) operate the technical workflow — reception, processing, embedding, microtomy, routine staining — and at advanced levels (advanced practitioner BMS) report defined specimen categories under consultant supervision. Medical laboratory assistants (MLAs) support reception and slide preparation. Mortuary technicians (anatomical pathology technicians, APTs) support autopsy practice. Histopathology secretaries handle report transcription, distribution, and clinical liaison. The candidate should recognise that the diagnostic report at the end of the chain is the product of an integrated workflow, not an isolated consultant act.

Multidisciplinary team (MDT) meetings represent the principal external clinical interface. The histopathologist presents the morphological findings, integrates them with radiology and clinical context, and supports a treatment recommendation. Preparation discipline matters: cases are reviewed in advance, ancillary tests reviewed, and any equivocal findings explicitly flagged. The MDT record is itself a documented clinical entity, and an inconsistency between the histology report and the MDT minute is a recognised source of complaint.

Antigen retrieval principles

Aldehyde cross-linking, useful as it is for architectural preservation, masks many antibody epitopes by sequestering them within rigid protein networks. Antigen retrieval — also called epitope retrieval — reverses this masking and is now a near-universal pre-treatment step before immunohistochemistry. Two families dominate. Heat-induced epitope retrieval (HIER) places the section in a buffered solution heated to high temperature (typically a pressure cooker at 121 °C, microwave at 95 °C, or commercial PT module). The heat partially hydrolyses methylene bridges and restores epitope conformation. Buffer chemistry tunes the result: citrate at pH 6.0 is the classical workhorse, suitable for the majority of routine antibodies, while TRIS-EDTA at pH 9.0 is reserved for difficult nuclear antigens including many transcription factors and proliferation markers.

Proteolytic-induced epitope retrieval (PIER) uses enzymes — trypsin, pepsin, proteinase K, or pronase — to cleave the cross-linked peptide backbone. PIER is used for a small number of antibodies, including some basement-membrane targets (collagen IV, laminin) and a few cytokeratins, where HIER produces over-retrieval and background. Many modern protocols combine a brief PIER pre-treatment with HIER. The candidate should remember that retrieval is empirically optimised for each antibody clone — a manufacturer-recommended protocol is the starting point, and laboratory-level validation against known positive and negative tissues is required before deployment.

Over-retrieval produces non-specific staining, loss of tissue from the slide, and degraded morphology. Under-retrieval produces weak or absent staining despite a viable epitope. The internal positive control on every immunohistochemistry slide — an in-built tissue element known to express the antigen, such as normal squamous mucosa for p63 or normal endothelium for CD31 — is the day-to-day check that retrieval has succeeded.

Antigen retrieval — buffer selection at a glance

Citrate pH 6.0: default for cytokeratins, hormone receptors, most cytoplasmic markers.

TRIS-EDTA pH 9.0: nuclear targets — Ki-67, TTF-1, p63, p40, MyoD1, transcription factors broadly.

EDTA pH 8.0: middle ground, used by some vendors for proliferation and oncogene targets.

Proteolytic (PIER): collagen IV, laminin, some basement-membrane and matrix antibodies.

None (omit): a small set of antibodies (occasional CD45 clones) actually deteriorate after retrieval; vendor protocol applies.

1.3 Decalcification

Calcified tissue — bone, calcified valves, dystrophic calcification in tumours — cannot be sectioned at the routine four to five micrometre thickness without shattering the blade. Decalcification removes calcium salts from the tissue before processing, and the agent chosen has direct consequences for downstream staining and molecular work.

Strong mineral acids — nitric and hydrochloric acid — decalcify rapidly (hours) but destroy nuclear basophilia and degrade nucleic acids. They are reserved for emergency frozen-section settings where speed dominates. Formic acid, weaker and slower (one to several days), preserves morphology better and is the workhorse for routine bone biopsies in many laboratories. EDTA, a chelating agent rather than an acid, is the gentlest option: it preserves antigens for immunohistochemistry, retains DNA suitable for FISH and PCR, and is the agent of choice for bone marrow trephines and orthopaedic specimens destined for translocation testing. The price is time — EDTA may take one to three weeks for a large resection — and a long turnaround is the principal limitation in busy services.

Microwave-assisted decalcification accelerates EDTA action and is now standard in many academic centres. Surface decalcification, a manual technique in which a partly-blocked specimen is briefly bathed in acid to soften the cut face, is a useful rescue for occult calcium encountered at microtomy.

1.4 Tissue processing

Stages and chemistry

Processing converts fixed, water-laden tissue into a paraffin-infiltrated block suitable for microtomy. The classical schedule has four stages: dehydration, clearing, infiltration, and embedding. Dehydration uses graded alcohols — typically seventy, eighty, ninety-five, and one hundred per cent ethanol — to displace water from the tissue. Direct transfer to pure alcohol would cause sudden osmotic shrinkage and tissue distortion; the ascending series is deliberately gentle.

Clearing replaces alcohol with a solvent that is miscible with both alcohol and paraffin. Xylene is the traditional clearing agent, named for the optical clearing it produces as tissue refractive index approaches that of the surrounding solvent. Xylene is hepatotoxic, neurotoxic, and a sensitiser; many laboratories now use xylene substitutes (limonene-based clearants, isoparaffinic solvents) that reduce occupational exposure at the cost of slightly slower clearing.

Infiltration replaces the clearing agent with molten paraffin wax (melting point 56–58 °C). The wax permeates the tissue, providing the support that allows thin sectioning. Modern paraffins are polymer-blend formulations — DMSO additives improve infiltration of dense tissue and reduce sectioning chatter. After infiltration the tissue is embedded in a metal mould, orientated as required, and allowed to cool. The finished block — tissue surrounded by wax, mounted on a cassette — is ready for the microtome.

Processor types and schedules

Two architectures dominate. Closed (vacuum) processors, exemplified by the Sakura Tissue-Tek VIP and the Leica ASP series, pump reagents through a sealed retort and rotate baskets through a fixed schedule. Open carousel processors — older, larger, slower — are largely obsolete in modern services but persist where rapid throughput is not needed.

Schedules are graded by length. An overnight schedule (twelve to fourteen hours) suits routine surgical specimens. A rapid schedule (one to four hours), used in microwave-assisted processors, supports same-day reporting of small biopsies. A long schedule (twenty-four hours or more) is reserved for fatty tissue (breast, lipoma) where slow penetration prevents core fat retention. Schedule mismatch is the commonest processing error — fatty tissue placed on a rapid schedule yields the classic Swiss-cheese chatter on cutting, where adipocyte cavities are unsupported by wax.

Reagent rotation and processor validation

Processor reagents — alcohols, clearing agent, and paraffin — degrade with use. Alcohols become dilute as they accumulate water from the previous tissue; clearing agent accumulates residual alcohol; paraffin becomes contaminated with carry-over wax and water. A reagent rotation schedule moves the least-contaminated bottle to the first position and discards the most-contaminated, with a fresh bottle introduced at the end of the chain. The frequency of rotation depends on tissue volume and is validated against specific gravity (for alcohols), water content (Karl-Fischer titration in advanced laboratories), and visual inspection.

Validation of a new processor schedule follows the ISO 15189 verification pathway: parallel running of test and control schedules on matched specimens, comparison of section quality, IHC reactivity, and downstream molecular yields. A processor that has been changed (new schedule, new reagent supplier, new wax) is not signed off until validation evidence is logged. This discipline matters because a silent processing fault propagates through every block in a batch and can yield a cluster of unexplained equivocal reports before it is detected.

Processing failures — bench recognition

Soft, holey core: under-fixation reached the processor; alcohol failed to displace residual water. Re-fix and re-process.

Brittle, crumbling block: over-dehydration or exhausted alcohols. Soak in glycerol-water before re-cutting.

Greasy, poorly-supported fat: rapid schedule applied to fatty tissue. Re-process on extended schedule.

Black formalin pigment: acidic formalin with haemorrhagic tissue. Treat with picric acid in alcohol to bleach the pigment.

Refractile mercury granules: Zenker or B5 residue. Treat with Lugol iodine, then sodium thiosulphate, before staining.

1.5 Embedding and microtomy

Orientation at embedding determines what the pathologist sees down the microscope. Skin shave biopsies are embedded on edge to display the epidermal-dermal junction; small bowel biopsies are orientated to give a longitudinal cut through villi; lymph nodes are bisected through the hilum. Multi-fragment specimens (endometrial pipelles, prostate cores) are embedded so that every fragment lies in the same plane.

Microtomy at four to five micrometres is the routine section thickness. Sections are floated on a warm water bath (40–45 °C) to flatten the wax ribbon, picked up on slides, and dried at 60 °C for thirty minutes before staining. Common microtomy artefacts include chatter (parallel fine ridges, often from a worn blade or a partly-fixed core), knife marks (single deep scratches along the cutting axis, from a nicked blade), and floaters (small tissue fragments from a previous block contaminating the water bath). Floaters are a recognised cause of misdiagnosis — a stray fragment of well-differentiated carcinoma on an otherwise benign block can mislead the unwary observer; suspicion arises when the fragment sits in a different focal plane from the surrounding tissue.

Frozen sections — covered in detail in Chapter 4 — use a cryostat to section unfixed tissue at minus 20 °C without prior processing. Ice-crystal artefact, in which water freezes into intracellular vacuoles that distort nuclei, is the dominant pitfall and is mitigated by rapid freezing in isopentane chilled with liquid nitrogen.

Slide adhesion and section recovery

Sections detach from slides during heat-pretreatment for antigen retrieval, especially with TRIS-EDTA at pH 9 and a pressure cooker cycle. The defence against this is a charged-slide surface that binds the section by electrostatic attraction. Three adhesives are commonly used. Poly-L-lysine coated slides, the classical preparation, work well for routine H&E but adhere less reliably to small or fragmented biopsies. Silane-coated slides (3-aminopropyltriethoxysilane, APES) bond more firmly and are preferred for difficult specimens such as endomyocardial biopsies and small renal cores. Commercial Plus and Superfrost Plus slides use a proprietary positive-charge surface and are now the default in most accredited services.

Despite all precautions, section loss does occur. Recovery options are limited — a recut from the block is the simplest answer, provided depth permits. When a unique section is lost and recut is impossible, the laboratory documents the loss, informs the reporting pathologist, and undertakes the next-block deeper level. The clinical team is informed of any delay. Block exhaustion, in which the lesion of interest has been entirely consumed, is now uncommon with modern conservation discipline but remains a possibility on tiny needle biopsies — a sobering reason for careful first-cut planning.

1.6 Routine staining: haematoxylin and eosin

Chemistry and rationale

The haematoxylin and eosin stain — universally abbreviated H&E — has been the foundation of histopathology for more than a century. Its survival reflects a happy chemistry: haematoxylin binds basophilic structures (nuclei, ribosomes, calcium deposits) in royal blue to purple, while eosin tints cytoplasm, collagen, and most secretions in shades of pink. The colour contrast, combined with the trained eye, encodes a remarkable density of architectural and cytological information.

Haematoxylin alone has no affinity for tissue — it is the oxidised derivative haematein, bound to a metal mordant, that gives the colour. Aluminium mordants (Mayer, Harris, Gill formulations) produce the familiar blue-purple stain; iron mordants (Weigert haematoxylin) yield a black nuclear stain resistant to subsequent acidic counterstains and are preferred when an acid stain such as Van Gieson follows. Eosin Y is an acidic xanthene dye; the addition of a small amount of phloxine in Eosin-Phloxine formulations sharpens the contrast of cytoplasm and connective tissue.

The four sequential steps of a routine H&E are deparaffinisation in xylene, rehydration through graded alcohols, nuclear staining, and counterstaining with eosin, followed by dehydration, clearing, and mounting. Progressive haematoxylin formulations (Mayer) stain to a defined endpoint and need no differentiation. Regressive formulations (Harris) overstain and then require an acid alcohol differentiation step, with blueing in ammonia or lithium carbonate water to develop the final blue colour. Both approaches yield identical microscopic results when properly controlled.

Common H&E faults

Weak nuclear staining indicates an exhausted haematoxylin solution, a missed blueing step, or a section that was overheated during drying. Pink nuclei suggest inadequate blueing — the haematein-aluminium complex remains red-brown rather than developing its true blue colour. Patchy staining points to incomplete deparaffinisation, leaving residual wax that excludes aqueous stains. Edge-of-section pallor reflects insufficient flotation time or a section that has not fully adhered to the slide.

Automated and rapid H&E

Almost all routine H&E is now performed on automated linear staining instruments. The Leica Autostainer XL and Sakura Tissue-Tek Prisma are representative platforms — a rack of slides progresses through a defined sequence of dip baths under microprocessor control, with timing, agitation, and reagent renewal logged for audit. Automation has two practical consequences. First, batch-to-batch reproducibility is excellent, and the manual variability of older bench-stained H&E has largely disappeared in accredited laboratories. Second, when a fault does occur, it tends to affect every slide in the batch simultaneously; diagnostic vigilance at first slide review is therefore the early-warning step. Rapid H&E protocols compress staining time into ten to twelve minutes, supporting same-day frozen-section feedback and intraoperative review.

Mounting and coverslipping complete the slide workflow. Mountant — usually a synthetic resin (DPX or its commercial equivalents) — joins the dehydrated, cleared section to the coverslip and provides the optical match that lets the microscope objective focus through to the tissue. Air bubbles, trapped mountant droplets, and inadequate clearing produce optical artefacts that are easy to misread as cytoplasmic vacuolation or refractile pigment. Automated coverslippers, replacing manual application, are now the norm and reduce both artefact rate and operator exposure to xylene vapour.

1.7 Special stains

Special stains — also termed histochemical stains — exploit specific chemical reactions to demonstrate substances that H&E alone cannot resolve. The major families are carbohydrate stains, connective tissue stains, microorganism stains, pigment stains, and amyloid stains. Each has a defined indication, a positive and negative control, and a recognisable failure mode.

Carbohydrate stains

Periodic acid–Schiff (PAS) demonstrates neutral mucins, glycogen, basement membranes, and fungal cell walls. The reaction oxidises 1,2-glycol groups to aldehydes, which then react with Schiff reagent to yield magenta. Diastase digestion (PAS-D) removes glycogen, allowing distinction between glycogen-rich and mucin-rich material — a glycogen-rich tumour such as clear cell renal cell carcinoma loses its PAS positivity after diastase, whereas a mucin-secreting adenocarcinoma retains it. Alcian blue at pH 2.5 stains acidic (sulphated and carboxylated) mucins, and the combined Alcian blue / PAS sequence is the workhorse for goblet-cell mucin in intestinal metaplasia. Mucicarmine stains epithelial mucin red and is classically used to confirm cryptococcal capsule.

Connective tissue stains

Masson trichrome demonstrates collagen (blue or green, depending on dye choice) against muscle and cytoplasm (red), making it the standard stain for hepatic fibrosis staging. Van Gieson highlights collagen pink and muscle yellow; elastic Van Gieson (EVG) adds Verhoeff iron haematoxylin to stain elastic fibres black, the standard for vascular pathology and for highlighting elastic-tissue invasion in lung carcinoma. Reticulin (Gomori silver) demonstrates type III collagen, indispensable for hepatic architectural assessment — preservation of the reticulin framework distinguishes regenerative nodules from hepatocellular carcinoma, and trabecular thickening greater than two cells supports malignancy.

Microorganism stains

Ziehl-Neelsen demonstrates acid-fast bacilli — mycobacteria — as red rods against a methylene blue background; the auramine-rhodamine fluorescent variant offers greater sensitivity for screening. Grocott methenamine silver (GMS) stains fungal cell walls black and is preferred over PAS for sparse fungal organisms because the silver precipitate is darker and more readily detected at low power. Giemsa demonstrates Helicobacter pylori, parasites, and lymphoid chromatin; modified Steiner and Warthin-Starry silver stains are alternatives for spirochaetes and other slender bacteria.

Pigment and mineral stains

Perls Prussian blue demonstrates ferric iron (haemosiderin) by reaction with potassium ferrocyanide in acid, yielding a vivid blue precipitate. It is essential in haemochromatosis (parenchymal iron in hepatocytes) and in iron-deficiency assessment in bone marrow. Fontana-Masson silvers reduce melanin and argentaffin granules — useful for melanocytic lesions and for Cryptococcus, whose capsule contains a melanin precursor that reacts positively. Von Kossa demonstrates calcium phosphate by silver deposition; it stains the anion (phosphate) rather than the cation, so a positive result confirms phosphate-bound calcium but does not specifically prove calcium itself, a distinction occasionally raised in MCQ stems.

Amyloid stains

Congo red is the classical amyloid stain — it binds the beta-pleated sheet structure of amyloid fibrils, producing a salmon-pink stain in bright field and pathognomonic apple-green birefringence under crossed polarisers. The birefringence, not the bright-field colour, makes the diagnosis; a candidate who reports a positive Congo red without confirming birefringence has produced an incomplete observation. Thioflavin T and S yield fluorescent positivity and offer higher sensitivity at the cost of needing fluorescence microscopy.

Special stain controls — a non-negotiable

Positive control: A known-positive section run in parallel on every batch. Failure invalidates the test slide.

Negative control: Omit the dye, or use a section known to lack the target. Confirms non-specific staining is absent.

Internal control: An adjacent normal structure on the same slide (e.g. bile duct in liver for cytokeratin). The first quality check at the microscope.

Daily log: Reagent lot, control result, technician initials. Required for ISO 15189 and audit.

Failure protocol: Repeat with fresh reagent, escalate to senior BMS, document in non-conformance log.

Special stain panels by clinical context

Special stains are rarely ordered singly in modern practice; the clinical question usually demands a panel. In medical liver biopsy, the standard panel is Masson trichrome (fibrosis), reticulin (architecture), PAS-D (alpha-1 antitrypsin globules and Kupffer-cell digestion patterns), Perls (iron), and orcein or Victoria blue (copper-associated protein and hepatitis B surface antigen). In a chronic gastritis biopsy the workhorse panel is modified Giemsa or Warthin-Starry for Helicobacter, and Alcian blue / PAS for intestinal metaplasia. In suspected infection in an immunocompromised patient, the standard infection panel runs ZN, GMS, Gram (Brown-Hopps), and a Giemsa or Warthin-Starry for spirochaetes. The candidate who can name the panel by clinical scenario is performing at sign-out level.

1.8 Digital pathology and slide scanning

Whole-slide imaging — WSI — captures the entire glass slide as a multi-resolution digital file viewable on a workstation. WSI adoption has accelerated since FDA primary-diagnostic clearance in 2017 and the United Kingdom national digital pathology programme. The FRCPath examination now uses digital images in its image-SBA component, and a working knowledge of the workflow is examinable in its own right.

Scanning combines bright-field optics, a motorised stage, and an automated focus and tiling algorithm. The slide is divided into thousands of small fields of view, each captured at the chosen objective magnification (typically 20× or 40× equivalent), then computationally stitched into a pyramidal multi-resolution image stored in a vendor-specific or DICOM-aligned format. File sizes per slide range from several hundred megabytes to several gigabytes, and the storage architecture is a non-trivial part of the implementation cost.

Quality control of WSI extends the principles of analogue slide QC. Pre-scan inspection rejects slides with cracked coverslips, large air bubbles, or smeared mountant. Post-scan validation checks every image for focus uniformity, stitching artefacts, and tissue coverage. Routine calibration uses a tissue micro-array or a dedicated phantom slide. ISO 15189 has been amended to address digital pathology, and the Royal College of Pathologists has published specific guidance on the validation pathway required before a scanner is used for primary diagnosis. Inter-scanner reproducibility, colour-management profiles, and monitor calibration of the reporting workstation all enter the audit trail.

Common WSI artefacts deserve recognition. Tile-boundary stitching errors produce thin visible lines across the image, and out-of-focus tiles produce circular blurred zones where the auto-focus failed on a tissue void. A red-green or magenta-cyan colour cast usually reflects a monitor calibration drift rather than a tissue or stain problem; the practical check is to compare the digital image against the original glass slide on a microscope.

Digital pathology validation — RCPath summary

Validation set: A minimum of sixty cases spanning the case mix of the service, reported on glass and on WSI by the same pathologist with a washout interval.

Concordance threshold: Intra-observer agreement of at least ninety-five per cent for major diagnoses; discrepancies investigated and documented.

Scanner and monitor: Calibration to a documented colour profile; phantom slide checks at defined intervals; monitor luminance and resolution recorded.

Workflow audit trail: Slide barcoding, scan QC, image-to-case linkage, and reporting workstation all entered into the laboratory information system.

Ongoing assurance: Continued inclusion of WSI cases in EQA and discrepancy review; re-validation after scanner replacement or major software change.

1.9 Artefacts

Artefacts are histological features generated by handling rather than by disease, and their recognition is examinable at every level. Crush artefact compresses small round-cell tumours into smears of streaky chromatin — recognised in small bowel and lymph-node biopsies, and a recurring trap in lymphoma stems. Cautery artefact, from diathermy at the resection margin, produces eosinophilic smudging and nuclear elongation that can mimic spindle-cell malignancy; the giveaway is the linear distribution at the cut edge. Drying artefact — clear vacuolation of cytoplasm — appears when a section sits uncovered before mounting.

Pigment artefacts deserve specific recognition. Formalin pigment (acid haematin), as introduced earlier, is brown, granular, and birefringent; it accumulates in heavily haemorrhagic tissue fixed in unbuffered formalin and is removed by picric-alcohol treatment. Mercury pigment, from Zenker or B5 residue, is black, refractile, and removed by Lugol iodine followed by sodium thiosulphate. Malarial pigment (haemozoin) is golden-brown, birefringent, and concentrated in macrophages of spleen and Kupffer cells; it should be distinguished from formalin pigment by clinical context and birefringence pattern. Carbon (anthracotic) pigment is jet-black, non-refractile, and abundant in hilar lymph nodes — endemic in urban populations and unrelated to fixation.

A subset of artefacts can be diagnostically misleading. Floaters — extraneous tissue picked up from the water bath — are recognised by their different focal plane, different staining intensity, and absence from serial sections. Telescoping, in which one segment of bowel is pushed into the next during transit, mimics intussusception and is distinguished by the absence of true ischaemic change at the entry point. Pseudocalcification, where formalin reacts with carbonate to deposit basophilic granules, mimics genuine calcification but is removed by acid decalcification in seconds — a behaviour that true calcification does not show.

Transit and handling artefacts complete the catalogue. Compression artefact follows narrow-bore biopsy passes; the cores show squashed glands at one end with normal architecture at the other, and the candidate should recognise that the squashed end represents the entry point of the trocar. Retraction artefact — the apparent clear halo around tumour nests in some basal cell carcinomas — is a fixation-and-processing phenomenon rather than a true lymphovascular space, and the unwary trainee may report it as lymphovascular invasion. Ink-bleed artefact occurs when surgical inking is applied without adequate drying or to a wet specimen; the ink tracks along tissue planes and falsely suggests margin involvement at points it never reached.

Staining and mounting artefacts include eosinophilic precipitate (an exhausted or contaminated eosin solution), basophilic powder (haematoxylin precipitate from incomplete filtration), refractile mountant droplets that mimic intracellular vacuoles, and air-bubble artefact under the coverslip that locally distorts polarisation findings. These are all recognised by their non-tissue distribution — they cross cell boundaries indifferently and do not respect histological architecture, which is the diagnostic clue that distinguishes artefact from genuine lesion.

Artefact triage at the microscope

Distribution clue: Artefact crosses cell boundaries and ignores histological architecture; genuine lesion respects them.

Edge versus diffuse: Cautery, ink-bleed, and compression cluster at margins or tissue edges; processing failures are typically diffuse.

Floaters: Different focal plane, different staining intensity, absent from serial sections. Recut to confirm.

Pigments: Site plus refractility plus birefringence: formalin (brown, birefringent, removed by picric alcohol), mercury (black, refractile, Lugol then thiosulphate), malarial (golden, birefringent, in macrophages), carbon (jet black, non-refractile, hilar nodes).

Misleading mimics: Retraction halo ≠ lymphovascular invasion; telescoping ≠ intussusception; pseudocalcification disappears on brief acid decalcification.

1.10 Quality control and external assessment

Quality in histopathology operates on three planes: internal quality control (IQC), internal quality assurance (IQA), and external quality assessment (EQA). IQC is the day-to-day discipline of run-by-run controls — positive special-stain controls, daily reagent checks, and microtome blade-life records. IQA includes peer review of difficult cases, departmental discrepancy meetings, and double-reporting of selected case mixes (for example, all skin lesions reported by trainees). EQA is the externally-administered scheme, in the United Kingdom run by the UK NEQAS network, in which laboratories receive blind cases or stained slides for assessment against a reference standard.

Accreditation to ISO 15189 — the standard for medical laboratories — formalises these activities into a documented quality management system. Key requirements include a designated quality manager, traceability of every result back to the original specimen, a documented turnaround-time policy, an error and incident log, and an annual management review. Pre-analytical and post-analytical phases (specimen reception and report delivery) attract as much auditor attention as analytical performance, reflecting the well-established observation that most laboratory errors occur outside the analyser.

Reporting error in histopathology is broadly classified into interpretive errors (the wrong diagnosis from the correct slides), pre-analytical errors (wrong specimen, wrong block, lost orientation), and clerical errors (typographical, transcription, addressing). Audit data from large UK series consistently identify clerical errors as the most frequent category — a humbling reminder that vigilance at sign-out is not optional.

UK NEQAS schemes for histopathology

The UK National External Quality Assessment Service (UK NEQAS) administers several histopathology-relevant schemes, including general histopathology, immunohistochemistry and in-situ hybridisation, gynaecological cytopathology, and digital pathology. Participating laboratories receive circulated unstained sections (for IHC schemes) or pre-stained slides and corresponding case information, and return reports or staining scores by a defined deadline. Returns are graded against a consensus or reference standard, and consistent poor performance triggers a graduated response — written feedback, mentoring visit, suspension of accreditation, and in serious cases referral to the regulatory body. Participation in a recognised EQA scheme is a UKAS requirement for ISO 15189 accreditation; non-participation is a critical non-conformity.

Root cause analysis and never events

When a serious error is identified — a wrong-patient report, a missed cancer diagnosis, a transfusion of incompatible blood — the laboratory undertakes a root cause analysis (RCA). The RCA technique, drawn from human factors engineering, asks the five-whys question repeatedly until a systemic rather than individual cause is identified. The output is an action plan with named owners and review dates. The discipline matters because a culture that blames the individual at the sharp end fails to fix the system that allowed the error, and the same error recurs.

Specific high-consequence errors are designated as never events in NHS terminology — events that should never occur if defined safety systems are in place. Examples relevant to histopathology include misidentification of a patient leading to wrong-site or wrong-patient diagnosis, retained surgical specimen later discovered in fixative, and loss of a unique specimen during transit. Each never event triggers mandatory external reporting and external review. The candidate is not asked to recite the full list, but is expected to know that the term denotes a class of high-consequence pre-analytical failure with regulatory weight.

Turnaround time and the reporting pathway

Turnaround time (TAT) is the elapsed time from specimen reception to authorised report. National key performance indicators in the United Kingdom set TAT targets by specimen category: small biopsies within seven calendar days for 80 per cent of cases, resections within ten calendar days for the same threshold, and cytology specimens within three to five days depending on subtype. TAT is audited continuously, with monthly departmental review against trajectory, and persistent breaches trigger root-cause review of workflow bottlenecks (cut-up capacity, processing queue, ancillary test delays, consultant validation throughput).

The reporting pathway after slide arrival splits into primary report (consultant or trainee), peer review (where applicable), ancillary test ordering, and final authorisation. Pre-sign-out double-reporting — a second consultant reviewing every case before authorisation — is the standard in some subspecialty services (gynaecological cancer, paediatric pathology) and is now recommended by RCPath for all primary cancer diagnoses in many tumour streams. Reflex ancillary testing (HER2 reflex on every breast carcinoma, MMR immunohistochemistry on every colorectal carcinoma, BRAF reflex on all melanomas above a defined Breslow thickness) is coordinated through standing orders to minimise turnaround impact.

Diagnostic discordance and second-opinion practice

Diagnostic discordance — disagreement between observers reviewing the same case — is a recognised feature of histopathological practice rather than an aberration. Major discrepancy (differing diagnosis affecting clinical management) is rare but is the focus of discrepancy review meetings; minor discrepancy (differing grade, differing nodal count, alternate phrasing) is more frequent and is the basis of audit and education. The Royal College of Pathologists publishes a recommended classification (Cases of Note categorisation, with grades 1 to 4 reflecting clinical impact) that frames the local response, and a recurring pattern of grade 3 or 4 discrepancy triggers individual performance review.

Second-opinion practice — sending a case to a specialist external reviewer — is the formalisation of subspecialist consultation. Cases sent on second opinion follow a documented pathway: the slides and blocks are sent with relevant clinical information, the external opinion is received in writing, the local pathologist either incorporates or notes divergence in the final report, and the recipient is invoiced or supported through NHS reciprocal arrangements. The trainee should know that asking for help is encouraged and that no consultant works at a uniform level of confidence across the breadth of modern histopathology.

1.11 Tissue banking and consent under the Human Tissue Act

Surplus tissue from a diagnostic specimen — material remaining after diagnostic blocks have been taken — is a valuable resource for translational research, biomarker discovery, and tumour banking. In the United Kingdom, the use of such tissue is governed by the Human Tissue Act 2004 (HTA), administered by the Human Tissue Authority. The default position is that any tissue used outside the original diagnostic purpose requires appropriate consent, and many research uses additionally require a project-specific ethics approval and an HTA-licensed storage facility.

Three points are examinable. First, residual tissue stored in a wax block is exempt from the HTA storage licensing requirement when held for clinical care, but is captured by the Act if extracted for research. Second, broad consent for future research can be obtained at the time of the original surgical consent and is recommended practice; specific consent for an identified research project is otherwise required. Third, a Designated Individual at each HTA-licensed facility is legally responsible for compliance, and audit visits assess consent documentation, traceability of stored material, and disposal records. International equivalents (the United States Common Rule, the EU Biobanking and Biomolecular Resources Research Infrastructure framework) follow similar principles with jurisdictional variation.

1.12 Key points

Chapter 1 — key points

Fixation: 10% neutral buffered formalin is the default. Cross-links proteins by methylene bridges. Penetrates passively (Medawar square-root rule); volume ten-fold the specimen; pre-cut large resections.

Decalcification: EDTA chelates calcium and preserves DNA and antigens; required for trephines destined for FISH. Strong acids hydrolyse nucleic acids.

Processing: Dehydration → clearing → wax infiltration. Soft holey core means under-fixation reaching the processor; brittle block means over-dehydration.

Staining: H&E remains the workhorse; special stains run with positive, negative, and internal controls. Congo red requires apple-green birefringence to confirm amyloid.

Digital pathology: RCPath validation pathway: sixty cases, ≥95% concordance, scanner and monitor calibration, audit trail.

Artefacts: Recognised by non-tissue distribution. Crush, cautery, drying, pigments, floaters, telescoping, retraction, ink-bleed.

Quality and HTA: ISO 15189 + UK NEQAS; never events trigger RCA. Surplus tissue for research falls under the Human Tissue Act 2004.

1.13 Chapter SBAs

Q1.1. Cross-linking of basic amino acid residues by methylene bridges is the dominant fixation mechanism for the universal default fixative in surgical pathology. A breast lumpectomy is received intact in a small volume of 10% neutral buffered formalin at the laboratory after a sixteen-hour transit. On sectioning the next day, the central tumour zone is pale, soft, and pulls away from surrounding tissue at the microtome. Which single feature of this scenario is the most likely cause of the central artefact?

A. Acidic, unbuffered formalin generated formalin pigment in the tumour core.

B. Inadequate fixative volume and intact specimen prevented formaldehyde penetration to the core.

C. Excessive cross-linking by prolonged formalin caused masking of nuclear epitopes.

D. Specimen was inadvertently fixed in Bouin solution rather than 10% NBF.

E. Tissue processor used a rapid schedule unsuited to a fatty specimen.

Answer: B

Formaldehyde penetrates tissue by passive diffusion, and the depth reached in a given time follows the Medawar square-root relationship. An intact breast lumpectomy with a thick fatty rim presents a long diffusion path; combined with an inadequate fixative volume — the working rule is ten-fold tissue volume — the formaldehyde concentration at the core falls below the threshold needed for effective cross-linking. The result is a soft, under-fixed centre that chatters and tears during microtomy and yields a pale, smudged appearance with a sharper outer rim. This is the classical pattern of under-fixation reaching the processor, and the remedy is pre-cut bread-loafing of large resections so that fixative reaches all surfaces.

Option A is wrong because formalin pigment is brown granular acid haematin, not pallor and softness. Option C describes over-fixation, which masks epitopes for IHC but does not produce a soft, holey core. Option D, Bouin, would generate yellow staining of tissue and uniform fixation rather than a central defect. Option E is plausible in fatty tissue but produces Swiss-cheese chatter through the entire block, not a localised central pale zone.

Q1.2. Chelation of calcium ions, in preference to acid demineralisation, preserves antigenicity and nucleic acid integrity in calcified tissue. A bone marrow trephine from a patient with suspected multiple myeloma requires decalcification before sectioning, and the haematology team has additionally requested FISH for cyclin D1 rearrangement. Which decalcification agent should the laboratory select?

A. Concentrated nitric acid for one to two hours.

B. Concentrated hydrochloric acid for two hours.

C. Ten per cent formic acid for forty-eight hours.

D. Ethylenediaminetetraacetic acid (EDTA) for several days.

E. Surface decalcification with acid at the block face only.

Answer: D

EDTA is a chelating agent that sequesters calcium ions without exposing tissue to the acidic environment that hydrolyses DNA and denatures protein epitopes. In a trephine destined for FISH, DNA integrity is non-negotiable — strong-acid decalcification will fragment the targets and produce uninterpretable hybridisation signals. EDTA also preserves antigens for the immunohistochemistry panel that typically accompanies plasma-cell work-up (CD138, kappa and lambda, cyclin D1). The trade-off is time: EDTA decalcification of a trephine takes several days, and laboratories supporting myeloma services plan turnaround accordingly.

Options A and B are strong mineral acids that decalcify rapidly but destroy nucleic acids and damage many antibody epitopes. Option C, formic acid, is intermediate and is acceptable for routine bone biopsies but is not preferred when FISH is planned. Option E, surface decalcification, is a microtomy rescue technique for occult calcium at the block face and is inappropriate for a trephine where the entire core requires uniform decalcification.

Q1.3. Binding of dye molecules to the beta-pleated sheet conformation of fibril proteins underlies the histochemical detection of amyloid deposits in tissue. A renal biopsy from an elderly patient with proteinuria shows pink-staining acellular material expanding the mesangium on H&E. Congo red staining of a serial section shows salmon-pink mesangial deposits in bright field. Which observation is required to confirm the diagnosis of amyloidosis?

A. Strong Periodic acid–Schiff positivity of the deposits.

B. Apple-green birefringence of the deposits under crossed polarisers.

C. Loss of staining after diastase pre-treatment of a serial section.

D. Positivity of the deposits with Perls Prussian blue.

E. Negative staining with Masson trichrome of a serial section.

Answer: B

The diagnostic test in Congo red histochemistry is not the bright-field colour but the apple-green birefringence seen when the section is rotated under crossed polarisers. Congophilic salmon-pink staining alone can be produced by a number of non-amyloid substances, including dense collagen and some elastic deposits; the polarisation behaviour reflects the orderly beta-pleated sheet arrangement of amyloid fibrils and is essentially specific. A trainee who reports Congo red positivity without examining polarisation has produced an incomplete observation, and many examination stems test exactly this distinction.

Option A, PAS positivity, is non-specific in the mesangium — diabetic nodules, light-chain deposition disease, and many glomerulopathies show PAS-positive expansion. Option C is the diastase manoeuvre for distinguishing glycogen from mucin, irrelevant to amyloid. Option D, Perls, demonstrates haemosiderin iron and is unrelated. Option E, trichrome negativity, is non-specific and provides no positive confirmation.

1.14 Chapter EMQ

EMQ 1.1. Artefact recognition. For each scenario below, select the single most likely artefact from the option list. Each option may be used once, more than once, or not at all.

A. Floater

B. Cautery (diathermy) artefact

C. Crush artefact

D. Formalin pigment (acid haematin)

E. Mercury pigment

F. Retraction artefact

G. Ice-crystal artefact

H. Ink-bleed artefact

I. Pseudocalcification

J. Telescoping

(1) A skin biopsy of a basal cell carcinoma shows islands of basaloid tumour cells separated from the surrounding stroma by clear acellular spaces, prompting the trainee to consider lymphovascular invasion. The clear spaces do not contain endothelial cells or red cells and follow the contour of every tumour nest. **Answer: F**

(2) A frozen section of a melanoma sentinel lymph node shows large clear vacuoles distorting nuclear contour. The section was prepared on a cold day without using isopentane chilled in liquid nitrogen. **Answer: G**

(3) A liver biopsy from a patient with falciparum malaria, fixed in unbuffered formalin for forty-eight hours during transit, shows abundant brown granular birefringent material at the periphery of haemorrhagic foci. **Answer: D**

(4) An otherwise benign-appearing endometrial pipelle biopsy contains a small fragment of well-differentiated adenocarcinoma that is sharply demarcated from surrounding tissue and sits in a focal plane distinctly different from the rest of the section. **Answer: A**

(5) A colonic polypectomy specimen shows India ink (black) and acetic-acid eosin (red) appearing on both the polyp surface and along the deep submucosal plane, despite an apparently uninvolved deep margin on H&E. The inking was performed on an unblotted, wet specimen at cut-up. **Answer: H**

Chapter 2 — Immunohistochemistry: principles, antibody panels, and controls

Immunohistochemistry (IHC) is the technique that brought antigen-specific staining into the diagnostic pathology workflow, and over four decades it has reshaped what the morphologist can claim from a glass slide. A tumour that is morphologically ambiguous becomes lineage-defined; a poorly-differentiated carcinoma of unknown primary becomes a candidate organ of origin; a sarcoma of uncertain category becomes a translocation candidate; a breast carcinoma becomes a biomarker-stratified treatment plan. The FRCPath Part 1 examiners expect a candidate to know the principle of each step, the pitfalls that mimic disease, and the panel that answers a defined clinical question. This chapter covers the chemistry, controls, and clinical panels that underpin contemporary IHC practice.

2.1 Antibody types and clone nomenclature

Polyclonal, monoclonal, and recombinant antibodies

Antibodies used in diagnostic IHC fall into three structural categories. Polyclonal antibodies are raised by immunising a host species (commonly rabbit) with the target antigen, then harvesting the resulting heterogeneous serum. The serum contains immunoglobulins directed at multiple epitopes on the antigen, which gives polyclonal reagents high sensitivity but variable specificity between batches. Polyclonals remain useful where epitope variation is expected — for example, immunoglobulin heavy and light chains in plasma cell work-up — but their lot-to-lot variability is the major drawback in an accredited service.

Monoclonal antibodies are generated by the Kohler-Milstein hybridoma technique, in which an antibody-producing B cell is fused with an immortalised myeloma line. The resulting hybridoma secretes a single antibody species directed at a single epitope — and that delivers excellent reproducibility and specificity. The trade-off is the binary nature of the binding: if the chosen epitope is masked by fixation or absent in a tumour variant, the monoclonal can yield false negatives. Each monoclonal carries a unique clone designation — for example, ER clone SP1, p63 clone 4A4, HER2 clone 4B5 — and clone identity is logged on every report because clone-specific scoring thresholds and validation data attach to the clone, not to the target alone.

Recombinant antibodies represent the third generation. The variable regions of a chosen monoclonal are cloned into an expression vector and produced in cell culture, eliminating the live hybridoma and the animal welfare and supply-chain limitations that accompanied it. Recombinant rabbit monoclonals are now common and combine the affinity of rabbit immunisation with the reproducibility of recombinant production.

Antibody types — practical summary

Polyclonal: multi-epitope, high sensitivity, batch variation. Examples: rabbit anti-IgG, anti-CD3 polyclonal (now less used).

Monoclonal: single epitope, reproducible. Most diagnostic antibodies. Clone identity matters for scoring.

Recombinant: vector-expressed monoclonals. Reproducible supply, defined sequence.

Clone nomenclature: clone designation logged on report. ER SP1, p63 4A4, HER2 4B5, PD-L1 22C3 and 28-8 and SP142 and SP263 are not interchangeable.

Antibody validation in the diagnostic laboratory

Every new antibody, every new clone, and every change of validated protocol triggers a laboratory-level validation procedure. The RCPath and UK National Quality Assessment Network for IHC (IQN-Path) guidance specifies the steps: a range of known positive and negative tissues are stained in parallel, retrieval and dilution are optimised, and the protocol is compared against a reference standard (a UK NEQAS reference slide, a published gold-standard tissue, or in-house cases with previous concordant results). For predictive biomarker antibodies — HER2, hormone receptors, PD-L1, mismatch repair — the validation is more rigorous because clinical decisions depend on the result; a minimum panel of approximately twenty cases spanning the dynamic range of expression is the accepted norm.

Tissue micro-arrays (TMAs) are widely used in validation. A TMA core block carries dozens or hundreds of small tissue cores in a single section — allowing simultaneous staining of a calibrated reference set. TMAs streamline validation, support inter-laboratory comparison, and are the substrate for many UK NEQAS distributions.

2.2 Detection chemistry

Direct, indirect, and amplified detection

Detection chemistry converts the binding of an antibody to its antigen into a visible chromogenic deposit. The simplest schema is direct detection — in which the primary antibody is conjugated to a reporter enzyme (horseradish peroxidase, HRP, or alkaline phosphatase, AP); the enzyme then catalyses chromogen deposition at the site of binding. Direct detection is fast and gives low background but has limited sensitivity because each antigen molecule yields only one chromogen deposit.

Indirect detection introduces a second-step antibody. The primary antibody is unlabelled; a labelled secondary antibody — raised against the immunoglobulin species of the primary — then binds the primary. Each primary can be bound by several secondaries — amplifying signal. The avidin-biotin complex (ABC) method, popular in the 1980s and 1990s, exploits the high-affinity avidin-biotin bond: a biotinylated secondary is followed by an avidin-HRP complex that delivers many enzyme molecules per primary binding event. ABC remains in use but has been largely displaced by polymer-based detection.

Polymer-based detection (the EnVision system from Agilent-Dako, the PowerVision and BondPolymer systems from competing vendors) replaces the avidin step with a dextran or polymer backbone carrying numerous secondary antibody molecules and HRP enzymes. The polymer delivers very high sensitivity, eliminates the background that endogenous biotin causes (notably in kidney and liver), and is the workhorse of modern automated platforms. Tyramide signal amplification (CSA, catalysed signal amplification) adds a further amplification step using HRP-catalysed deposition of tyramide-conjugated reporter, useful for low-abundance antigens and increasingly for multiplex IHC.

Chromogen selection

Diaminobenzidine (DAB) is the universal default chromogen for HRP-based detection. The HRP oxidises DAB to a brown insoluble precipitate that is stable, permanent, and contrasts well against haematoxylin counterstain. Alkaline phosphatase systems use a different chromogen palette: Fast Red, Vector Red, and AP-blue. Red chromogens are useful when the target tissue has abundant pigment that obscures DAB — melanin in melanoma, anthracosis in lung, lipofuscin in liver — and red staining superimposes more readily on these backgrounds. AEC (aminoethylcarbazole) was once popular as a red HRP chromogen but is alcohol-soluble and incompatible with conventional dehydration and mounting; it is now rarely used.

Automated IHC platforms

Almost all diagnostic IHC is now performed on automated platforms: the Ventana BenchMark and DISCOVERY (Roche), Leica BOND, Agilent-Dako Omnis, and Biocare intelliPATH are representative instruments. Each handles deparaffinisation, retrieval, primary antibody application, detection, counterstaining, and dehydration in a single closed run, with full audit trail of reagent lot, retrieval profile, and operator. Automation has improved reproducibility, reduced operator variability, and is a precondition for UKAS ISO 15189 accreditation in IHC services. Manual IHC persists in research settings and for unusual antibodies that have not been adapted to platform protocols, but in routine diagnostics it is now the exception.

2.3 Controls

A stained slide without controls is uninterpretable. Three families of controls are deployed in routine IHC. The positive control demonstrates that the entire run worked on tissue known to express the antigen. The negative control demonstrates absence of non-specific binding from the secondary system. The internal control — present on the test slide itself — verifies that the run worked on that particular section. Each family addresses a distinct failure mode — none is redundant.

Positive controls: on-slide and off-slide

On-slide internal positive controls exploit normal tissue elements adjacent to the lesion. Normal endothelium is the internal control for CD31 and CD34; normal squamous epithelium for p63 and p40; normal hepatocytes for HepPar-1 in liver tumour assessment; normal smooth muscle for desmin and SMA. The trained observer scans these elements before reading the test result — a negative CD31 in a vascular tumour means little if the adjacent normal endothelium also fails to stain, because the run itself has failed.

Off-slide positive controls are run on a separate dedicated control slide containing tissue known to express the target. A multi-tissue control block — often a composite paraffin block containing tonsil, appendix, liver, kidney, breast, and prostate — provides a built-in positive control for the majority of antibody targets in a single section. Multi-tissue blocks are now standard in accredited laboratories and reduce the cost and complexity of dedicated single-tissue controls.

Negative controls

Three approaches to negative control are described, with different rigour. The no-primary control omits the primary antibody and detects non-specific binding of the secondary detection system; it is the most commonly used. The isotype control replaces the primary with an irrelevant antibody of the same immunoglobulin class and concentration, controlling for non-specific Fc-mediated binding. The omission control simply runs through the protocol without any antibody and confirms that chromogen deposition is antibody-dependent. The omission control is the bare minimum and is now considered insufficient for accredited practice; on-slide internal negative tissue (normal lymphocytes in a CK panel, or normal stromal cells in an epithelial marker run) provides the most clinically meaningful negative check.

Control families — a clinical summary

On-slide internal positive: scan adjacent normal tissue first; failure of the internal positive invalidates the test result.

Off-slide positive: multi-tissue block run with every batch. Records reagent and platform performance.

On-slide internal negative: non-target normal cells on the same section. Confirms specificity in that particular tissue.

No-primary negative: controls non-specific binding of secondary system.

Isotype negative: controls non-specific Fc-mediated binding; used in research and selected diagnostic contexts.

2.4 In-situ hybridisation as an adjacent technique

In-situ hybridisation (ISH) is the cousin technique to IHC — instead of detecting a protein with a labelled antibody, ISH detects a nucleic acid sequence (DNA or RNA) with a labelled complementary probe. The result, like IHC, is a chromogenic or fluorescent signal localised to the cell or subcellular compartment of interest. ISH is essential for several diagnostic questions that IHC alone cannot resolve, and the two techniques are routinely interpreted side-by-side on the same case.

Fluorescence in-situ hybridisation (FISH) uses fluorophore-labelled probes — typically a target probe in one colour and a control centromere or break-apart probe in a second colour — visualised on a fluorescence microscope. FISH is the gold standard for HER2 amplification testing in breast and gastric cancer, for translocation testing in soft-tissue sarcomas (EWSR1 break-apart in Ewing sarcoma family, SS18 in synovial sarcoma, FUS in low-grade fibromyxoid sarcoma, DDIT3 in myxoid liposarcoma), and for ALK and ROS1 rearrangements in lung adenocarcinoma. Chromogenic and silver in-situ hybridisation (CISH, SISH) deliver the same biological information on bright-field microscopy — a particular advantage when fluorescence microscopy is not available and when slides need to be archived under conventional storage.

RNA in-situ hybridisation (RNAscope) detects messenger RNA transcripts with high specificity using a paired-probe technology — two adjacent probes are required for signal amplification, dramatically reducing background. RNAscope is increasingly used for diagnostic questions where the protein antibody is unreliable, including HPV-related oropharyngeal carcinoma (high-risk HPV E6/E7 mRNA), Epstein-Barr virus-associated lymphoma and nasopharyngeal carcinoma (EBER-1 ISH), and for selected viral and chimeric transcripts. The technique is technically more demanding than DNA-ISH and requires careful tissue handling to preserve RNA integrity — a poorly-fixed or long-archived block can yield false-negative RNAscope results.

The candidate should know which question is best answered by which technique. Protein expression — IHC. Gene amplification (HER2, MYCN, MET) — FISH or CISH. Gene rearrangement or translocation — break-apart FISH. Viral RNA expression — RNAscope or EBER-ISH. Methylation status — methylation-specific PCR or pyrosequencing rather than ISH. Mutation detection — Sanger sequencing or targeted next-generation sequencing.

Choosing the technique for the question

Protein presence/absence: IHC — fast, cheap, available everywhere.

Gene amplification: FISH or CISH dual-probe — HER2/CEP17, MYCN, MET.

Gene rearrangement: break-apart FISH — EWSR1, SS18, ALK, ROS1, FUS, NTRK.

Viral RNA: EBER-ISH for EBV; high-risk HPV mRNA for oropharyngeal carcinoma.

Specific mutation: targeted PCR, Sanger, or NGS — IHC surrogates (BRAF V600E, IDH1 R132H) exist for selected mutations.

2.5 Multiplex immunohistochemistry

Multiplex IHC (mIHC) stains a single section with two or more antibodies simultaneously, displaying their patterns in different colours. The technique answers questions that sequential single-stain slides cannot — for example, co-localisation of two markers in the same cell, spatial relationships between tumour and immune compartments, or quantitative ratios within a defined tissue zone. Two technical strategies are in routine diagnostic use.

Sequential chromogenic multiplex runs antibodies one after another, each with a different chromogen (DAB followed by Fast Red, followed by a third chromogen if needed). The result is a bright-field slide readable on a standard microscope. Sequential multiplex is limited to three or four markers before chromogen overlap becomes ambiguous, and the order of staining matters because earlier rounds can be partially eluted or masked by later steps.

Tyramide-based multiplex (Opal, Akoya Biosciences) uses HRP-catalysed deposition of a tyramide-fluorophore conjugate, followed by stripping of the primary antibody complex before the next round. The same secondary detection system can therefore be reused across six or seven markers, each tagged with a different fluorophore. The resulting multiplex slide is read on a multispectral fluorescence platform with image-analysis software that unmixes the spectra. Tyramide multiplex is the dominant research-grade approach and is finding diagnostic applications in PD-L1 immune-cell quantification and in tumour-immune microenvironment characterisation.

Newer methods extend multiplexing to higher dimensions. Imaging mass cytometry, codetection by indexing (CODEX), and multiplexed ion beam imaging (MIBI) can interrogate forty or more markers on a single section but remain research tools at the time of writing. The FRCPath candidate is not expected to operate these platforms but should know that they exist and that the principle is sequential or simultaneous detection of many antibodies with isotope or fluorophore tagging.

2.6 Antibody panels by clinical question

In routine practice IHC is rarely ordered as a single antibody. Instead — panels are constructed around a defined differential diagnosis. The candidate who can construct the panel from the clinical question — rather than reflexively staining for everything — is operating at consultant level. The following subsections set out the panels examined most frequently at Part 1.

Carcinoma of unknown primary

Carcinoma of unknown primary (CUP) is the classical panel question — and remains the foundation example. The first-line panel orients the lineage and source. Cytokeratin 7 and cytokeratin 20 anchor the algorithm: CK7+/CK20- favours lung, breast, thyroid, gynaecological tract, and salivary gland; CK7-/CK20+ favours colorectal and Merkel cell; CK7+/CK20+ favours pancreatobiliary, gastric, urothelial, and ovarian mucinous tumours; CK7-/CK20- favours hepatocellular, renal cell, prostate, adrenocortical, and some squamous and neuroendocrine tumours. Lineage-specific transcription factors then refine the location: TTF-1 (lung adenocarcinoma, thyroid), GATA3 (breast, urothelial), CDX2 (intestinal), PAX8 (gynaecological, thyroid, renal), p63 and p40 (squamous and urothelial), SALL4 (germ cell), HepPar-1 and arginase-1 (hepatocellular).

A useful general principle is that a tumour with a strong organ-restricted transcription factor positivity (TTF-1, CDX2, PAX8) is much more likely to represent that organ than a tumour with only a positive cytokeratin pattern. The 2024 ICCR guidance for CUP recommends a stepwise approach: morphology and CK7/CK20 first, then lineage transcription factors, then organ-restricted markers, with molecular testing reserved for cases that remain unresolved after IHC. A subset of CUP cases (around 10 per cent) remain unclassifiable despite a broad panel.

Lymphoma initial work-up

Lymphoma work-up begins with confirmation of haematopoietic lineage — and lineage subtyping. The first-line panel is CD45 (LCA, pan-leucocyte), CD20 (B cell), CD3 (T cell), CD79a (B cell, retained in plasma cells), and CD30 (Hodgkin lymphoma, anaplastic large cell, embryonal carcinoma). A negative CD45 with positive cytokeratin redirects to a non-haematopoietic diagnosis — carcinoma, melanoma, or sarcoma. Once B- or T-lineage is established, second-line markers identify specific lymphoma subtypes — BCL2, BCL6, MUM1, CD10 for diffuse large B-cell lymphoma cell of origin; CD5, CD23, cyclin D1 for mantle cell and small lymphocytic lymphomas; CD138, MUM1, kappa, lambda for plasma cell neoplasms. Detailed lymphoma classification is covered in the Vol 2 lymphoid chapter; the present text covers only the initial orientation panel.

Spindle cell and round cell tumour panels

Spindle cell tumours demand a panel that excludes the four common categories — sarcomatoid carcinoma, melanoma, lymphoma, and sarcoma. The standard first-line panel runs cytokeratins (broad-spectrum AE1/AE3 plus a second cytokeratin), S100 and SOX10 (melanoma and nerve sheath), CD45 (lymphoma), and one or two soft-tissue markers (desmin or smooth muscle actin for smooth muscle; CD34 for vascular and dermatofibrosarcoma protuberans). A positive cytokeratin reorients to sarcomatoid carcinoma; positive S100 and SOX10 reorient to melanoma or nerve sheath; positive CD45 reorients to lymphoma. Negative all-four positions the lesion as soft-tissue sarcoma and triggers a second-tier soft-tissue panel.

Round cell tumour panels follow a similar logic, distinguishing small round blue cell tumours into lymphoma, neuroblastoma, Ewing sarcoma family, embryonal rhabdomyosarcoma, desmoplastic small round cell tumour, and small cell carcinoma. The orientation panel includes CD45, cytokeratin, synaptophysin and chromogranin (neuroendocrine), CD99 (Ewing family, membranous), desmin and myogenin (rhabdomyosarcoma), and WT1 (desmoplastic small round cell tumour, dot-like). Molecular confirmation is increasingly part of the work-up for the translocation-defined sarcomas.

Melanoma confirmation

Melanoma is diagnosed morphologically when classical features are present but requires IHC support when atypical or amelanotic. The standard melanoma panel includes S100 (sensitive but not specific — also stains nerve sheath, chondrocytes, myoepithelial cells), SOX10 (nuclear, more specific than S100 in routine diagnostic settings), HMB-45 (cytoplasmic, premelanosomal protein gp100), Melan-A (cytoplasmic, MART-1), and tyrosinase. SOX10 is the most reliable single marker for melanocytic lineage including spindle and desmoplastic variants in which HMB-45 may be negative. A panel of SOX10 plus HMB-45 or Melan-A is the day-to-day workhorse, with S100 added for spindle and desmoplastic cases.

Thyroid epithelial tumours

Thyroid follicular-derived tumours have a focused panel — TTF-1 and PAX8 confirm thyroid lineage (positive in papillary, follicular, poorly-differentiated, and anaplastic carcinomas, plus follicular adenoma), thyroglobulin supports differentiated origin (positive in follicular and papillary, often lost in poorly-differentiated and anaplastic), and BRAF V600E IHC (clone VE1) serves as a surrogate for the V600E mutation in papillary carcinoma. Medullary carcinoma, of parafollicular C-cell origin, shows positive calcitonin, chromogranin, synaptophysin, and CEA — and is negative for thyroglobulin, which is the discriminating combination. Anaplastic thyroid carcinoma frequently loses thyroglobulin and may be PAX8-positive only; a panel of cytokeratin, PAX8, and TTF-1 confirms thyroid origin in an otherwise undifferentiated mass.

Prostate carcinoma panel

Prostate carcinoma diagnosis on biopsy turns on the absence of a basal cell layer in a small focus of suspicious glands, supported by IHC. The classical prostate biopsy panel — often run as a triple cocktail — is high-molecular-weight cytokeratin (HMWCK, 34BE12 clone) and p63 to mark basal cells, with AMACR (P504S) as a positive tumour marker. Benign glands show a continuous basal cell layer (positive HMWCK and p63); high-grade prostatic intraepithelial neoplasia retains a discontinuous basal layer; and invasive adenocarcinoma loses the basal layer entirely and is positive for AMACR. PIN-4 (a commercial cocktail of HMWCK, p63, and AMACR in different chromogens) delivers the panel in a single slide. PSA and PSAP confirm prostatic origin in a metastatic deposit. NKX3.1 is a sensitive nuclear marker for prostate lineage and is retained even in poorly-differentiated and treated tumours where PSA is lost.

Neuroendocrine differentiation

Neuroendocrine tumours, from any organ, share a defining panel — chromogranin A, synaptophysin, and INSM1. Chromogranin is the more specific marker (cytoplasmic granular staining); synaptophysin is more sensitive but slightly less specific. INSM1, a nuclear transcription factor, is now the third routine marker and is particularly valuable in poorly-differentiated tumours and small cell carcinomas where chromogranin may be weak or focal. CD56 is added in some panels but is less specific and stains a wider range of tumours. Once neuroendocrine differentiation is confirmed, the next question is grade, classically expressed as Ki-67 proliferation index — under three per cent for grade 1 (well-differentiated), three to twenty per cent for grade 2, and over twenty per cent for grade 3 (WHO 2019 GEP-NEN classification) or for neuroendocrine carcinoma.

Soft-tissue tumour second-tier markers

Once a soft-tissue tumour is positioned as a sarcoma rather than carcinoma, melanoma, or lymphoma, the second-tier panel narrows the subtype. Smooth muscle markers — desmin, h-caldesmon, smooth muscle actin (SMA) — define leiomyosarcoma and gastrointestinal stromal tumour. Skeletal muscle markers — desmin, myogenin (MyoG, clone F5D), MyoD1 — define rhabdomyosarcoma; nuclear myogenin positivity is the most specific marker for skeletal muscle differentiation. Vascular markers — CD31, CD34, ERG, FLI-1 — define angiosarcoma and vascular tumours; ERG is the most specific nuclear vascular marker and is preferred over CD34 (which also stains spindle cell lipoma, dermatofibrosarcoma protuberans, solitary fibrous tumour, and many others). Adipocytic markers are limited — S100 stains adipocytes weakly, MDM2 and CDK4 mark well-differentiated and dedifferentiated liposarcoma via gene amplification. The IHC panel is increasingly integrated with FISH and molecular testing because translocation-defined sarcomas (synovial, Ewing family, alveolar soft part, clear cell, myxoid liposarcoma) have specific fusion partners detectable on break-apart FISH.

2.7 Mismatch repair immunohistochemistry

Mismatch repair (MMR) IHC interrogates loss of expression of the four MMR proteins — MLH1, MSH2, MSH6, and PMS2. These proteins function as heterodimers — MLH1-PMS2 and MSH2-MSH6, and loss of one partner typically destabilises the other in the same dimer. Loss of MLH1 with concurrent loss of PMS2 is the commonest pattern and represents MLH1 promoter hypermethylation (sporadic) or germline MLH1 mutation (Lynch syndrome). Loss of MSH2 with concurrent loss of MSH6 represents MSH2 mutation; isolated MSH6 or PMS2 loss indicates a mutation in the unpaired protein.

MMR IHC is now performed reflexly on all newly diagnosed colorectal carcinomas in the United Kingdom (NICE guidance) and on selected endometrial carcinomas. Loss of any one protein triggers a sequential algorithm: BRAF V600E testing or MLH1 methylation testing to triage sporadic versus germline cases, with germline candidates referred to clinical genetics. The IHC interpretation depends critically on a reliable internal positive control, since loss is defined by complete absence of nuclear staining in tumour with retained staining in adjacent stromal lymphocytes and normal epithelium. A weak or patchy positive does not equate to loss, and a heterogeneous tumour with both retained and lost zones may reflect intratumoural mosaicism that complicates interpretation.

MMR loss patterns and downstream actions

MLH1/PMS2 loss: commonest sporadic pattern. Reflex MLH1 methylation or BRAF V600E. Germline if methylation negative.

MSH2/MSH6 loss: Lynch syndrome until proven otherwise; refer to clinical genetics.

Isolated MSH6 loss: MSH6 mutation. Germline MSH6 carriers have a milder phenotype and later cancer onset.

Isolated PMS2 loss: PMS2 mutation. The least common pattern; clinical genetics referral.

All retained: MMR-proficient; no Lynch indication from IHC. MSI testing reserved for selected cases.

2.8 HER2 and hormone receptor immunohistochemistry

HER2 in breast and gastric carcinoma

Human epidermal growth factor receptor 2 (HER2) IHC is the gateway test for HER2-targeted therapy in breast and gastric cancer. The ASCO/CAP 2018 (updated 2023) guidance for breast HER2 defines a four-tier scoring system. Score 0 represents no staining or membrane staining incomplete and faint in up to 10 per cent of tumour cells. Score 1+ represents incomplete and faint staining in more than 10 per cent of cells. Score 2+ (equivocal) represents weak-to-moderate complete membrane staining in more than 10 per cent of cells, or intense complete membrane staining in 10 per cent or fewer cells; this score triggers reflex in-situ hybridisation. Score 3+ (positive) represents intense complete membrane staining in more than 10 per cent of cells.

Gastric HER2 scoring follows a distinct algorithm, reflecting the lateral and basolateral staining pattern of gastric tumours that often spares the apical membrane. The biopsy threshold permits a positive score with as few as five clustered tumour cells showing intense membrane staining, recognising the focal nature of HER2 expression in gastric carcinoma. Pathologists familiar with breast HER2 must remember that gastric scoring uses different rules and that direct translation across organs is incorrect.

The 2023 update to ASCO/CAP breast HER2 guidance introduced the HER2-low concept, defined as IHC 1+ or 2+ ISH-negative tumours. HER2-low status now drives eligibility for antibody-drug conjugates such as trastuzumab deruxtecan, making the distinction between IHC 0 and IHC 1+ clinically actionable — a distinction that previously had no consequence and was therefore often under-emphasised. The candidate should be alert to the pre-analytical sensitivity of this distinction: under-fixation or over-decalcification of a breast core can shift a low-expressing tumour between scores.

HER2 in-situ hybridisation algorithm

A HER2 IHC score of 2+ (equivocal) triggers reflex in-situ hybridisation. The dual-probe ISH algorithm enumerates HER2 signals (red) and chromosome 17 centromere signals (CEP17, green) in twenty representative tumour nuclei, then calculates two parameters — the HER2/CEP17 ratio and the average HER2 copy number per cell. The 2018 ASCO/CAP guidance, retained in the 2023 update, classifies the result into five groups. Group 1 (HER2/CEP17 ratio at least 2.0 and average HER2 copy number at least 4.0) is HER2-positive. Group 5 (ratio under 2.0 and copy number under 4.0) is HER2-negative. Groups 2, 3, and 4 are intermediate and trigger an additional concurrent review with the IHC slide and a recount by a second observer — each intermediate group has a defined resolution pathway that ends with a binary positive or negative call.

Common pitfalls in HER2 ISH include scoring of non-tumour cells (lymphocytes, stromal cells), miscounting in chromosome 17 polysomy, and failure to identify the invasive tumour focus rather than carcinoma in situ. Internal control is the surrounding normal breast epithelium — diploid HER2 and CEP17 signals — and a run that fails to demonstrate diploid control invalidates the test. ISH on small biopsy specimens can be technically demanding when only a handful of invasive tumour cells are present; a re-test on the excision is the recommended approach when biopsy yield is insufficient.

Hormone receptors: ER, PR, AR

Oestrogen receptor (ER) and progesterone receptor (PR) status are reported on every breast carcinoma and on selected gynaecological tumours. The standard scoring schemes are the Allred score (proportion plus intensity, totalling 0 to 8) and the percentage-positive scheme (continuous variable from 0 to 100 per cent). Both yield the same clinical action: ER positivity above the 1 per cent threshold supports endocrine therapy, although the 2020 ASCO/CAP guidance noted that tumours expressing ER at 1 to 10 per cent (ER-low) have intermediate prognosis and treatment benefit. Internal positive control is normal breast lobular and ductal epithelium; loss of internal positivity invalidates the result. Androgen receptor (AR) is increasingly assessed in triple-negative breast cancer where AR-positive disease may benefit from selected hormonal manipulation.

PD-L1 in immunotherapy selection

Programmed death-ligand 1 (PD-L1) IHC is the predictive biomarker for immune checkpoint inhibitor therapy — non-small cell lung cancer, urothelial carcinoma, triple-negative breast cancer, head and neck squamous carcinoma, and others. The challenge for the histopathologist is that multiple validated clones (22C3, 28-8, SP142, SP263) are tied to specific drug indications and to specific scoring algorithms — and they are not interchangeable. The tumour proportion score (TPS), used in lung cancer for pembrolizumab eligibility, counts the percentage of viable tumour cells with partial or complete membrane staining at any intensity. The combined positive score (CPS), used in head and neck and urothelial cancer, counts both tumour cells and immune cells (lymphocytes, macrophages) showing membrane staining, divided by total viable tumour cells and multiplied by 100. The immune cell score (IC), used historically in SP142 trials in lung, scores only the proportion of tumour area occupied by PD-L1-positive immune cells.

Clinical scoring thresholds depend on the indication: TPS at least 50 per cent for first-line monotherapy in advanced lung cancer; TPS at least 1 per cent for second-line; CPS at least 1 in head and neck; CPS at least 10 in gastric. The pathologist reports the score against the specified threshold and identifies the clone used. UK NEQAS and the IQN-Path scheme run regular PD-L1 schemes because inter-observer variability remains a recognised problem; experienced reporters and frequent calibration improve agreement.

PD-L1 — clones, indications, and scoring

22C3 (pharmDx): pembrolizumab. Lung TPS, head and neck CPS, urothelial CPS, gastric CPS.

28-8: nivolumab. Lung TPS, head and neck CPS, urothelial.

SP142: atezolizumab. Lung IC (historical), triple-negative breast IC.

SP263: durvalumab. Lung TPS, urothelial.

Scoring discipline: identify the clone, identify the algorithm, identify the threshold. Do not interchange.

2.9 Pitfalls and artefacts in IHC

IHC is rich in artefacts that mimic disease — and the experienced reporter learns each one. Edge effect describes intensified staining at the periphery of a tissue section, where fixation and processing are most complete and antibody penetration is maximal; the centre of a large block may appear falsely negative by comparison. Edge effect is particularly troublesome for large resections fixed intact, and pre-cut bread-loafing during cut-up is the prophylaxis.

Endogenous biotin is the classical pitfall of avidin-biotin detection systems, which is one of several reasons polymer-based detection has displaced ABC in modern laboratories. Liver and kidney parenchyma contain abundant endogenous biotin that the avidin reagent binds non-specifically, producing strong false-positive cytoplasmic staining indistinguishable from genuine antibody binding. Endogenous biotin is overcome by a blocking step (avidin followed by biotin) or, more reliably, by using a polymer-based system that does not depend on the avidin-biotin bond. Endogenous peroxidase, abundant in red blood cells, neutrophils, and eosinophils, presents the parallel problem in HRP-based systems and is blocked by pre-treatment with hydrogen peroxide.

Pigment confusion is a common trap in melanoma and liver pathology. Melanin pigment is brown and granular, indistinguishable from DAB chromogen on bright-field microscopy. The discipline is to scan an H&E section for melanin before reading a DAB-stained IHC slide, and to switch to a red chromogen (Fast Red) when melanin is heavy. Lipofuscin, the wear-and-tear pigment of long-lived cells (cardiac myocytes, hepatocytes, neurons), is yellow-brown and can also confuse DAB interpretation; it is autofluorescent under UV illumination, which is the discriminating feature in mIHC platforms. Formalin pigment, as covered in Chapter 1, is brown and birefringent.

Cross-reactivity refers to a primary antibody recognising an unintended target — one with similar epitope sequence. S100 stains melanocytes (intended) but also Schwann cells, chondrocytes, myoepithelial cells, dendritic cells, and adipocytes (unintended for melanoma diagnosis). A clinician asking whether a small spindle cell tumour is melanoma versus schwannoma cannot answer the question with S100 alone — the panel must include SOX10 (positive in both, less useful) and HMB-45 or Melan-A (positive in melanoma, negative in schwannoma). The candidate should know the expected cross-reactivity profile of every routinely-used antibody.

Floaters with positive staining are particularly hazardous because the diagnostic mind tends to trust positive findings. A small fragment of strongly positive tumour cells in an otherwise negative background, sitting in a different focal plane from the surrounding section, should be regarded as a floater until proven otherwise. Confirmation requires recutting at a deeper level and demonstrating absence of the positive fragment.

2.10 Quantitative scoring and image analysis

Manual scoring schemes

Quantitative IHC scoring takes several established forms. The Allred score combines proportion of positive tumour cells (0 to 5) with average intensity (0 to 3) for a total score of 0 to 8. The H-score combines staining intensity with proportion to yield a continuous variable from 0 to 300, calculated as the percentage of cells stained at each intensity multiplied by intensity (3, 2, or 1) and summed. The percentage-positive scheme is simpler — the proportion of tumour cells showing any membrane or nuclear staining (depending on the target) above a defined threshold.

Ki-67 proliferation index is conventionally reported as the percentage of tumour cell nuclei showing any positive staining, counted across a representative high-power area (200 to 500 cells minimum). The Ki-67 result is sensitive to counting technique, hotspot selection, and inter-observer variability; international working groups have published standardised counting protocols (the International Ki-67 in Breast Cancer Working Group) but the practical reproducibility remains modest.

Digital image analysis

Image analysis software — vendor-supplied and open-source — increasingly supports quantitative IHC scoring on whole-slide images. Algorithms segment tumour from stroma, identify positive nuclei or membranes, and produce a numerical readout. Image analysis improves reproducibility for Ki-67 and HER2, but requires careful validation against manual scoring and is not yet a stand-alone replacement for the pathologist's eye. The FRCPath candidate should know the principle and the validation requirement; detailed software operation is not examined at Part 1.

Tumour-infiltrating lymphocyte scoring

Tumour-infiltrating lymphocyte (TIL) scoring has emerged as a prognostic and predictive marker in several tumour types — most established in triple-negative breast cancer and HER2-positive breast cancer, with growing data in colorectal, melanoma, and lung. The International TILs Working Group consensus methodology assesses the percentage of stromal area occupied by mononuclear inflammatory cells (lymphocytes and plasma cells), evaluated on a single representative H&E slide of the invasive tumour at 200 to 400 times magnification. Categories are low (under ten per cent), intermediate (ten to forty per cent), and high (over forty per cent). The score is reported as a percentage and a category. TIL assessment is morphological on H&E — IHC is not required for routine TIL scoring, although CD3 and CD8 staining can refine the composition of the infiltrate when needed.

Frozen-section IHC limitations

Selected intraoperative questions — for example, confirmation of parathyroid tissue, lineage assessment of an unexpected metastasis — can be answered by rapid IHC on a frozen section. Rapid IHC protocols compress retrieval, primary, secondary, and chromogen steps into under thirty minutes. The trade-offs are real: rapid protocols sacrifice some sensitivity and specificity, controls are minimal, and the morphological substrate (a frozen section) is already compromised compared with paraffin. Intraoperative IHC is therefore reserved for tightly defined questions where the answer changes surgical management — a permanent paraffin section with full retrieval and platform staining is the gold standard for any non-urgent question.

2.11 External quality assessment in IHC

The UK NEQAS Immunocytochemistry and In-Situ Hybridisation scheme is the principal external quality assessment programme for diagnostic IHC in the United Kingdom and is widely subscribed internationally. Participating laboratories receive unstained sections of a defined tissue, stain them in their routine workflow, and return slides for central assessment. The assessment is undertaken by a panel of subspecialty pathologists who score each slide for technical and interpretive quality against a published reference standard. Returns yielding consistently poor scores trigger graduated feedback, mentoring visits, and in extreme cases scheme suspension.

The IQN-Path consortium runs additional schemes for predictive biomarkers (HER2, ER/PR, MMR, PD-L1) with stricter quantitative criteria reflecting their clinical impact. Participation in a recognised scheme is a UKAS requirement for ISO 15189 accreditation; non-participation is a critical non-conformity that places the accreditation at risk.

2.12 Cost-effectiveness and reflex testing

IHC is the most expensive routine ancillary test in histopathology by reagent cost per slide. A panel of ten antibodies on a single case represents a non-trivial budgetary impact when scaled across departmental throughput, and laboratory directors are accountable for cost-effective utilisation. Reflex testing — automatic ordering of defined antibody panels at cut-up for certain specimen categories — improves turnaround and embeds clinical guidance into workflow. Common reflexes include MMR on all colorectal carcinomas, HER2 and hormone receptors on all invasive breast carcinomas, TTF-1 and napsin A on all non-small cell lung carcinomas, and PD-L1 on selected indications. Each reflex protocol is documented, has a defined trigger, and is reviewed annually against utilisation and clinical impact data.

A simple worked example illustrates the budgetary scale. A medium-sized UK department reporting 15,000 cases per year, with an average of 1.5 IHC slides per case at a fully-loaded cost of £20 per slide (reagent, technical time, consumables, platform amortisation), spends approximately £450,000 per year on routine IHC alone. Reflex panels add predictable spend (around 150 colorectal MMR panels at £80 each adds £12,000), but un-reflexed ad-hoc requests are the main driver of cost variance. Departmental audit of IHC utilisation — comparing observed panels against ICCR-recommended panels for each specimen category — identifies the cases that drive excess spend and triggers educational interventions.

Trainee QC of an IHC slide at sign-out

The trainee approaching an IHC slide for the first time should follow a fixed quality sequence before interpreting the test result. First, identify the internal positive control on the slide — normal tissue known to express the antigen, adjacent to or within the lesion. Second, scan the negative regions and confirm absence of non-specific background and absence of chromogen precipitate. Third, identify the lesion and assess the stain pattern (nuclear, cytoplasmic, membranous, dot-like, perinuclear, paranuclear). Fourth, score the result against the published threshold or scheme for that antibody. Fifth, document the clone, retrieval, and detection system on the report if relevant to interpretation. A slide that fails the first two checks is uninterpretable and is rejected rather than reported.

2.13 Key points

Chapter 2 — key points

Antibody types: Polyclonal (high sensitivity, batch variation), monoclonal (reproducible, clone matters), recombinant (defined sequence). Clone identity logged on report — ER SP1, HER2 4B5, PD-L1 22C3/28-8/SP142/SP263 not interchangeable.

Antigen retrieval: Citrate pH 6.0 for cytoplasmic markers; TRIS-EDTA pH 9.0 for nuclear targets; proteolytic for matrix antibodies.

Controls: On-slide internal positive is the first check; failure invalidates the run. Off-slide multi-tissue block, no-primary, and isotype controls complete the framework.

MMR IHC: Reflex on every CRC. MLH1/PMS2 loss → BRAF V600E or MLH1 methylation; MSH2/MSH6 loss → genetics. Loss = complete absence with retained internal control.

HER2 and hormone receptors: ER and PR as percentage positive; HER2 by IHC (0/1+/2+/3+) with reflex ISH for 2+. Standardised ASCO/CAP scoring.

Molecular surrogates: BRAF V600E (VE1), IDH1 R132H (H09), ALK (D5F3), ROS1 (D4D6), pan-TRK, SDHB, INI1 (SMARCB1), BRG1 (SMARCA4).

Pitfalls: Edge artefact, endogenous biotin, melanin, pigment masking. Always read with an internal positive in view.

2.14 Chapter SBAs

Q2.1. Heterodimerisation of MMR proteins with destabilisation of the unpaired partner generates the characteristic dual-loss patterns seen on MMR immunohistochemistry. A 68-year-old man with a sigmoid adenocarcinoma has reflex MMR IHC. The tumour shows complete absence of nuclear staining for MLH1 and PMS2 in tumour cells, with retained nuclear staining of MSH2 and MSH6 in tumour, and retained staining of all four proteins in adjacent stromal lymphocytes. Which single next step is the most appropriate?

A. Refer directly to clinical genetics for Lynch syndrome assessment.

B. Repeat the IHC panel — the loss is likely technical.

C. Order BRAF V600E testing or MLH1 promoter methylation analysis.

D. Report as MMR-proficient since MSH2 and MSH6 are retained.

E. Request next-generation sequencing of the tumour for MMR pathway mutations.

Answer: C

Loss of MLH1 with concurrent loss of PMS2 in the tumour, with retained staining in stromal cells (the internal control), is a valid and interpretable MMR-deficient result. The dominant cause of this pattern is sporadic MLH1 promoter hypermethylation, which is in turn often associated with the BRAF V600E mutation. The next step in the NICE-endorsed algorithm is therefore reflex BRAF V600E testing or direct MLH1 methylation analysis to triage sporadic from germline disease. A BRAF V600E-mutant or MLH1-hypermethylated tumour does not need genetics referral; a BRAF V600E-wild-type and MLH1-unmethylated tumour represents likely germline MLH1 mutation and is referred for Lynch syndrome assessment.

Option A is premature — direct genetics referral without triage burdens the service and concerns the patient unnecessarily for what is most often sporadic disease. Option B is incorrect because the internal positive control is valid (retained staining in stroma) and the loss is real. Option D misinterprets MMR loss: any single protein loss defines MMR-deficiency regardless of which proteins are retained. Option E is disproportionate at this stage and is not part of the reflex algorithm for newly diagnosed CRC.

Q2.2. Membrane proportion plus intensity threshold, defined by clone-specific scoring algorithms, governs the interpretation of HER2 IHC in invasive breast carcinoma. A breast core biopsy shows invasive ductal carcinoma. HER2 IHC (clone 4B5) shows weak-to-moderate complete circumferential membrane staining in 40 per cent of tumour cells. Which single most appropriate next step should be recommended?

A. Report as HER2 positive (score 3+) and recommend trastuzumab.

B. Report as HER2 score 2+ (equivocal) and request reflex in-situ hybridisation.

C. Report as HER2 score 1+ (HER2-low) and discuss antibody-drug conjugate eligibility.

D. Report as HER2 negative (score 0) and recommend endocrine therapy if ER positive.

E. Repeat HER2 IHC on the excisional biopsy when available.

Answer: B

The 2018 ASCO/CAP scoring system, retained in the 2023 update, defines HER2 score 2+ (equivocal) as weak-to-moderate complete membrane staining in more than 10 per cent of tumour cells. The described pattern — weak-to-moderate complete circumferential staining in 40 per cent of cells — meets this definition precisely. The recommended action for an equivocal IHC result is reflex in-situ hybridisation (FISH, CISH, SISH, or DDISH) to assess HER2 gene amplification by enumerating HER2 signals and the chromosome 17 centromere control. The ISH result determines the final HER2 status: amplified (HER2 positive) or non-amplified (HER2 negative). HER2-low classification (IHC 1+ or 2+ ISH-negative) becomes available after the ISH result.

Option A overcalls the result — score 3+ requires intense complete membrane staining in more than 10 per cent of cells, not weak-to-moderate. Option C undercalls — score 1+ requires incomplete and faint staining. Option D ignores the membrane positivity entirely. Option E delays the result unnecessarily; equivocal core biopsy IHC is correctly resolved by ISH reflex on the same biopsy without waiting for excision.

Q2.3. Non-specific binding of avidin reagents to endogenous biotin produces a recognisable false-positive pattern in tissues rich in this cofactor. A trainee reviews a renal core biopsy stained for a putative cytoplasmic antigen using an avidin-biotin complex (ABC) detection system. The tumour shows strong granular cytoplasmic staining, but the adjacent normal renal tubules also show strong granular cytoplasmic staining. The off-slide multi-tissue positive control stains as expected. Which single explanation is the most likely?

A. The antibody is performing correctly and the normal tubules express the antigen.

B. Endogenous biotin in renal tubular cells has bound the avidin reagent and produced false-positive staining.

C. Antigen retrieval was over-aggressive and damaged the normal tubular epitope.

D. The negative control was omitted from the run and cannot be assessed.

E. Pigment confusion from lipofuscin in renal tubules has mimicked positive staining.

Answer: B

Renal tubular epithelium and hepatocyte cytoplasm contain abundant endogenous biotin, which binds the avidin component of an ABC detection system with high affinity. The result is false-positive granular cytoplasmic staining in these tissues that is indistinguishable from genuine antibody binding by appearance. The diagnostic clue is that the staining appears in tissues known to carry endogenous biotin, regardless of the primary antibody used. The remedy in legacy ABC protocols is an avidin-biotin blocking step before the primary; the modern solution is to switch to a polymer-based detection system, which does not depend on the avidin-biotin bond and is unaffected by endogenous biotin.

Option A is unlikely because the staining is in normal tubules as well as tumour, and a putative cytoplasmic antigen distributed identically in normal and neoplastic tissue is a red flag for technical rather than biological positivity. Option C describes antigen retrieval damage which weakens or eliminates staining rather than enhancing it. Option D may be true as a separate observation but does not explain the positive pattern in tissues with known endogenous biotin. Option E is incorrect because lipofuscin is yellow-brown and granular but does not behave like a true chromogen — it is autofluorescent and is recognised by its presence on the unstained section.

2.15 Chapter EMQ

EMQ 2.1. Antibody panel selection. For each clinical scenario, select the single most useful next-line antibody or marker from the option list. Each option may be used once, more than once, or not at all.

A. SOX10

B. TTF-1

C. CDX2

D. PAX8

E. GATA3

F. Cyclin D1

G. WT1 (nuclear)

H. Synaptophysin

I. HepPar-1

J. p40

(1) A spindle cell tumour of the back in a 55-year-old man shows weak focal S100 staining. The morphology is suspicious for desmoplastic melanoma. The next antibody to confirm melanocytic lineage is required. **Answer: A**

(2) A 65-year-old woman has a peritoneal nodule. Morphology shows small round blue cells with prominent dot-like cytoplasmic staining on a putative marker. Confirmation of desmoplastic small round cell tumour is sought. **Answer: G**

(3) A lung mass biopsy from a 70-year-old smoker shows a poorly-differentiated tumour. CK7 is positive and CK20 is negative. The next single marker to support a lung adenocarcinoma diagnosis is needed. **Answer: B**

(4) A liver mass biopsy in a patient with cirrhosis shows trabecular tumour with hepatoid morphology. CK7 negative, CK20 negative. The single best lineage confirmation marker is sought. **Answer: I**

(5) A poorly-differentiated carcinoma in a 50-year-old woman shows CK7 positive, CK20 negative pattern. The differential includes urothelial and breast primary. The single most useful next marker to support a breast (or urothelial) origin is needed. **Answer: E**

Chapter 3 — Molecular pathology: extraction, PCR, NGS, and variant interpretation

Molecular pathology has moved from a research-laboratory curiosity to a core diagnostic discipline within a single career span. The morphologist now signs out a colorectal carcinoma with MMR IHC and reflex BRAF/KRAS/NRAS profiling, a lung adenocarcinoma with EGFR, ALK, ROS1, and broad-panel NGS, a melanoma with BRAF V600E and NRAS — and is expected to integrate the result into a report that drives treatment decisions. The FRCPath Part 1 examiners assess principle, not pipette technique — what each test measures, what it cannot measure, how the result is validated, and how it is interpreted alongside morphology and IHC. This chapter sets out the techniques, the workflow, and the variant-interpretation framework that underpin clinical molecular pathology in 2026.

3.1 Sample requirements and pre-analytical considerations

Molecular tests carry sample requirements that the morphologist controls at cut-up. The two dominant variables are tumour cellularity — the proportion of viable tumour nuclei in the tested area — and total nucleic acid yield. A test platform calibrated to detect a variant at five per cent allele frequency requires a tumour cellularity of at least ten per cent, since each tumour cell contributes two alleles and dilution by stromal and immune cells lowers the detectable signal. The reporting pathologist marks a region of interest on an H&E slide, estimates tumour cellularity, and instructs the laboratory accordingly. Macrodissection — scraping the marked region from an unstained section — raises tumour cellularity above the surrounding tissue baseline. Laser-capture microdissection refines the technique further but is reserved for cases with very small tumour foci.

Fixation conditions matter as much as cellularity. Formalin cross-links DNA and degrades RNA, so a poorly-fixed or long-archived block will yield fragmented nucleic acids that fail amplification or library preparation. The standard quality metrics are DIN (DNA Integrity Number, from 1 to 10) and DV200 (the percentage of RNA fragments longer than 200 nucleotides). A DIN below 4 or a DV200 below 30 per cent flags a sample unlikely to give a reliable result, and the laboratory may decline the test or hedge the report. Fresh tissue collected in RNAlater or fresh-frozen tissue gives the best nucleic acid yield and is the substrate of choice when broad molecular profiling is planned in advance.

Pre-analytical discipline for molecular pathology

Tumour cellularity: estimate on H&E — at least 10–20% for routine testing; higher for high-sensitivity assays.

Block age: FFPE blocks remain usable for several years but yield degrades — recent blocks preferred.

Fixation: 10% NBF for 6–48 h optimal; Bouin destroys nucleic acids — never used for molecular targets.

Decalcification: EDTA preserves nucleic acids; strong acids hydrolyse DNA.

Macrodissection: scrape marked tumour-rich area to raise effective cellularity.

Storage: blocks at room temperature; extracted nucleic acids at −80 °C in aliquots.

3.2 Nucleic acid extraction from FFPE

Extraction begins with deparaffinisation — xylene or proprietary deparaffinisation agents dissolve the wax — followed by proteinase K digestion to release nucleic acids from the cross-linked protein matrix. The lysate is purified through silica column or magnetic bead chemistry, with selective elution of DNA, RNA, or total nucleic acid depending on protocol. Yields from FFPE are an order of magnitude lower than from fresh tissue, and the extracted DNA is fragmented — typical fragment lengths fall between 100 and 500 base pairs, which limits the size of amplicon that can be reliably amplified. The laboratory quantifies the extracted material by fluorometry (Qubit) for total nucleic acid and by automated electrophoresis (Bioanalyzer, TapeStation, or LabChip) for size distribution before proceeding to downstream assays.

3.3 PCR-based techniques

Conventional and real-time PCR

Polymerase chain reaction (PCR) amplifies a target DNA sequence between two primers using a thermostable DNA polymerase, most commonly Taq polymerase from Thermus aquaticus, through cycles of denaturation, primer annealing, and extension. Real-time quantitative PCR (qPCR) tracks amplification in real time using a fluorescent reporter, either a sequence-specific TaqMan probe or an intercalating dye (SYBR Green). qPCR underpins clinical assays for KRAS, NRAS, BRAF, and EGFR hotspot mutations — Cobas, therascreen, and Idylla platforms are widely used at point-of-care or in centralised molecular laboratories. The assays are fast (results within hours), highly sensitive (allele frequency detection down to one per cent), and limited to the hotspot variants specifically interrogated by the assay primers.

Sanger sequencing

Sanger dideoxy sequencing — the chain-termination method introduced by Fred Sanger in 1977 — remains the routine technique for confirming variants of uncertain significance and for sequencing small targets where mutation location is known. The principle uses dideoxynucleotide triphosphates that terminate chain extension, generating a population of fragments whose terminal nucleotide is identified by fluorescence on capillary electrophoresis. Sanger has a detection limit of around 20 per cent allele frequency, meaning that variants below this threshold may be missed in low-cellularity tumour samples. This sensitivity floor is the principal reason that Sanger has been displaced by NGS for routine tumour profiling, but it remains the orthogonal confirmation method for clinically actionable variants identified by NGS.

Pyrosequencing

Pyrosequencing, a sequencing-by-synthesis method that detects pyrophosphate release on nucleotide incorporation, sits between Sanger and NGS in sensitivity and throughput. It is the standard clinical method for MLH1 promoter methylation analysis (triaging MLH1-deficient colorectal carcinomas into sporadic versus germline) and for MGMT promoter methylation in glioblastoma (predicting temozolomide response). Pyrosequencing reads are short (typically 30 to 60 bases) and the platform is well-suited to targeted methylation interrogation; whole-genome methylation profiling uses array or sequencing-based methods covered later.

Multiplex PCR and reverse-transcription PCR

Multiplex PCR amplifies several targets in a single reaction by pooling primer pairs in defined concentrations. The technique underpins many of the rapid hotspot panels used in routine practice (Idylla cartridges run multiple PCR reactions in a closed device) and is the foundation of amplicon-based NGS library preparation. Reverse-transcription PCR (RT-PCR) reverse-transcribes RNA into complementary DNA (cDNA) using reverse transcriptase, then amplifies the cDNA by standard PCR. RT-PCR is the established method for fusion transcript detection in haematological malignancies (BCR-ABL1 monitoring in chronic myeloid leukaemia, PML-RARA in acute promyelocytic leukaemia) and remains widely used where the target fusion partners are well-defined.

PCR artefacts and amplification pitfalls

PCR is susceptible to a small but important set of artefacts. Allele dropout describes the preferential amplification of one allele over another, generating an apparent homozygous result from a heterozygous sample; the cause is usually a primer-site polymorphism or degraded template at one allele. Primer-dimer formation generates short amplicons that compete with the intended target. Cross-contamination between samples or from environmental DNA produces false positives, particularly problematic in highly sensitive assays; the discipline of separate pre-PCR and post-PCR workspaces is universal in molecular laboratories. Polymerase error rates are low but non-zero, and high-cycle reactions amplify rare polymerase-induced substitutions to detectable frequencies — high-fidelity polymerases (Q5, Phusion) reduce this background and are preferred for clinical applications.

3.4 Next-generation sequencing

Library preparation strategies

Next-generation sequencing (NGS) parallelises the sequencing of millions of DNA fragments, generating gigabases of data per run. Two library preparation strategies dominate clinical practice. Amplicon-based panels (Ion AmpliSeq, Illumina TruSeq Amplicon) amplify defined target regions with primer pools, then sequence the products. The strategy is fast and tolerant of low input nucleic acid (down to 10 ng), making it well-suited to small FFPE biopsies, but it cannot detect copy number changes accurately and is limited to the specifically-targeted regions. Hybrid-capture panels (Illumina TruSight Oncology, Agilent SureSelect) shear genomic DNA, attach adapters, and use biotinylated probes to capture target regions for sequencing. Hybrid capture handles much larger panels (several hundred to several thousand genes), detects copy number and structural variants better than amplicon, and is the substrate for broad-panel genomic profiling — but requires more input DNA (typically 50 to 100 ng) and longer turnaround.

Panel size scales with clinical scope. Hotspot panels (under 50 genes, often around 50 hotspot variants) suit routine treatment-decision testing — KRAS, NRAS, BRAF, EGFR, ALK, ROS1, MET, RET, BRCA1/2, and a handful of others. Targeted broad panels (200 to 500 genes) interrogate the major druggable pathways, tumour suppressors, and DNA repair genes for broader treatment matching. Whole-exome sequencing (WES) captures all protein-coding regions, and whole-genome sequencing (WGS) captures the entire genome including non-coding regulatory regions. WGS is now offered through national programmes — the UK Genomic Medicine Service provides WGS for selected cancers — and is the long-term direction of travel.

Sequencing chemistry and platforms

The dominant sequencing-by-synthesis chemistry is the Illumina platform: short-read (150 to 300 base pairs), high-accuracy, and high-throughput. Illumina sequencers (MiSeq, NextSeq, NovaSeq) underpin most clinical molecular pathology laboratories. Long-read platforms (Pacific Biosciences SMRT, Oxford Nanopore) generate reads of thousands to tens of thousands of base pairs at lower per-base accuracy and are increasingly used for structural variant detection, fusion calling, and methylation analysis in a single workflow. Nanopore sequencing is particularly attractive for rapid intraoperative methylation classification of brain tumours; the Heidelberg DKFZ rapid Nanopore classifier produces a methylation-based diagnosis in under an hour.

3.5 Bioinformatics and variant interpretation

From raw reads to annotated variants

Sequencing platforms output base-called reads, typically as FASTQ files, which are then aligned to a reference genome (currently GRCh38 in most clinical workflows). Variant calling identifies positions where the sample differs from reference, distinguishing germline and somatic variants by comparing tumour and matched normal where available. Quality metrics on every variant include read depth (how many sequencing reads cover the position), variant allele frequency (VAF, the proportion of reads supporting the variant), and base quality scores. A confidently called clinical variant typically requires a minimum depth of 100 to 500 reads — depending on the assay sensitivity — and a VAF consistent with the expected tumour cellularity.

Annotation translates the genomic coordinate into a clinically meaningful description: the affected gene, the protein-level consequence (missense, nonsense, frameshift, splice-site), the functional domain, and the known clinical and population-frequency databases (ClinVar, gnomAD, COSMIC, OncoKB, CIViC). The bioinformatics workflow filters out artefacts (sequencing errors, alignment artefacts at homopolymer regions, contamination signals) and produces a curated variant call file for clinical review.

Variant nomenclature

Standardised variant nomenclature follows the Human Genome Variation Society (HGVS) recommendations. The c. notation describes a variant at the coding DNA level (c.1799T>A for the BRAF V600E mutation), with numbering relative to a defined reference transcript. The p. notation describes the protein-level consequence (p.Val600Glu, often abbreviated V600E in clinical practice).

The g. notation describes the genomic position on a reference assembly. A complete variant report includes the gene symbol, the reference transcript identifier (NM accession number), the c. and p. notations, the genomic position, and the variant type (substitution, deletion, insertion, duplication, inversion). Departure from HGVS conventions is a recognised reporting failure that compromises downstream interpretation and database submission.

Tumour-only versus tumour-normal paired sequencing

Two workflow models exist in clinical somatic sequencing. Tumour-only sequencing analyses tumour DNA alone, using population frequency databases (gnomAD) and tumour-specific knowledge bases (COSMIC, OncoKB) to filter out likely germline polymorphisms. The approach is faster and cheaper, but cannot reliably distinguish somatic from germline variants — particularly important for cancer susceptibility genes (BRCA1/2, MMR genes, TP53, PTEN) where germline variants carry heritable implications. Tumour-normal paired sequencing analyses a matched germline sample (typically peripheral blood) alongside the tumour, allowing definitive distinction of somatic from germline. Paired sequencing is the gold standard for broad profiling and is increasingly the norm in academic laboratories and in the UK Genomic Medicine Service. The trade-offs are cost, logistics, and the requirement to consent the patient for germline analysis with its potential incidental findings.

Variant classification and clinical tiering

A clinical variant report categorises each variant by both biological significance and clinical actionability. Biological classification (germline variants) follows the ACMG/AMP 2015 five-tier scheme: pathogenic, likely pathogenic, variant of uncertain significance (VUS), likely benign, and benign. Somatic variant tiering follows the joint AMP/ASCO/CAP 2017 scheme — Tier I (strong clinical significance), Tier II (potential clinical significance), Tier III (unknown clinical significance), Tier IV (benign or likely benign).

The ESMO Scale for Clinical Actionability of molecular Targets (ESCAT) is the European framework specifically for cancer-related variants. It categorises a tumour-variant-drug-indication triplet into tiers I to X — Tier I represents prospective clinical evidence of clinical benefit (companion diagnostic with regulatory approval), Tier II represents prospective evidence but for a different indication, Tier III represents retrospective or limited evidence, Tier IV represents preclinical evidence, Tier V represents biological rationale only. A clinically useful report identifies which tier each actionable variant occupies and links the variant to specific treatment options where applicable.

Variant tiering at a glance

ACMG/AMP (germline): P, LP, VUS, LB, B — five tiers, based on evidence categories.

AMP/ASCO/CAP (somatic): Tier I (strong clinical), II (potential), III (unknown), IV (benign).

ESCAT (cancer-specific): I (companion Dx), II (off-label evidence), III (limited evidence), IV (preclinical), V (rationale only).

VAF interpretation: compare with tumour cellularity — VAF much higher suggests germline; VAF below cellularity suggests subclonal somatic.

Report discipline: variant, gene, consequence, VAF, tier, clinical relevance, recommended action.

3.6 Fusion gene detection

Fusion genes — formed by chromosomal translocations, inversions, or deletions joining two previously separate genes — define many sarcomas, several haematological malignancies, and an expanding list of solid tumours. Detection strategies fall into three families. Break-apart fluorescence in-situ hybridisation (FISH), as covered in Chapter 2, uses two probes flanking a known partner gene; separation of the signals indicates a rearrangement. FISH is reliable, paraffin-compatible, and works well for the established translocations (EWSR1 in Ewing sarcoma family, SS18 in synovial sarcoma, ALK in lung and ALCL, ROS1 in lung). It is partner-agnostic — the assay confirms an EWSR1 rearrangement but does not identify the fusion partner.

DNA-based NGS detects fusions through analysis of split reads and discordant read pairs that span the breakpoint. Hybrid-capture panels with intronic baiting flank the recurrent breakpoint regions and capture the fusion junction. The advantage over FISH is that DNA-NGS identifies the specific partner and the exact breakpoint, supports detection of novel partners, and is integrated into a broad panel. The limitation is that not all fusions are detectable by DNA-only NGS — fusions with very large intronic regions or with diverse breakpoint distributions may evade hybrid capture.

RNA-based fusion detection — anchored multiplex PCR (Archer FusionPlex) or hybrid-capture RNA panels — sequences the transcribed fusion RNA directly, detecting the actual chimeric transcript regardless of intronic breakpoint location. RNA-based methods are the most sensitive for detecting fusions with diverse partners (NTRK1/2/3, ALK, RET, ROS1, FGFR1/2/3, BRAF) and are now the standard for solid tumour fusion screening. The trade-off is RNA quality — degraded RNA from old or poorly-fixed FFPE may fail. Many laboratories deploy a layered approach — IHC screen for ALK, ROS1, or pan-TRK protein, with reflex FISH or RNA-NGS for IHC-positive cases.

3.7 Immunohistochemical surrogates for molecular alterations

Several molecular alterations are reliably detectable on routine IHC, providing a fast and inexpensive screening tool that triggers reflex molecular confirmation when needed. The candidate should know which IHC surrogates exist, what they screen for, and where their limitations lie. The classical example is BRAF V600E IHC (clone VE1) is a mutation-specific antibody that recognises only the V600E mutant protein. A positive VE1 supports BRAF V600E mutation with high concordance to PCR or sequencing in melanoma, papillary thyroid carcinoma, hairy cell leukaemia, and selected colorectal and brain tumours; non-V600E variants are missed and a negative result does not exclude BRAF mutation more broadly.

Other established IHC surrogates include IDH1 R132H (clone H09) addresses the commonest IDH1 mutation in glioma and is useful in adult diffuse glioma WHO grade 2 to 4 classification, with the limitation that rarer IDH1 and IDH2 variants are not detected and require sequencing in IHC-negative cases. ALK D5F3 antibody for ALK rearrangement in lung adenocarcinoma and anaplastic large cell lymphoma is a recognised companion diagnostic with FDA approval. ROS1 antibody (D4D6) for ROS1 rearrangement in lung adenocarcinoma is similarly used as a screen. Pan-TRK antibody screens for NTRK1, NTRK2, and NTRK3 fusions across many tumour types, with positive cases reflexed to RNA-based confirmation. Beta-catenin nuclear and cytoplasmic accumulation indicates CTNNB1 mutation or APC pathway alteration, a surrogate widely used in desmoid tumour, solid-pseudopapillary pancreatic tumour, and selected hepatocellular and adrenocortical entities.

Loss-of-expression IHC indicates a different class of molecular alteration. SDHB loss indicates a germline or somatic mutation in any subunit of succinate dehydrogenase, with strong predictive value in hereditary paraganglioma-pheochromocytoma syndromes and in SDH-deficient gastrointestinal stromal tumours. INI1 (SMARCB1) loss indicates SMARCB1 mutation or deletion in epithelioid sarcoma, malignant rhabdoid tumour, and atypical teratoid rhabdoid tumour; BRG1 (SMARCA4) loss in SMARCA4-deficient thoracic sarcomas; MTAP loss as a surrogate for CDKN2A homozygous deletion in mesothelioma and selected other tumours; ATRX loss as a surrogate for ATRX mutation in IDH-mutant astrocytoma. p53 immunohistochemistry shows a characteristic mutant pattern (strong diffuse nuclear positivity, or complete null pattern with internal control retained) that indicates TP53 mutation with high concordance; the wild-type pattern (heterogeneous moderate positivity) does not exclude TP53 mutation entirely.

IHC molecular surrogates — high-yield list

BRAF V600E (VE1): melanoma, PTC, hairy cell, CRC, brain. Misses non-V600E variants.

IDH1 R132H (H09): glioma. Misses rarer IDH1/2 variants.

ALK (D5F3), ROS1 (D4D6), Pan-TRK: lung and other solid tumour fusion screens.

Nuclear beta-catenin: CTNNB1 / APC pathway — desmoid, SPN pancreas, HCC subtypes.

p53 mutant pattern: strong diffuse or complete null with internal control retained → TP53 mutation likely.

Loss patterns: SDHB → SDH mutation; INI1 → SMARCB1; BRG1 → SMARCA4; MTAP → CDKN2A del; ATRX → ATRX mutation.

3.8 Methylation analysis

DNA methylation — addition of a methyl group to the cytosine of a CpG dinucleotide — regulates gene expression and is a stable epigenetic mark that survives FFPE processing. Three clinical methylation assays are routine. Methylation-specific PCR (MS-PCR) treats DNA with bisulphite (converting unmethylated cytosine to uracil), then amplifies with primer pairs specific for methylated or unmethylated sequence; band presence or qPCR signal indicates methylation status. Pyrosequencing on bisulphite-treated DNA quantifies methylation at specific CpG positions and is the clinical method for MGMT promoter methylation in glioblastoma and for MLH1 promoter methylation in MMR-deficient colorectal carcinoma.

Genome-wide methylation arrays — the Illumina EPIC array covers around 850,000 CpG sites — produce a methylation profile that can be matched against a reference classifier to assign a tumour diagnosis. The Heidelberg DKFZ methylation classifier for central nervous system tumours, now incorporated into the WHO 5th edition CNS classification, illustrates the power of the approach — methylation profile assigns a diagnostic class with high confidence in cases where morphology alone is ambiguous. Methylation classifiers are emerging for sarcomas (the Heidelberg sarcoma classifier), renal tumours, and selected paediatric tumour groups.

3.9 Copy number variation and tumour mutational burden

Copy number variation

Copy number variation (CNV) — gain or loss of genomic segments — is detected by FISH (single-locus, gold standard for HER2 and MYCN amplification), by SNP arrays (genome-wide, sensitive to small amplifications and deletions), and increasingly by hybrid-capture NGS through analysis of read-depth signal. NGS-based CNV requires careful normalisation against a reference population of normal samples and is influenced by tumour cellularity and sample quality. The clinical utility includes HER2 amplification in breast and gastric cancer, MYCN amplification in neuroblastoma, MET amplification in lung adenocarcinoma, CDKN2A homozygous deletion in glioma and mesothelioma, and chromosome 1p/19q co-deletion in oligodendroglioma.

Tumour mutational burden

Tumour mutational burden (TMB) is the count of non-synonymous somatic mutations per megabase of sequenced DNA. TMB-high tumours, defined as at least 10 mutations per megabase in the FoundationOne and similar clinical panels, are predictive of response to immune checkpoint inhibitor therapy across multiple tumour types. The FDA tissue-agnostic approval of pembrolizumab for TMB-high tumours was a landmark in pan-cancer biomarker use. TMB calculation is panel-dependent — different panel sizes and bioinformatic workflows produce different absolute TMB values for the same tumour — so cross-platform calibration and harmonisation efforts (the Friends of Cancer Research TMB Harmonization Project) are ongoing. The candidate should know the principle and the platform-dependence of TMB rather than memorise specific numerical thresholds.

3.10 Microsatellite instability and homologous recombination deficiency

Microsatellite instability

Microsatellite instability (MSI) — the accumulation of length variation in short tandem repeat sequences (microsatellites) — is the signature of mismatch repair deficiency. MSI testing complements MMR IHC and provides an orthogonal confirmation in selected settings. The classical PCR-based assay (the Bethesda or Promega panels) amplifies five or more mononucleotide microsatellite markers (BAT-25, BAT-26, NR-21, NR-24, MONO-27) and compares allele lengths in tumour and matched normal. Instability at two or more markers defines MSI-high; one marker defines MSI-low (a category of uncertain clinical significance); zero markers defines microsatellite stable. NGS-based MSI assessment, integrated into broad panels, evaluates many more microsatellite loci and is now the routine approach in many laboratories. Concordance between MMR IHC and MSI testing is over 95 per cent, and discordant cases — IHC-deficient with MSS, or IHC-retained with MSI — trigger orthogonal confirmation and germline testing where appropriate.

Homologous recombination deficiency

Homologous recombination deficiency (HRD) — loss of function in the homologous recombination DNA repair pathway — predicts response to platinum chemotherapy and PARP inhibitor therapy in ovarian, breast, prostate, and pancreatic cancer. HRD is assessed by direct gene mutation testing (BRCA1, BRCA2, PALB2, RAD51C, RAD51D, and other HR pathway genes) and by genomic scar scoring — measuring patterns of large-scale state transitions, loss of heterozygosity, and telomeric allelic imbalance that result from defective recombination repair. The combined HRD score (Myriad myChoice, Foundation HRD) integrates mutation status and genomic scar; HRD-positive tumours are eligible for PARP inhibitor maintenance therapy in advanced ovarian cancer regardless of BRCA mutation status.

3.11 Liquid biopsy and circulating tumour DNA

Circulating tumour DNA (ctDNA) — fragmented tumour-derived DNA released into the bloodstream by apoptotic or necrotic tumour cells — provides a minimally-invasive substrate for molecular profiling. Plasma ctDNA assays detect actionable mutations in lung, breast, colorectal, prostate, and other cancers, with established clinical utility in three settings. First, when tissue biopsy is impractical or contraindicated, plasma ctDNA serves as the substrate for treatment-decision profiling — EGFR T790M detection in lung adenocarcinoma at progression on first-line EGFR-TKI is the classical example. Second, minimal residual disease (MRD) testing after curative-intent therapy uses tumour-informed personalised ctDNA panels to detect microscopic residual disease, predicting recurrence months before radiological progression. Third, early-cancer detection (the multi-cancer early detection field — Galleri and competing assays) uses methylation and mutation signatures in plasma to detect cancer signal across multiple tumour types.

The technical challenge of ctDNA is signal-to-noise — ctDNA represents a small and variable fraction of total cell-free DNA, dominated by haematopoietic-cell-derived background. Detection of variants at allele frequencies below one per cent requires highly sensitive methods — droplet digital PCR (ddPCR) for single-target assays, deep-sequencing NGS panels with unique molecular identifiers (UMIs) for multi-gene profiling. False positives from clonal haematopoiesis of indeterminate potential (CHIP) — clonal expansion of haematopoietic stem cells carrying somatic mutations — complicate interpretation, particularly for DNMT3A, TET2, ASXL1, and TP53 mutations that are common to both CHIP and solid tumours.

Digital PCR — principle and applications

Droplet digital PCR (ddPCR) partitions a PCR reaction into tens of thousands of nanolitre-scale droplets, each containing zero, one, or a few template molecules. After amplification, each droplet is read as positive or negative for the target sequence, and the absolute concentration of starting template is calculated by Poisson statistics. The advantage over quantitative PCR is independence from a standard curve, giving absolute rather than relative quantitation and exceptional sensitivity for rare variants. ddPCR is the workhorse of ctDNA assays for single targets and for MRD monitoring once a tumour-specific variant has been identified. Limitations include the per-assay design effort for each target and the limited multiplexing capacity (typically four or fewer targets per reaction).

Mutational signature analysis

Mutational signatures — characteristic patterns of base substitutions across the genome — record the mutagenic processes a tumour has experienced. The Catalogue of Somatic Mutations in Cancer (COSMIC) mutational signature framework (version 3 onwards) defines around 80 single-base substitution signatures with biological interpretation. The clinically relevant signatures include the UV signature (predominantly C-to-T at dipyrimidines, characteristic of skin cancers), the tobacco-smoking signature (C-to-A transversions, characteristic of lung adenocarcinoma in smokers), the APOBEC signature (T-to-C and T-to-G in TpC contexts, common in bladder and breast cancer), the homologous recombination deficiency signature (Signature 3, supporting HRD positivity), and the mismatch repair deficiency signatures. Signature analysis requires whole-exome or whole-genome sequencing and is not yet routine in small-panel diagnostic NGS, but it is emerging as a tissue-agnostic biomarker.

Turnaround time in molecular pathology

Turnaround time targets for molecular tests are tighter than for many histopathological assays because the result drives time-sensitive treatment decisions. Reflex hotspot mutation testing on a lung biopsy typically targets 7 to 10 calendar days; broader NGS profiling targets 14 to 21 days; broad-panel genomic profiling and whole-genome sequencing target 28 days. The bottleneck steps are tissue allocation at cut-up, nucleic acid extraction, library preparation and sequencing, and bioinformatic analysis with multidisciplinary variant review. Streamlined workflows in academic centres now deliver actionable variants within 10 days of biopsy in many lung adenocarcinoma cohorts, supporting first-line therapy decisions at the initial oncology consultation.

3.12 Reporting and incidental germline findings

A molecular pathology report carries three sequential responsibilities — what was tested, what was found, and what it means clinically. The standard structure identifies the assay, sample, tumour cellularity, gene targets, variants found with VAF and tier, clinically relevant negative findings, limitations of the assay, and recommended next steps. Variants of uncertain significance are reported but accompanied by an explicit caveat that they should not currently drive treatment decisions.

Tumour-only sequencing can detect variants that are in fact germline — and some of these have heritable implications for the patient and family. The American College of Medical Genetics maintains a list of genes for which incidental findings should be returned to patients (the ACMG SF list, now in version 3.2). In molecular pathology practice, BRCA1, BRCA2, MLH1, MSH2, MSH6, PMS2, TP53, and selected others may be identified in the course of tumour profiling; suspected germline findings are flagged for clinical genetics referral, with germline confirmation testing on a blood or buccal sample. The pre-test counselling pathway and the post-test return-of-results pathway are both auditable elements of an accredited molecular service.

3.13 Quality control in the molecular laboratory

Molecular pathology is among the most quality-intensive disciplines in the diagnostic laboratory. Each assay requires a defined positive control (known mutated cell line or reference standard), a defined negative control (no-template control to detect contamination), and a sample-level quality check (nucleic acid quantity and integrity). Run-level QC tracks sequencing depth, on-target rate, duplication rate, and uniformity of coverage. Sample-level QC tracks contamination signal, sample swap detection (typically through a panel of fingerprinting SNPs), and turnaround time. The laboratory participates in external quality assessment schemes — EMQN and IQN-Path operate the dominant European schemes — and a poor return triggers root-cause analysis and corrective action.

Validation of a new assay follows a structured pathway. Analytical validation establishes accuracy, precision, sensitivity, specificity, and reportable range against reference materials and against an orthogonal method (Sanger or qPCR) for clinically actionable variants. Clinical validation establishes that the result correlates with the intended clinical outcome. Verification is the abbreviated process for an established assay being adopted by a new laboratory — a smaller cohort confirms that local performance matches published expectations. ISO 15189 accreditation requires documented validation or verification for every clinical assay.

3.14 Integration with morphology and IHC

The molecular result is not the diagnosis — it is one piece of evidence integrated with morphology and IHC to produce a coherent report. A KRAS G12C lung carcinoma is first an adenocarcinoma with TTF-1 positivity and KRAS-mutant disease driving treatment options. An NTRK fusion sarcoma is first a soft-tissue tumour with appropriate morphology and IHC pattern, with the fusion explaining the entity and directing TRK inhibitor therapy. The Part 1 candidate is expected to know when to order molecular testing — IHC surrogates can predict the mutation, the morphology suggests the relevant target, and the clinical setting demands targeted therapy or treatment matching. The reverse is equally important — knowing when not to order is part of cost discipline and clinical relevance.

Integrated reporting — a single report incorporating morphology, IHC, and molecular findings — is the gold standard. The reporting pathologist coordinates the workflow, ensures that the molecular result is interpreted in the morphological context, and resolves any apparent discordance (a triple-negative IHC with a HER2-amplified ISH, a CDX2-positive carcinoma with an unexpected KRAS-wild-type pattern). The MDT meeting is the formal venue for this integration, where surgical, oncological, and radiological context complete the clinical picture.

Tumour heterogeneity and subclonal architecture

Solid tumours are clonally heterogeneous, with subclones evolving under selection pressure from therapy and from the local microenvironment. A small biopsy samples one part of one tumour at one time, and the variants identified represent the dominant subclone at that location. Spatial heterogeneity is well-documented in renal cell carcinoma, glioblastoma, and lung adenocarcinoma; temporal heterogeneity manifests as treatment-resistant subclones emerging at progression. The variant allele frequency on a molecular report carries information about clonality — a VAF markedly below the level expected from tumour cellularity suggests a subclonal variant, while a VAF close to expected suggests a clonal driver. Interpretation of subclonal variants is nuanced; the variant may represent a treatment-resistance mechanism, a sampling artefact from contaminating normal cells, or a true biological subpopulation with prognostic implications.

Structured reporting and integrated MDT communication

Structured reporting templates are now standard in molecular pathology, providing a predictable order of information and enabling extraction of data for audit and research. The IRSCC (International Registry of Standardised Cancer Datasets) maintains templates aligned with the ICCR histopathology datasets, ensuring that molecular findings sit alongside staging and biomarker data in a consistent format. The molecular section of an integrated report identifies the assay, the gene targets, the variants found, their tier, and their clinical implications — and explicitly notes negative findings for clinically relevant targets (KRAS wild-type, EGFR wild-type, ALK negative) that inform treatment decisions just as positive findings do.

3.15 Companion diagnostics by tumour type

A companion diagnostic is a test that supports the safe and effective use of a paired therapeutic agent. The pathologist applies companion diagnostics every day, and a working knowledge of the major indications anchors much of the Part 1 syllabus. The following overview groups the most common indications by tumour type without exhausting the rapidly-expanding list.

Lung adenocarcinoma

Lung adenocarcinoma is the most molecularly-stratified solid tumour in routine practice. Reflex testing on biopsy at diagnosis covers EGFR (TKI selection — first, second, and third generation inhibitors), ALK rearrangement (alectinib, brigatinib, lorlatinib), ROS1 rearrangement (entrectinib, crizotinib), BRAF V600E (dabrafenib plus trametinib), MET exon 14 skipping and MET amplification (capmatinib, tepotinib), RET fusion (selpercatinib, pralsetinib), NTRK fusion (larotrectinib, entrectinib), KRAS G12C (sotorasib, adagrasib), HER2 mutation and amplification (trastuzumab deruxtecan), and PD-L1 (immune checkpoint inhibitor selection). Most laboratories deploy a hybrid-capture or amplicon NGS panel covering the recurrent variants in a single test, with reflex RNA-NGS for fusion confirmation.

Colorectal carcinoma

Colorectal carcinoma reflex testing includes MMR IHC on every case (with reflex MLH1 methylation if MLH1/PMS2 loss), KRAS and NRAS hotspot mutation testing (anti-EGFR antibody eligibility — wild-type is required), BRAF V600E (prognostic and predictive of poorer anti-EGFR response, with encorafenib plus cetuximab as a targeted option), and NTRK fusion screening in MMR-deficient cases (larotrectinib eligibility). HER2 amplification is increasingly tested in selected metastatic colorectal cancers (trastuzumab deruxtecan, tucatinib plus trastuzumab). Microsatellite instability or MMR-deficient status itself is now a tissue-agnostic indication for pembrolizumab.

Breast carcinoma

Breast carcinoma reflex testing includes ER, PR, and HER2 status on every invasive case, with reflex HER2 ISH for IHC 2+ equivocal results. BRCA1/2 germline testing is offered in metastatic or triple-negative disease for olaparib and talazoparib eligibility. PIK3CA mutation testing on metastatic ER-positive disease informs alpelisib eligibility. ESR1 mutation testing in metastatic ER-positive disease on aromatase inhibitor progression informs elacestrant eligibility. The 21-gene Oncotype DX and 70-gene MammaPrint expression assays inform adjuvant chemotherapy decisions in early-stage hormone-receptor-positive disease.

Melanoma, GIST, ovarian, and prostate

Melanoma reflex testing covers BRAF V600 (and selected non-V600 variants) and NRAS — directing BRAF and MEK inhibitor or immune checkpoint inhibitor selection. Gastrointestinal stromal tumour (GIST) testing covers KIT and PDGFRA mutation analysis (imatinib sensitivity is exon- and codon-specific), with reflex SDH IHC and germline testing in KIT/PDGFRA wild-type disease (SDH-deficient GIST). Ovarian high-grade serous carcinoma reflex testing covers BRCA1/2 mutation status (somatic and germline) and HRD score (PARP inhibitor maintenance eligibility). Prostate adenocarcinoma reflex testing on metastatic disease covers BRCA1/2 and broader HRD pathway analysis (olaparib eligibility), with mismatch repair testing for selected indications.

3.16 Molecular integration in WHO 5th edition classifications

The WHO 5th edition tumour classifications, published from 2019 onwards, integrate molecular alterations into the diagnostic framework as required defining features rather than as ancillary information. The pattern recurs across organ systems. In adult diffuse glioma, the integrated diagnosis combines histology, IDH status, 1p/19q co-deletion (oligodendroglioma), ATRX (astrocytoma), TERT promoter mutation, and CDKN2A homozygous deletion (high-grade astrocytoma) — yielding entities such as oligodendroglioma IDH-mutant 1p/19q-codeleted and astrocytoma IDH-mutant CNS WHO grade 4. A morphologically identical glioma now carries a different name and clinical implication depending on its molecular profile.

Soft-tissue tumours follow the same trajectory. Fusion-defined sarcomas are diagnostic entities defined by their characteristic translocation — synovial sarcoma SS18-SSX, Ewing sarcoma EWSR1-FLI1 (and variants), alveolar rhabdomyosarcoma PAX3/7-FOXO1, alveolar soft part sarcoma ASPSCR1-TFE3, clear cell sarcoma EWSR1-ATF1. Haematolymphoid tumours integrate cytogenetics, immunophenotype, and morphology in the WHO 5th and ICC 2022 classifications — myeloid neoplasms with defining genetic abnormalities (CBF leukaemias, NPM1-mutant AML, RUNX1-mutant AML), lymphomas categorised by translocation (mantle cell with t(11;14), follicular with t(14;18), Burkitt with MYC translocation). The candidate is expected to know, at Part 1, the recurrent translocations and the diagnostic combinations they define.

3.17 Key points

Chapter 3 — key points

Pre-analytical: FFPE in 10% NBF, 6–48 h fixation, recent block, ≥10–20% tumour cellularity; macrodissection raises yield.

Techniques: Sanger for confirmation; real-time qPCR; allele-specific PCR; digital PCR for low VAF; NGS for breadth. Bouin and strong-acid decal destroy targets.

Variant interpretation: ACMG/AMP five-tier (germline); AMP/ASCO/CAP four-tier (somatic); ESCAT for clinical actionability. VAF vs tumour cellularity distinguishes germline from somatic.

Fusion detection: Break-apart FISH for EWSR1, SS18, ALK, ROS1, NTRK; RNA NGS for partner identification.

MSI and TMB: MSI by PCR (five mononucleotide markers) or NGS; aligns with MMR IHC. TMB threshold (10 mut/Mb) for pembrolizumab eligibility.

Liquid biopsy: ctDNA from plasma for tracking known variants at low VAF; complements but does not replace tissue.

Reporting: Variant, gene, consequence, VAF, tier, action. Incidental germline findings disclosed per consent framework.

3.18 Chapter SBAs

Q3.1. Detection of a somatic variant depends on the proportion of tumour-derived reads at the variant position — which in turn depends on tumour cellularity and assay sensitivity. A small endobronchial biopsy of a lung adenocarcinoma is reflexed for NGS profiling. The pathologist estimates tumour cellularity at 8 per cent on H&E. The reporting panel has a validated detection limit of 5 per cent variant allele frequency. Which single statement best describes the consequence for the result?

A. The sample is suitable and any variant detected will be reliably called.

B. The sample yields a maximum expected variant allele frequency of around 4 per cent, below the detection limit — a negative result cannot exclude a clinically actionable mutation.

C. Tumour cellularity does not affect variant calling if read depth is sufficient.

D. Macrodissection cannot improve the result because the tumour is too small.

E. The variant allele frequency for any somatic mutation will be 100 per cent of tumour reads.

Answer: B

A heterozygous somatic mutation contributes one altered allele out of two per tumour cell, so the maximum theoretical VAF equals half the tumour cellularity — in this case around 4 per cent, below the 5 per cent assay limit. A negative result therefore cannot exclude a clinically actionable mutation, and the pathologist should report the limitation explicitly. Mitigation options include macrodissection (scraping a tumour-rich area to raise effective cellularity), re-biopsy of a larger lesion if clinically feasible, or use of a more sensitive orthogonal assay (Idylla or ddPCR) targeted at the most likely actionable variants. Reporting a clean negative on an under-cellular sample is the unforced error to be avoided.

Option A is incorrect because cellularity is the rate-limiting variable — read depth alone cannot compensate. Option C is the same misconception phrased differently. Option D is incorrect because macrodissection is widely available and is often the right next step. Option E confuses VAF (a proportion of reads) with mutation status (a property of the tumour cell).

Q3.2. Detection of gene fusions in solid tumours is technique-dependent, with each approach having defined strengths and pitfalls relating to breakpoint diversity, intronic length, and RNA quality. A poorly-differentiated soft-tissue tumour from the deep thigh of a 25-year-old shows monomorphic spindle cells. The morphology suggests synovial sarcoma, and SS18 break-apart FISH is positive. Which single statement best describes what the FISH result has established?

A. The tumour has an SS18-SSX1 fusion suitable for treatment matching.

B. The tumour has a rearrangement of the SS18 gene; the specific fusion partner has not been identified by this assay.

C. The result excludes synovial sarcoma because break-apart FISH is non-specific.

D. Further testing is required because break-apart FISH is unreliable in soft-tissue tumours.

E. The tumour has both SS18 and SSX rearrangements identified by the assay.

Answer: B

Break-apart FISH uses two probes flanking a single gene (here SS18 on chromosome 18q11), one labelled in each colour. In a normal cell the probes lie adjacent and the signals appear fused; in a rearranged cell the probes separate and the signals appear apart. The assay is therefore partner-agnostic — it confirms an SS18 rearrangement without identifying the partner. Synovial sarcoma fuses SS18 (chromosome 18) with SSX1, SSX2, or rarely SSX4 (chromosome X); identification of the specific partner requires RNA-based sequencing (anchored multiplex PCR or RNA-NGS) and may be relevant for clinical correlation but is not provided by break-apart FISH alone.

Option A overclaims — partner identification requires additional testing. Option C is incorrect because break-apart FISH is well-validated for SS18 rearrangement and is morphologically supportive. Option D is incorrect — FISH remains a reliable technique in soft-tissue diagnosis. Option E describes a dual-fusion FISH design which is a different probe configuration than a break-apart assay.

Q3.3. Methylation analysis of tumour suppressor gene promoters provides predictive and triage information that complements mutation testing. A 70-year-old man with a left-sided colonic adenocarcinoma has reflex MMR IHC showing loss of MLH1 and PMS2 with retained MSH2 and MSH6. BRAF V600E IHC (clone VE1) is negative. Which single next test is the most appropriate?

A. Repeat MMR IHC on a different block.

B. Refer directly to clinical genetics for Lynch syndrome assessment.

C. MLH1 promoter methylation analysis (typically by pyrosequencing).

D. Whole-genome sequencing of the tumour.

E. Microsatellite instability testing on a different platform.

Answer: C

The MMR IHC pattern (MLH1 and PMS2 loss) most often reflects sporadic MLH1 promoter hypermethylation, which is in turn often (but not always) associated with the BRAF V600E mutation. When BRAF V600E is absent, the next discriminator between sporadic and germline disease is direct MLH1 promoter methylation analysis. A methylated promoter supports sporadic disease and reduces the priority of genetics referral; an unmethylated promoter strongly supports germline MLH1 mutation and triggers clinical genetics referral for confirmatory germline testing. The two-step algorithm (BRAF first, then methylation if BRAF wild-type) is now widely encoded in national guidance.

Option A is unnecessary — the IHC pattern is clear and internal control is implied retained in the stem. Option B is the action that follows an unmethylated promoter result; it is premature here. Option D is disproportionate at this stage. Option E does not discriminate sporadic from germline disease; concordance of MSI testing with MMR IHC is expected.

3.19 Chapter EMQ

EMQ 3.1. Molecular test selection. For each clinical scenario, select the single most appropriate molecular technique from the option list. Each option may be used once, more than once, or not at all.

A. Sanger sequencing

B. Pyrosequencing

C. Real-time quantitative PCR (Idylla or therascreen)

D. Amplicon-based NGS panel (small)

E. Hybrid-capture NGS panel (large)

F. Break-apart FISH

G. RNA-based fusion panel

H. Methylation array (Illumina EPIC)

I. Droplet digital PCR (ddPCR)

J. Whole-genome sequencing

(1) A urgent BRAF V600E result is required within 24 hours for a metastatic melanoma patient awaiting targeted-therapy decision. The laboratory has access to point-of-care molecular platforms. **Answer: C**

(2) A glioblastoma resection requires MGMT promoter methylation status to inform temozolomide eligibility. **Answer: B**

(3) A central nervous system tumour resected from a 12-year-old child is morphologically equivocal between several embryonal entities. Methylation-based classification has been requested to refine the diagnosis. **Answer: H**

(4) A poorly-differentiated lung tumour shows aberrant pan-TRK IHC positivity, but no specific fusion partner has been identified. Confirmation and partner identification are required. **Answer: G**

(5) Plasma is collected from a metastatic colorectal carcinoma patient at progression. The clinical question is detection of a known RAS variant at very low allele frequency to triage further targeted therapy. **Answer: I**

Chapter 4 — Frozen sections and intraoperative diagnosis

Frozen-section diagnosis sits at the busiest intersection of surgical and pathological practice. A surgeon is at the operating table, a patient is anaesthetised, a decision has to be made within minutes, and the histopathologist is the one who has to make it. The diagnostic substrate is imperfect, the controls are limited, the morphology is degraded by ice and rapid handling, and the consequences of an error are immediate. The FRCPath Part 1 examiners assess frozen-section knowledge at principle level: when to use the technique, when to refuse, how to communicate the result, and how to recognise the artefacts that mimic disease. This chapter sets out the workflow, the indications and contraindications, the language of intraoperative reporting, and the quality framework that holds it together.

The technique itself has a long history. William Welch performed the first intraoperative frozen section at Johns Hopkins in 1891 at William Halsted's request, and Thomas S. Cullen, also at Hopkins, published a formalin-fixed frozen technique in 1895; Louis B. Wilson at the Mayo Clinic standardised the modern unfixed workflow in 1905 (Journal of the American Medical Association, December 1905) — using a carbon-dioxide freezing microtome and methylene blue staining to deliver intraoperative diagnosis on tissue from the operating table within minutes. The clinical adoption was rapid, and within a decade frozen-section diagnosis was a routine adjunct in cancer surgery on both sides of the Atlantic. The modern cryostat — a microtome enclosed in a refrigerated chamber — is a direct lineal descendant of those early designs, and the underlying principles of rapid freezing, thin sectioning, and rapid staining have changed remarkably little.

Frozen-section laboratory layout and hardware

The frozen-section laboratory is typically a small dedicated space located close to operating theatres — proximity matters because transport time is part of the turnaround. The core hardware is the cryostat, supported by a fume cabinet for staining, an anti-roll plate or brush, slide warmers, and a microscope at the bench. The cryostat microtome is most often a rotary microtome with a disposable blade; older sliding microtomes persist in some laboratories. The anti-roll plate — a small transparent acetate or glass plate positioned just above the blade — catches the section as it is cut and prevents the section from curling on the blade edge. Sections that escape the anti-roll plate curl and are difficult to pick up flat; the operator threads the section under the plate during the cut.

Modern cryostats include features that have improved the workflow — pre-set programs for rapid cool-down, automated knife-stroke speed control, ultraviolet decontamination cycles, and integrated specimen identification systems. Some platforms support digital image capture from a slide-mounted camera, enabling telepathology streaming directly from the cryostat. The capital cost of a cryostat is high — a typical clinical unit costs in the order of £20,000 to £60,000 — and laboratories audit utilisation against the volume of intraoperative requests to justify the investment.

Biosafety in the cryostat

Frozen tissue is unfixed and therefore infectious. The standard biosafety framework treats every frozen specimen as a potential biohazard, with universal precautions throughout the workflow — gloves, lab coat, eye protection, and a fume cabinet for staining. Containment level 3 specimens (suspected tuberculosis, viral haemorrhagic fever, prion disease) require specific protocols. Tuberculosis is managed by minimising aerosol generation, using sealed sectioning where possible, and decontaminating the cryostat after each suspected case. Prion disease — Creutzfeldt-Jakob disease, variant CJD, and the broader transmissible spongiform encephalopathies — is an absolute contraindication to routine cryostat use because prions resist conventional decontamination; dedicated single-use equipment with subsequent incineration is the only acceptable approach, and frozen-section examination is generally declined in suspected prion cases.

4.1 Indications and contraindications

Legitimate indications

A frozen section should be ordered only when the result will change intraoperative management. The accepted indications group into four families. The first is margin assessment — confirmation that a resection has cleared a tumour with adequate clearance, allowing the surgeon to extend resection if margins are positive. Examples include breast lumpectomy cavity margin shaves, head and neck mucosal margins (oral cavity, larynx), gastrointestinal anastomotic margins, and hepatobiliary bile duct margins. The second is identification of tissue — confirmation that the surgeon has obtained the intended structure. Parathyroid identification during four-gland exploration is the classical example, and the rapid intraoperative parathyroid hormone assay has largely but not entirely replaced it. The third is diagnosis of an unexpected or unknown lesion — for example, a mass encountered during laparotomy of presumed appendicitis, a pulmonary nodule, or a lymph node found during oncological surgery. The fourth is staging — sentinel lymph node assessment in breast and melanoma surgery, where positive nodes change the planned extent of axillary or basin dissection.

Contraindications and inappropriate requests

Frozen section is contraindicated when the answer cannot reliably be given on a frozen, when the answer does not change the operation, or when there is insufficient tissue for both intraoperative and permanent diagnosis. Specific contraindications include very small biopsies where freezing exhausts the tissue and precludes permanent diagnosis (small endoscopic biopsies, core needle biopsies under 1 cm), heavily fatty tissue that does not section well frozen (open breast biopsies in patients with adipose-rich tissue), calcified or bony tissue (the cryostat blade will not cut bone reliably), and any situation where definitive diagnosis depends on assays not available on a frozen section (oestrogen and progesterone receptor status, HER2, molecular testing, or detailed immunophenotyping for lymphoma).

Inappropriate frozen-section requests are common and the histopathologist has both the right and the responsibility to decline. A request for primary diagnosis of a thyroid nodule on a frozen section is generally inappropriate — the distinction between follicular adenoma, minimally invasive follicular carcinoma, and the non-invasive follicular thyroid neoplasm with papillary-like nuclear features (NIFTP) depends on careful assessment of capsular and vascular invasion that is unreliable on a frozen. A request for definitive diagnosis of lymphoma on a frozen is similarly inappropriate, since classification depends on immunophenotyping and molecular work. The pathologist who declines a frozen request explains why and proposes an alternative pathway — usually permanent section diagnosis with a defined turnaround.

Indications and contraindications — quick reference

Use frozen for: margin clearance, tissue identification (parathyroid), unexpected mass diagnosis, sentinel node staging.

Do not use frozen for: very small biopsies, fatty tissue without lesion, calcified tissue, lymphoma primary diagnosis, thyroid follicular lesion classification, biomarker assessment.

Decline politely: explain why; offer permanent diagnosis pathway with defined turnaround.

Always confirm: clinical question, expected impact on operation, who is making the call back to surgeon.

4.2 Cryostat workflow

Specimen receipt and handover

Specimen receipt at the frozen-section bench is the most error-prone phase of the workflow. The standard sequence is verification of patient identifier (two identifiers, name plus hospital number or date of birth), verification of specimen identifier matching the request, clarification of the clinical question, and clarification of the specific tissue requested for frozen (whole specimen, designated margin, or a designated lymph node). The histopathologist receives the specimen by hand from the theatre runner or via a pneumatic tube, examines it grossly, and selects the area to be frozen. Photography of the gross specimen, with annotations marking the frozen-section area, is now routine and is the chain-of-evidence record for any subsequent dispute.

Cryostat principles

The cryostat is a refrigerated chamber typically maintained at minus 18 to minus 25 °C, housing a microtome. Fresh tissue is embedded in optimal cutting temperature (OCT) compound — a water-soluble glycol and polyvinyl alcohol matrix — and frozen in a metal mould placed on the cryostat chuck. The freezing rate is critical. Slow freezing allows ice crystals to grow within cells and produces the classical ice-crystal artefact: cytoplasmic vacuolation that distorts nuclei and obscures architecture. Rapid freezing in isopentane (2-methylbutane) chilled with liquid nitrogen, or in commercial freezing sprays, produces a glassy ice that preserves morphology much better. Critical specimens — small lymph nodes, kidney biopsies, muscle biopsies — are flash-frozen in isopentane before mounting; routine surgical frozens are typically frozen directly on the cryostat chuck with a slower freeze that is acceptable for margin and tumour identification.

Sectioning and staining

Sections are cut at 4 to 8 micrometres, picked up on charged slides, and immediately fixed in alcohol or acetone before rapid haematoxylin and eosin staining. The rapid H&E protocol compresses the staining sequence into 1 to 3 minutes per step: fixation, water rinse, haematoxylin, blueing, eosin, dehydration in two alcohols, clearing in xylene, and mounting. Total time from cryostat to slide-on-microscope is typically 6 to 10 minutes in an experienced laboratory. Toluidine blue is an alternative single-step stain used in some neuropathological frozen workflows for rapid demonstration of nuclei. Mounting uses a temporary aqueous mountant for rapid review, with a permanent coverslip applied later if the slide is to be retained.

4.3 Sentinel lymph node assessment

Sentinel lymph node biopsy is the staging procedure for breast cancer and melanoma. Intraoperative assessment historically used frozen sections cut at multiple levels across the bisected node, with rapid H&E examination for tumour deposits. The trade-offs are well-documented. Frozen-section sensitivity for sentinel node metastasis in breast cancer is around 70 to 80 per cent, missing micrometastases and isolated tumour cells. False positives from displaced benign epithelium and from intraductal cells from the breast track during dissection have been reported. The 2011 Z0011 trial and subsequent practice changes — selective omission of completion axillary dissection in patients with one or two positive sentinel nodes — have shifted many centres away from routine intraoperative frozen-section sentinel node assessment in breast cancer, since the result no longer drives immediate operative change in that cohort.

Melanoma sentinel node assessment differs. The depth of dissection required for completion lymphadenectomy historically depended on sentinel node status, and intraoperative diagnosis influenced the surgical plan. The MSLT-II trial demonstrated that completion node dissection does not improve melanoma-specific survival over careful observation in sentinel-node-positive disease, and many centres now defer melanoma sentinel node assessment to permanent sections with multilevel cuts and S100/SOX10 IHC, achieving higher sensitivity than frozen-section examination. Frozen-section sentinel node assessment continues in selected centres and selected indications, and the candidate should know both the technique and the current debate around its role.

Sentinel node intraoperative assessment — sensitivity and pitfalls

Breast frozen-section sensitivity: 70–80% for any deposit; lower for micrometastases (<2 mm) and isolated tumour cells.

Melanoma sentinel node: permanent with S100/SOX10 IHC outperforms frozen-section examination.

Touch imprint cytology: alternative or adjunct to frozen-section examination; preserves the node for permanent diagnosis.

Reporting language: describe size and number of foci; defer micrometastasis vs isolated tumour cell to permanent.

Z0011 effect: sentinel-positive breast cancer not always followed by completion axillary dissection — intraoperative result may not change surgery.

4.4 Specific intraoperative scenarios

Breast lumpectomy margins

Intraoperative margin assessment in breast lumpectomy aims to confirm clearance and reduce re-excision rates. The standard frozen-section workflow examines shave margins from the lumpectomy cavity walls or examines bread-loafed slices of the lumpectomy specimen itself. Reported sensitivity for invasive carcinoma at the margin is around 80 to 90 per cent; ductal carcinoma in situ is harder to recognise on frozen and sensitivity drops correspondingly. Alternatives include intraoperative imaging (specimen radiograph, intraoperative ultrasound), touch imprint cytology of margin surfaces, and radiofrequency or other margin-detection technologies. The choice between approaches depends on local expertise and on the proportion of cases in which the result is expected to change the operation; centres with high re-excision rates benefit most from intraoperative margin assessment.

Endocrine surgery

Parathyroid surgery is the dominant endocrine frozen-section indication. The surgeon resects a suspected parathyroid lesion and sends it for frozen confirmation. The pathologist identifies parathyroid tissue by recognising the characteristic chief cell and oxyphil populations, distinguishing them from thyroid follicles, lymph node tissue, ectopic thymus, and fibroadipose tissue. Parathyroid adenoma versus hyperplasia is generally not distinguished on frozen and is deferred to permanent. The intraoperative parathyroid hormone assay, with a 50 per cent drop within 10 minutes of removal indicating successful resection, has reduced the proportion of cases sent for frozen but has not eliminated the requirement, particularly when adenoma localisation by imaging is uncertain or in re-operative cases.

Thyroid surgery occasionally generates frozen-section requests. The classical question — papillary thyroid carcinoma versus benign nodule — is sometimes answered confidently on frozen when classical nuclear features (overlap, grooves, intranuclear pseudoinclusions, optically clear chromatin) are unequivocal. Follicular-patterned lesions are notoriously difficult on frozen because capsular and vascular invasion are not reliably assessed in the limited sample and frozen morphology is degraded. Many laboratories decline frozen diagnosis of follicular-patterned thyroid lesions and defer to permanent sections; the candidate should know the principle that follicular thyroid neoplasia is generally a deferred diagnosis.

Hepatobiliary and pancreatic surgery

Frozen-section examination of bile duct and pancreatic resection margins is routine in pancreaticoduodenectomy and proximal bile duct resection. The pathologist examines the proximal and distal margin slices for invasive carcinoma, intraductal papillary mucinous neoplasm (IPMN) with high-grade dysplasia, biliary intraepithelial neoplasia, and pancreatic intraepithelial neoplasia. The clinical significance of low-grade in-situ disease at the margin is debated and varies by centre; a positive margin for invasive carcinoma or high-grade in-situ disease typically prompts extension of the resection where anatomically feasible.

Neurosurgery

Intraoperative neuropathology has its own discipline. Frozen sections of brain tumour are typically smeared (a small portion of the tissue is squashed between two slides) and stained with toluidine blue or rapid H&E, alongside a frozen section of the remaining tissue. The combination of smear and frozen yields better cytological detail than frozen alone — the smear allows assessment of individual cell morphology without the freezing artefact that obscures detail on the frozen. The classical intraoperative questions are diagnosis (glioma versus lymphoma versus metastatic carcinoma versus infection versus demyelination) and adequacy (representative tumour tissue versus reactive gliosis). Definitive grading and molecular classification follow on permanent sections and molecular work-up, sometimes including rapid Nanopore methylation classification.

Mohs micrographic surgery

Mohs micrographic surgery is a specialised intraoperative pathology workflow for high-risk non-melanoma skin cancer, particularly basal cell carcinoma and squamous cell carcinoma on the face and other anatomically sensitive sites. The Mohs surgeon excises a thin layer of tumour with mapped orientation, the laboratory sections the excised tissue in en-face horizontal frozen sections, and the surgeon reads the slides personally for residual tumour at the deep and peripheral margins. Positive margins direct further targeted excision, with iterative passes until clearance is achieved. The technique delivers excellent local control while sparing maximal normal tissue. The pathologist's role is variable across centres — some Mohs surgeons read their own slides, others share interpretation with a pathologist; either way, the en-face frozen-section workflow is the defining feature.

Gastrointestinal and colorectal surgery

Frozen-section examination of colorectal resection margins is routine in low rectal anastomotic surgery — the distal margin of an anterior resection is examined for residual carcinoma, dysplasia, or inflammatory bowel disease activity, with positive findings prompting further resection. Anorectal squamous lesions at the dentate line raise the question of high-grade dysplasia versus invasive squamous cell carcinoma, sometimes deferred to permanent because of inherent morphological difficulty on frozen. Appendix specimens occasionally require intraoperative review — for example, a low-grade appendiceal mucinous neoplasm (LAMN) discovered at appendicectomy may prompt consideration of right hemicolectomy or peritoneal washout if invasive carcinoma is suspected, but definitive classification typically waits for permanent sections.

Pulmonary and pleural surgery

Lung wedge resections of indeterminate pulmonary nodules are common intraoperative consultations. The pathologist confirms malignancy or benign aetiology and — when malignancy is confirmed — sometimes attempts a primary versus metastatic distinction. The decision to proceed to lobectomy or pneumonectomy may depend on the frozen result; in many contemporary lung cancer pathways the decision is made on pre-operative biopsy rather than intraoperatively, and the frozen serves only as confirmation. Pleural-based masses raise the differential of mesothelioma versus carcinoma versus reactive mesothelial proliferation — a diagnostic question that frozen-section morphology alone cannot answer reliably. Mesothelioma diagnosis requires permanent sections and a defined IHC panel (calretinin, WT1, D2-40, CK5/6 versus carcinoma markers such as TTF-1, BerEP4, MOC-31), and frozen-section examination should not be used to commit to mesothelioma in the operating theatre.

Renal and urological surgery

Renal mass intraoperative diagnosis is now uncommon — most renal tumours are pre-operatively imaged, biopsied where appropriate, and operated on with a planned approach. The intraoperative question is more often margin status during partial nephrectomy — the parenchymal margin closest to the tumour is examined on frozen, with positive margin findings prompting extended resection or completion nephrectomy. Renal allograft biopsies during transplant surgery are not typically processed as frozen sections — the implantation biopsy is fixed and processed for permanent sections with electron microscopy and immunofluorescence as covered in Chapter 20.

Gynaecological surgery

Ovarian mass intraoperative diagnosis is the classical gynaecological frozen-section indication. The surgeon presents an unexpected ovarian mass at laparotomy for presumed benign disease, or a known ovarian mass with uncertain malignant potential, and asks whether radical surgery (staging, omentectomy, peritoneal sampling) is justified. The pathologist distinguishes broad categories — benign cystadenoma, borderline tumour, frankly invasive carcinoma — recognising that detailed subtyping (high-grade versus low-grade serous, mucinous versus seromucinous) often defers to permanent sections. Frozen-section sensitivity for invasive ovarian carcinoma is high (over 90 per cent); borderline tumour diagnosis on frozen is less reliable, particularly for the mucinous category where extensive sampling is the gold standard.

Endometrial cancer surgery occasionally generates intraoperative requests — assessment of myometrial invasion depth on hysterectomy specimens has been described as guiding the extent of lymphadenectomy. The technique is centre-dependent and falling out of favour as sentinel lymph node mapping and pre-operative MRI staging supplant intraoperative depth assessment in many services. Cervical cone biopsy margins occasionally require frozen-section examination when fertility-sparing surgery is planned. Trophoblastic disease — the differential between hydatidiform mole and choriocarcinoma — generally waits for permanent sections.

Reactive versus neoplastic — recurring frozen pitfalls

Several morphological patterns trip the unwary frozen-section reporter, and recognising them is part of the discipline. Reactive mesothelial cells in ascites and pleural fluid mimic carcinoma — they form papillary clusters, show variable nuclear size, and may be mistaken for primary peritoneal carcinoma. The discriminating features are the inflammatory background, the absence of true acinar architecture, and the cohesive sheet pattern rather than infiltrative growth. Squamous metaplasia in cervix and bronchus mimics squamous carcinoma when reactive nuclear atypia is marked; orientation matters — the metaplastic squamous epithelium retains a stratified pattern with surface differentiation, whereas carcinoma loses both. Granulomas mimic metastases in lymph nodes — Hodgkin lymphoma sometimes presents this way, and the differential between granulomatous inflammation and Hodgkin requires permanent sections with CD30 and CD15 immunohistochemistry. Crush artefact in small biopsies obscures distinction between lymphocyte and tumour cell — and is best resolved by careful examination of intact tissue at the section edge.

4.5 Frozen-section artefacts

Frozen-section morphology is degraded compared with paraffin morphology, and recognition of the dominant artefacts is essential for accurate interpretation. Ice-crystal artefact is the most common — water within cells freezes into intracellular vacuoles that displace organelles, distort nuclei, and lift sections from the slide. The artefact is reduced by rapid freezing in isopentane and by minimising tissue thickness, and it is recognised by the regular vacuolation pattern and the loss of fine nuclear detail. Freezing artefact in fatty tissue causes a holey, lacy pattern that can mimic lipoma or be misread as inflammation; the texture is often diagnostic when recognised.

Knife marks on frozen sections — fine parallel ridges across the section — indicate a nicked or worn blade and are corrected by changing the blade. Chatter, a less regular folded artefact, indicates a poorly-supported section or an inadequately frozen block, and is corrected by refreezing with better OCT support. Folds and tears arise from inappropriate sectioning angle or from over-handling at slide transfer. Detached and floating fragments contaminate the staining baths and become floaters on subsequent slides; the discipline of fresh baths for sentinel slides and for cases with sparse tumour reduces this risk.

Drying artefact, eosinophilic and refractile, appears at the edges of a section that has been allowed to dry between cutting and fixation. The artefact is minimised by immediate fixation and is recognised by its distribution at the periphery rather than throughout the section.

4.6 Reporting language and communication

Intraoperative reporting is a verbal act with permanent consequences. The discipline is closed-loop communication: the pathologist gives the report verbally to the named surgeon, the surgeon repeats the report back, and the pathologist confirms agreement. The conversation is documented on a dedicated frozen-section form with a timestamp, the names of both parties, the frozen-section diagnosis, and any caveats or deferred questions. A summary note is also entered into the laboratory information system.

Language choice matters. The frozen-section diagnosis is reported as one of three categories. The first is definitive — for example, 'invasive ductal carcinoma at margin, deep'. The second is descriptive with deferred conclusion — 'atypical cells suspicious for carcinoma; await permanent for definitive diagnosis'. The third is non-diagnostic — 'tissue insufficient for diagnosis on frozen; permanent will follow'. The choice depends on the confidence of the morphology and on the predictable impact of the call. The reporting pathologist should never overcall in the operating theatre, because the cost of a false-positive intraoperative call (over-extension of resection, removal of a normal structure) is high.

A deferred diagnosis is not a failure. Deferring a follicular-patterned thyroid nodule, a lymphoid lesion, or a small sentinel lymph node deposit is the correct response when frozen-section morphology cannot support a confident call. The surgeon proceeds with the planned operation, completion or extension decisions are made on the permanent report, and the patient is informed in due course. The histopathologist who feels pressured into giving a definitive call against their own judgement should resist; experienced surgeons respect a clear and reasoned defer.

Intraoperative report — discipline of language

Definitive: 'Invasive ductal carcinoma, present at deep margin.' Use when confident.

Descriptive with defer: 'Atypical glandular cells, suspicious for carcinoma; permanent required.' Use when leaning but not certain.

Defer: 'Cannot diagnose on frozen; permanent will follow.' Use when morphology does not support a confident call.

Insufficient: 'Tissue not representative; consider re-biopsy if clinically indicated.' Use when sampling fails.

Never: Give a definitive call you would not stand behind in a discrepancy review meeting.

4.7 Quality assurance and discordance

Frozen-section accuracy is audited continuously by comparison with the permanent diagnosis on the same specimen. Discordance is classified by impact. Major discordance is a difference between the frozen and the permanent that changes the operation or the management plan — for example, a frozen call of carcinoma at margin that is benign on permanent (false positive), or a frozen call of benign that is carcinoma on permanent (false negative). Minor discordance is a difference that does not change management — a benign-versus-benign reclassification, or a low-grade-versus-high-grade refinement that follows permanent IHC. The accepted major discordance rate target in accredited services is under 3 per cent, and persistent breach triggers individual and systems review.

The leading drivers of major discordance are sampling error (the frozen section did not include the lesion), interpretive error (the morphology was misread), and the inherent limitation of frozen morphology for certain entities (lobular carcinoma in breast, micrometastases in sentinel nodes, follicular thyroid neoplasia). Audit identifies recurring patterns and triggers targeted education and protocol change. The RCPath Cases of Note classification (introduced in Chapter 1) provides the framework for clinical impact grading.

Audit metrics and reporting

A rigorous frozen-section audit captures several metrics: total intraoperative requests, requests declined and the reasons, turnaround time from receipt to verbal report (target under 20 minutes for a single specimen), concordance rate with permanent diagnosis, major and minor discordance counts, false-positive and false-negative rates by specimen category, and deferred-to-permanent rate by case type. The metrics are reported quarterly at departmental governance meetings, with named individual responsibility for adverse-trend investigation. Anonymised league-table comparison across consultants and across institutions supports benchmarking — an outlier rate, in either direction, prompts review.

LIMS integration of frozen-section reporting is now standard. The frozen-section report is entered into the laboratory information system at the time of verbal communication and updated with the permanent diagnosis on completion. Linked records allow automated discordance flagging — when the permanent diagnosis differs from the frozen-section call in a defined way, the case is auto-routed to an audit queue for review. Manual flagging by reporting pathologists, who routinely review the permanent sections from their own frozens, remains the most reliable source of learning, and the discipline is built into trainee teaching.

Trainee supervision and out-of-hours cover

Frozen-section reporting is consultant-level work, and trainee involvement is supervised. The standard model in UK training has the trainee receive the specimen, perform the cut-up, review the slides, and propose a diagnosis to a supervising consultant who then signs out the case. The consultant remains responsible for the call. Out-of-hours and weekend frozen-section cover is provided by a consultant rota with named on-call individuals — typically dedicated cancer surgery lists are scheduled into hours, and the out-of-hours rota covers emergency intraoperative requests for trauma, neurosurgery, and unanticipated findings. Telepathology consultation has expanded the geographical reach of subspecialty cover and allows smaller hospitals to obtain expert opinion on difficult frozens within minutes.

Cost considerations frame the service. A typical frozen-section consultation has a fully-loaded direct cost of approximately £150 to £250 in UK practice — accounting for cryostat amortisation, reagent, technical time, and consultant time. The indirect cost is greater when out-of-hours pathways are activated. Departmental utilisation review compares the volume of intraoperative requests against the published evidence of clinical impact for each specimen category — categories with low clinical-impact rates (for example, intraoperative thyroid frozen for follicular lesions, where the call rarely changes operation) are candidates for protocol review and reduction.

4.8 Adjuncts and alternatives

Touch imprint cytology

Touch imprint cytology involves gentle pressing of a cut surface onto a slide, transferring cells without permanently altering the tissue. The slide is rapidly stained (Diff-Quik, toluidine blue, or rapid Papanicolaou) and read for malignant cells. Touch imprint is particularly useful for sentinel lymph node assessment, where it preserves the node for permanent step-section examination, and for hepatic and pulmonary nodules where the technique complements frozen-section diagnosis. Sensitivity is comparable to frozen for clear-cut malignancies and lower for micrometastases and small lesions.

Squash smear preparation

Squash smears, as introduced in the neurosurgery section above, spread a small fragment of fresh tissue between two slides to give cytological detail without freezing artefact. The technique is most useful for central nervous system tumours, lymph nodes (for cytological orientation), and small lesions where frozen morphology is unhelpful. Squash and frozen are routinely combined in neurosurgical intraoperative diagnosis.

Rapid IHC on frozens

Rapid intraoperative IHC has been developed for specific questions where the answer changes surgery. The most established example is cytokeratin staining of sentinel lymph nodes for breast cancer, where a frozen-section IHC protocol delivers a result in around 30 minutes and improves micrometastasis detection over rapid H&E alone. The technique is technically demanding, expensive, and limited to centres with the workflow capacity. Most laboratories do not deploy routine rapid IHC and rely on rapid H&E plus follow-up permanent sections with conventional IHC.

Telepathology for intraoperative consultation

Telepathology — remote viewing of a frozen slide by a consultant pathologist via a digital connection — has become routine in centres without on-site frozen-section cover, particularly out of hours and for subspecialty consultation. The slide is scanned on a rapid whole-slide imaging system or streamed live from a robotic microscope, and the reporting pathologist reviews it from another site. Validation of telepathology against on-site review is an accreditation requirement; published series report concordance over 95 per cent for routine intraoperative questions. The technique extends the reach of subspecialty expertise and supports out-of-hours frozen cover for smaller hospitals.

4.9 Key points

Chapter 4 — key points

Indications: Margin clearance, tissue identification (parathyroid), unexpected mass diagnosis, sentinel node staging.

Contraindications: Lymphoma primary diagnosis, follicular thyroid lesion classification, biomarker assessment, very small biopsies, fatty tissue without lesion.

Sentinel node: Breast frozen sensitivity 70–80% for any deposit; lower for micrometastases. Melanoma sentinel: permanent with S100/SOX10 outperforms frozen.

Closed-loop communication: Pathologist gives verbal report, surgeon repeats, pathologist confirms. Documented on dedicated form with timestamp and named parties.

Language discipline: Definitive, descriptive-with-defer, defer, or insufficient. Never give a call you would not stand behind at discrepancy review.

Artefacts of frozen: Ice crystals, freezing chatter, melt-around. Preserve a portion for permanent sections; permanent always trumps frozen.

4.10 Chapter SBAs

Q4.1. Intracellular water freezing into ice crystals during slow tissue cooling produces a characteristic morphological artefact that obscures nuclear detail and lifts sections from the slide. A renal biopsy is sent intraoperatively for assessment of a small mass. The cryostat operator places the fresh tissue directly on the cryostat chuck and freezes it over several minutes; the resulting section shows widespread vacuolation of cytoplasm and ragged nuclear outlines. Which single technique should reduce this artefact in subsequent cases?

A. Increase the cryostat chamber temperature to minus 10 °C.

B. Use isopentane chilled with liquid nitrogen for rapid initial freezing.

C. Section more thickly at 12 to 15 micrometres.

D. Stain with toluidine blue rather than haematoxylin and eosin.

E. Apply formalin to the tissue before freezing.

Answer: B

Ice-crystal artefact arises when intracellular water has time to organise into crystalline structures as the tissue cools. Slow freezing — for example, direct placement on a moderately cold cryostat chuck — allows the crystals to grow large enough to vacuolate cytoplasm and distort nuclei. Rapid freezing in isopentane chilled with liquid nitrogen drops the tissue temperature through the freezing zone fast enough that water vitrifies into a glassy, non-crystalline state, preserving morphology much better. The technique is standard for small specimens, kidney biopsies, muscle biopsies, and any tissue where cytological detail is critical. The trade-off is the additional time and equipment required, accepted in exchange for the morphological gain.

Option A worsens the problem — a warmer chamber slows the freeze and worsens crystal formation. Option C produces thicker sections that compound ice-crystal vacuolation rather than reducing it. Option D changes the stain but not the underlying morphological damage. Option E is incorrect because formalin fixation before freezing destroys the rationale for frozen-section examination and changes the assay entirely.

Q4.2. Verbal report of intraoperative findings to the operating surgeon, with confirmation by the surgeon, is the documented standard for intraoperative communication. A frozen section of a breast lumpectomy margin shows invasive ductal carcinoma at the deep margin. The pathologist telephones the operating theatre and gives the result to the on-call house officer answering the phone. Which single action represents the safest reporting practice?

A. Accept the house officer as the recipient and document the call.

B. Insist on speaking directly with the named operating surgeon and obtaining read-back confirmation.

C. Email the result to the theatre coordinator for the surgeon to read later.

D. Wait until the operation is complete and send the result by laboratory information system.

E. Defer the result entirely to the permanent section report.

Answer: B

Closed-loop verbal communication with the named operating surgeon is the accepted standard for intraoperative reporting. The surgeon making the operative decisions is the only person who can confirm receipt and integrate the result into the next operative step. The discipline of read-back confirmation — surgeon repeats the result back to the pathologist, who confirms agreement — prevents both mishearing and misattribution. Documentation on the frozen-section form with both names and a timestamp completes the record. Communication to a junior team member who is not making operative decisions risks delay or distortion of the message at the very moment when accuracy matters most.

Option A is sub-optimal because the house officer is not the decision-maker and may not relay the result accurately. Option C delays the result to a non-operative timeframe and defeats the purpose of intraoperative diagnosis. Option D is inappropriate because the surgeon is operating now and needs the result now. Option E is incorrect because the result has been generated and is actionable; refusing to communicate it harms the patient.

Q4.3. Sensitivity of frozen-section examination depends on the size of the lesion sought, the tissue type, and the number of levels examined. A 55-year-old woman has a sentinel lymph node biopsy at the time of breast lumpectomy. Frozen-section examination of one bisected node shows no metastasis. Permanent sections with step levels and cytokeratin IHC subsequently demonstrate an isolated tumour cell deposit (less than 0.2 mm) in one level. Which single statement best characterises this outcome?

A. A major discordance that should trigger root-cause analysis.

B. An expected limitation of frozen-section examination for very small deposits — not classed as a major discordance.

C. A reporting error by the frozen-section pathologist.

D. An indication that frozen-section examination should be abandoned for sentinel nodes.

E. An indication that the permanent IHC result is incorrect.

Answer: B

Isolated tumour cells (ITCs) are deposits under 0.2 mm and are at the limit of detection on frozen-section H&E. Sensitivity of frozen-section examination for ITCs is recognised to be poor — typically under 30 per cent — and the use of step sections plus cytokeratin IHC on permanent material is precisely how such deposits are identified. Missing an ITC on frozen is an inherent limitation of the technique rather than an error of the pathologist. ITCs in breast cancer are staged as pN0(i+) and the clinical significance is debated; in the post-Z0011 era, completion axillary dissection is not driven by isolated tumour cell findings, and the result rarely changes management. The case is not classed as a major discordance because no operative or management decision was harmed by the frozen-section result.

Option A overstates the impact; major discordance requires clinical management change. Option C wrongly attributes inherent technique limitation to operator error. Option D is too sweeping; sentinel node frozen examination retains a role for grossly evident metastases that do change operation in some institutions. Option E is incorrect because step sections plus IHC are the more sensitive technique by design.

4.11 Chapter EMQ

EMQ 4.1. Intraoperative requests and their appropriateness. For each scenario, select the single most appropriate response from the option list. Each option may be used once, more than once, or not at all.

A. Accept and provide a definitive frozen-section diagnosis

B. Accept and provide a descriptive frozen-section report with defer to permanent

C. Decline and offer permanent diagnosis pathway

D. Use touch imprint cytology in preference to frozen section

E. Use squash smear preparation in combination with frozen

F. Use Mohs en-face horizontal frozen-section workflow

G. Use intraoperative parathyroid hormone assay instead of frozen

H. Use rapid IHC on frozen section for cytokeratin

I. Telepathology consultation with subspecialist

J. Defer entirely to permanent sections with conventional IHC

(1) A 30-year-old woman undergoes a thyroid lobectomy for a 2 cm encapsulated follicular-patterned lesion. The surgeon requests an intraoperative diagnosis of follicular adenoma versus follicular carcinoma to decide on completion thyroidectomy. **Answer: C**

(2) A 65-year-old man undergoes a high-risk basal cell carcinoma excision on the temple. Maximum normal tissue sparing is required and the surgeon requests the appropriate intraoperative workflow. **Answer: F**

(3) A neurosurgeon resecting a posterior fossa tumour in a 45-year-old patient requests intraoperative diagnosis. The differential is metastatic carcinoma versus glioblastoma versus lymphoma. Cytological detail is needed for orientation. **Answer: E**

(4) A 70-year-old patient undergoes axillary surgery for breast cancer with multiple suspicious sentinel nodes. The breast surgeon requests intraoperative assessment but wishes to preserve all nodes intact for definitive multilevel IHC. **Answer: D**

(5) A district general hospital with no on-site frozen-section pathologist requires intraoperative diagnosis on a hepatic mass at 2 a.m. The nearest tertiary centre is 40 miles away. **Answer: I**

Chapter 5 — Reporting standards, quality assurance, and error management

A pathology report is the legal record of a diagnosis and the operational anchor for everything that follows — surgical management, oncological treatment, the multidisciplinary team meeting, the audit trail, and in some cases the courtroom record. The report has to be accurate, complete, intelligible to the clinical reader, structured for downstream extraction, and produced within a defined turnaround. These obligations are not aspirational — they are codified by the Royal College of Pathologists (RCPath), the International Collaboration on Cancer Reporting (ICCR), the American Joint Committee on Cancer / Union for International Cancer Control (AJCC/UICC) staging system, and the UK Care Quality Commission framework for clinical governance. The FRCPath Part 1 examiners assess the candidate's grasp of these frameworks and the discipline of error recognition and management that underpins them.

5.1 Structured reporting and cancer datasets

ICCR datasets and core data items

The International Collaboration on Cancer Reporting publishes structured reporting datasets that define the core data items required for each cancer specimen type — for example, breast invasive carcinoma, colorectal carcinoma, lung carcinoma, prostate radical prostatectomy. Each dataset specifies the items required in every report (core items) and the items that should appear when applicable (non-core items). Core items typically include the specimen type, the tumour site, the histological type, the histological grade, the tumour dimensions, the depth or extent of invasion, the resection margin status, lymph node status, lymphovascular invasion, perineural invasion, and the relevant biomarker results. Non-core items address findings of selective interest — for example, tumour budding in colorectal carcinoma or the Robson staging in renal cell carcinoma.

Synoptic reporting — the structured listing of core data items in a standardised order — is now the international norm. The synoptic block sits at the end of the report and is machine-readable for downstream extraction into cancer registries, audit databases, and clinical decision support tools. The RCPath cancer datasets, aligned with the ICCR specifications, are the UK-specific implementation and are referenced by NICE quality standards and by NHS cancer service specifications.

TNM staging — AJCC 8 / UICC 8

The TNM classification of malignant tumours, jointly maintained by the AJCC and UICC and currently in its 8th edition, is the universal staging framework for solid tumours. The system records the local extent of the primary tumour (T), the regional lymph node involvement (N), and distant metastases (M), with combinations grouped into prognostic stage groups (Stage I to IV). The 8th edition introduced organ-specific refinements — for example, separate categorisation of lung tumours by size in 1 cm increments up to 5 cm, integration of prognostic biomarkers (PSA, Gleason score) into prostate cancer staging, and clinical versus pathological staging distinctions in head and neck cancer.

The pathological stage (pT, pN, pM) is recorded on the histopathology report after resection, with the prefix p indicating pathological assessment. The clinical stage (cT, cN, cM) is recorded by the clinician before resection. The y prefix indicates post-neoadjuvant-therapy staging (ypT0 N0 indicating complete response). The r prefix indicates recurrent disease staging. The a prefix indicates staging at autopsy. The candidate is expected to know the principles of TNM rather than to memorise every organ-specific T category, but the major staging-defining anatomical features — peritoneal versus serosal involvement in colorectal cancer, capsular invasion in renal cell carcinoma, extracapsular extension in lymph nodes — are core knowledge.

Structured reporting essentials

ICCR datasets: international structured reporting standard, defining core and non-core items.

RCPath datasets: UK implementation, referenced by NICE and cancer service specifications.

Synoptic block: machine-readable structured list at end of report; underpins audit and registry extraction.

AJCC 8 / UICC 8: current TNM edition. Prefixes: p (pathological), c (clinical), y (post-neoadjuvant), r (recurrent), a (autopsy).

Core items: specimen type, histological type and grade, dimensions, margins, lymph nodes, lymphovascular and perineural invasion, biomarkers.

5.2 Report content and structure

A clinically useful histopathology report opens with patient and specimen identifiers and a clear statement of the clinical question or referral indication. The macroscopic description records what was received, how it was processed, and any orientation or marking. The microscopic description records the histological findings — entity, grade, extent, special features — in prose that is detailed enough to support the diagnosis but disciplined enough to avoid distracting the reader. The interpretation or comment integrates the findings with the clinical context, particularly when the diagnosis is unusual or when treatment implications need flagging. The diagnosis section provides the final summarised result, and the synoptic block provides the structured data items.

Several drafting principles improve report quality. Use clinical language that the surgeon or oncologist will recognise. Avoid jargon and Latin where plain English serves. State uncertainty explicitly — 'favoured to be benign' or 'cannot exclude carcinoma' is preferable to a definitive-sounding statement that obscures genuine doubt. Recommend the appropriate next step where it is clear — orthogonal IHC, molecular work-up, MDT review, clinical correlation. Comment on incidental findings that the clinician needs to know but might otherwise miss. Sign and date the report; in shared-reporting models, name both contributors.

Critical findings and urgent communication

Some pathological findings demand urgent verbal communication to the requesting clinician rather than reliance on the report alone. The accepted critical-finding list varies by institution but generally includes new diagnoses of malignancy in unexpected contexts, infections requiring isolation or contact tracing (tuberculosis, transmissible viral hepatitis), high-grade dysplasia or invasive cancer in pre-malignant lesions where management is time-sensitive, transplant rejection findings, and findings that materially change immediate management (placental abruption pattern in obstetric specimens, neonatal pathology that affects parents' decisions). Verbal communication is documented in the report with the recipient name and timestamp, and the formal report follows as quickly as practicable.

5.3 Internal quality assurance

Double-reporting and review

Internal quality assurance is built into the reporting workflow. Double-reporting (two-pathologist sign-out) is required for several specimen categories in UK practice — all prostatic biopsies positive for carcinoma, mismatch repair-deficient colorectal carcinomas, and selected complex cases at departmental discretion. Some departments operate prospective double-reporting on all cancer cases; others operate retrospective audit of randomly sampled cases. Slide review meetings (slide club, glass slide rounds) provide an additional layer of educational and quality oversight — interesting or difficult cases are presented for collective discussion, building the departmental knowledge base and the trainee curriculum.

Subspecialty sign-out — where consultants report only within their declared subspecialty — is the prevailing UK consultant model in larger services. Subspecialty practice raises diagnostic accuracy for difficult or rare entities and supports the use of structured datasets, but it requires service capacity and cross-cover arrangements for leave and out-of-hours work. Smaller services operate generalist sign-out with subspecialty consultation for difficult cases, often via telepathology.

Frozen-section versus permanent audit

As covered in Chapter 4, frozen-section versus permanent concordance is audited continuously. The same discipline applies to other intra-departmental discrepancies. Pre-MDT review identifies cases where the original report and the MDT-presented findings may diverge. Slide review at MDT — where the reporting pathologist or a subspecialty colleague re-reviews the slides in front of the MDT — sometimes identifies refinements or corrections. Issuing a supplementary report rather than a corrected report acknowledges these refinements transparently; a substantive change to the original diagnosis is issued as a corrected report with explicit explanation of what changed and why.

5.4 External quality assessment

External quality assessment (EQA) schemes test reporting performance across institutions using shared materials. The dominant UK schemes are operated by the Royal College of Pathologists (the RCPath EQA scheme), UK NEQAS (for technical IHC and ISH), and IQN-Path (for predictive biomarkers and molecular tests). Each scheme distributes test materials — typically virtual slide sets, glass slides, or molecular reference samples — and collects participant reports against a defined gold-standard answer. Performance is scored on diagnostic accuracy, completeness against published datasets, and adherence to reporting conventions.

Poor performance in EQA is the principal early warning of departmental or individual reporting weakness. Persistent poor return triggers structured feedback, mentoring, and in extreme cases referral to the General Medical Council. Participation in an appropriate EQA scheme is a UKAS ISO 15189 accreditation requirement, and non-participation places the laboratory's accreditation at immediate risk.

5.5 Error classification and management

Pre-analytical, analytical, and post-analytical errors

Pathology errors are conventionally classified by the phase in which they occur. Pre-analytical errors arise before the slide reaches the microscope — specimen mix-up at theatre, mislabelling, transcription error in the request form, inadequate fixation, lost specimen, inappropriate decalcification. Analytical errors arise in the laboratory — block mix-up at processing, slide mix-up at staining, floater contamination, technical processing failure. Post-analytical errors arise during reporting and communication — diagnostic interpretation error, transcription error in the report, miscommunication to the clinician, delay in report issue, failure to recognise a critical finding.

The relative frequency is well-documented. Pre-analytical errors are the most common in published audit series (around 60 to 70 per cent of laboratory errors overall), reflecting the complexity of specimen handover across teams and institutions. Analytical errors are next (around 15 to 25 per cent), and post-analytical errors are the least common but the most likely to harm the patient because they reach the clinical record. A rigorous error-management system addresses all three phases.

Cases of Note classification

The RCPath Cases of Note framework grades reporting errors by clinical impact. Grade A represents no clinical harm or potential harm from the error. Grade B represents potential for harm but no actual harm. Grade C represents minor actual harm. Grade D represents moderate actual harm. Grade E represents severe actual harm or death. The framework is applied prospectively to errors identified by audit or by post-issue review, and the resulting grade determines the depth of investigation — Grade A and B errors are typically managed within the department, while Grade C, D, and E errors trigger formal serious incident investigation under NHS England guidance.

Never events and serious incidents

Never events are defined incidents that should never occur in a properly-functioning healthcare system — and several apply to pathology. Misidentification of a patient or specimen leading to wrong-patient treatment is the canonical pathology never event; the consequence (mastectomy on the wrong patient, hysterectomy for a benign diagnosis) can be catastrophic. Specimen swap during processing is a related event with the same potential for harm. The duty of candour applies — patients (or families) must be informed of a never event, with full apology and a planned investigation. The serious incident framework (NHS England 2015, updated subsequently) defines the process for investigation, learning, and external reporting.

> **Error classification at a glance**
>
> **Pre-analytical (60–70%):** specimen mix-up, mislabelling, transcription, fixation, lost specimen.
> **Analytical (15–25%):** block or slide mix-up, floater, processing failure, slide quality.
>
> **Post-analytical (5–15%):** interpretation, report transcription, communication, delay, missed critical finding.
>
> **Cases of Note grade A:** no harm. Grade B: potential harm. Grade C–E: actual harm, escalating to severe / death.
>
> **Never events:** wrong-patient identification, specimen swap. Trigger duty of candour and serious incident investigation.

5.6 Root cause analysis and learning

Root cause analysis (RCA) is the structured investigation of a significant incident to identify the underlying causes and the system failures that allowed the incident to occur. The technique uses a sequence of questions — what happened, how did it happen, why did it happen, and what should change — to move beyond surface explanation to the system-level vulnerabilities. The aviation and high-reliability industries pioneered the technique; healthcare has adopted it across the NHS as the standard response to serious incidents. The RCA report identifies actions with named individual responsibility and deadlines, and follow-up audit verifies that the actions have been implemented and have prevented recurrence.

Significant event analysis (SEA) is the lighter-touch counterpart for events that did not rise to a serious incident but that nonetheless warrant departmental learning. A typical SEA reviews a small incident — for example, a transcription error caught at a final report check, or a near-miss in specimen handling — within the team that owns the process. The output is documented learning that may not require external reporting but does feed departmental improvement. SEAs are a routine part of clinical governance meetings.

Duty of candour

The duty of candour, statutory in England since 2014 and across the UK in similar form, requires healthcare organisations to be open and honest with patients (or their families) when something goes wrong. For pathology services, the duty applies to errors that have caused or could cause moderate harm or worse — for example, a missed cancer diagnosis that delayed treatment, or a wrong-patient report that led to inappropriate intervention. The discharging clinician (usually a member of the medical team caring for the patient) communicates with the patient, supported by the pathologist where appropriate. The communication is recorded in the patient's notes with the apology, the explanation, and the plan for further action.

5.7 Departmental governance

Departmental governance is the institutional framework that holds reporting standards, QA, and error management together. The standard structure includes a clinical governance lead, a quality manager, a designated UKAS coordinator, and named subspecialty leads. Monthly governance meetings cover EQA performance, audit findings, complaints, significant events, RCA progress, training compliance, mandatory standard reviews, and KPI tracking. The meeting minutes form the audit trail that UKAS and external review bodies examine during accreditation visits.

Key performance indicators (KPIs) track service delivery against standard targets. The dominant indicators are turnaround time (TAT, from receipt to authorised report — typically 7 days for routine biopsy, 14 days for complex resection), report completeness (proportion of cancer reports meeting RCPath dataset completeness), discrepancy rate (frozen-permanent, internal review), and complaint count. KPIs are reported quarterly with trend analysis; persistent breach triggers improvement action plans with named accountability.

UK regulatory and professional bodies

Several institutions provide the regulatory architecture within which UK histopathology services operate. The Royal College of Pathologists sets training standards, publishes datasets and good-practice guidance, operates EQA schemes, and certifies pathologists through the FRCPath examination. The General Medical Council licenses individual pathologists, sets fitness-to-practise standards, and revalidates each consultant every five years. UKAS (United Kingdom Accreditation Service) accredits laboratories against ISO 15189 — the standard for medical laboratory quality — through scheduled and unannounced visits. The Care Quality Commission inspects NHS trusts, including pathology services, against fundamental standards of safety and quality. NHS England (and parallel devolved bodies in Scotland, Wales, and Northern Ireland) publishes the operational specifications for cancer pathways, the serious incident framework, and the never-events list. The Medicines and Healthcare products Regulatory Agency (MHRA) regulates in-vitro diagnostic devices and tests, including molecular pathology assays used as companion diagnostics.

The audit cycle and PDSA

Clinical audit follows a structured cycle. The Plan stage defines the standard to be measured, the population, and the data items. The Do stage collects the data. The Study stage analyses performance against the standard. The Act stage implements change in response to findings. The cycle then repeats — re-audit verifies that the change has delivered the intended improvement. The Plan-Do-Study-Act (PDSA) cycle is the workhorse of quality improvement across UK healthcare and is taught at every level of clinical training. Department audits commonly cover dataset completeness, turnaround time, EQA performance, discrepancy rates, and adherence to local reporting protocols. Each audit has a named lead, defined endpoint, and a reporting cycle into governance.

MDT role of the pathologist

The multidisciplinary team meeting (MDT) is the operational hub of contemporary cancer care, and the pathologist is a core member. The pathologist's role at MDT includes presenting the pathology findings on each case, sharing relevant images on a high-resolution display, integrating the morphological diagnosis with the radiological, surgical, and oncological context, and supporting treatment-decision discussions. The discipline of pre-MDT slide review — examining the slides ahead of the meeting rather than reading them cold on the day — is the difference between a presenting role and a contributing role. Difficult or contentious cases benefit from prior subspecialty consultation, with the second opinion documented in the MDT record.

MDT outcomes are recorded in a structured MDT note that supplements the pathology report. Where the MDT discussion reveals a need for further pathology work — additional IHC, molecular testing, slide review by a subspecialist, or correction of an issued report — the pathologist takes named responsibility for the follow-up. The integrated outcome flows back into the patient's treatment plan and is recorded in the clinical record. The pathologist's contribution to MDT is recognised as continuing professional development time and is documented for revalidation.

5.8 Slide and report retention, storage, and retrieval

Slides, blocks, request forms, and electronic reports are part of the patient's medical record and are retained under defined retention rules. The RCPath retention guidance, aligned with the Health and Social Care Information Centre code, specifies the retention period for each material category. Slides and blocks are retained for ten years for adult cases, longer for paediatric and forensic cases, and indefinitely for selected categories including index cases of rare disease and cases with ongoing medico-legal interest. Request forms and electronic reports are retained according to the broader health-records retention schedule — typically thirty years from the last patient interaction for cancer cases.

Storage discipline supports retrieval. Slides are stored in numbered slide trays with a database link to the patient record. Blocks are stored similarly. The retrieval process is logged — every slide or block leaving the archive is signed out by name, and its return is signed back in. Slides loaned externally (for second opinion, for medico-legal review, for research with appropriate consent) are tracked through a loan register with defined return deadlines. Loss of a slide or block triggers an incident report and may, depending on circumstance, rise to the level of a significant event or serious incident.

Specimen tracking and chain of custody

Forward tracking — from theatre or clinic, through specimen receipt, accessioning, cut-up, processing, slide preparation, sign-out, and reporting — is the operational backbone of the laboratory. Modern LIMS platforms record each handover with timestamp and operator, generating a complete audit trail. Specimen tracking failures account for the bulk of pre-analytical errors, and the standard mitigations are barcode labelling at the point of acquisition (so the specimen is labelled before leaving the theatre), two-person verification at receipt, and reconciliation between request and specimen at cut-up. Chain-of-custody discipline is particularly important for forensic specimens, where any gap in the tracking record can compromise admissibility of evidence at trial.

Reporting style and common drafting pitfalls

Several drafting pitfalls recur in pathology reports. Equivocation — 'features could be consistent with' or 'cannot entirely exclude' — is sometimes appropriate but is over-used and erodes the clinical utility of the report. Excessive description without diagnostic synthesis leaves the reader to guess the bottom line. Failure to address the clinical question — the report focuses on incidental findings while not directly answering what the referring clinician asked — frustrates downstream care. Failure to recommend an action when one is needed — for example, suggesting MMR IHC reflex when MMR-deficient phenotype is suspected — misses a service opportunity. Each pitfall is addressed by structured drafting, by peer review, and by feedback from the multidisciplinary team.

5.9 Digital pathology and IT infrastructure

Contemporary histopathology depends on integrated IT infrastructure. The laboratory information management system (LIMS) records every step of the workflow — request receipt, accessioning, cut-up, processing, slide preparation, sign-out, and report distribution. The LIMS interfaces with the hospital electronic patient record so that results flow to the clinical team as soon as they are authorised. Whole-slide imaging (WSI) is increasingly integrated — slides are scanned at the time of sign-out, the digital image is stored alongside the report, and remote viewing supports MDT, telepathology, and slide sharing for second opinion. Digital reporting is now consultant-level practice in many UK centres and is the trajectory across the service.

Image management, storage capacity, network bandwidth, and cybersecurity are the operational concerns of a digital pathology service. A typical whole-slide image is one to several gigabytes; a fully-digital department generates tens of terabytes of imaging data per year. Backup, archive, and disaster recovery planning are governance items reviewed at departmental level. Cybersecurity incidents — ransomware attacks on NHS trusts — have demonstrated the operational vulnerability of digital pathology, and tested business-continuity plans for reverting to glass-slide workflow are an accreditation expectation.

5.10 Continuing professional development and revalidation

Continuing professional development (CPD) is the formal mechanism by which consultant pathologists maintain and develop their professional skills. The RCPath CPD scheme requires fifty credits per year, evenly distributed across clinical, professional, and research activities. CPD activities include attending courses and conferences, reviewing slides at slide club, participating in EQA, contributing to MDT, supervising trainees, undertaking audit, writing research papers and book chapters, and external teaching. CPD is documented in an annual portfolio that feeds into the appraisal and revalidation cycle.

Appraisal is an annual structured conversation between the consultant and a trained appraiser, reviewing the year's performance, identifying development needs, and confirming engagement with mandatory training, audit, and patient feedback. Revalidation is the five-yearly GMC process through which a consultant's licence to practise is confirmed; the appraisal portfolio is the principal evidence base. Failure to engage with appraisal or to demonstrate CPD compliance triggers escalation through the responsible officer route and may, in extreme cases, lead to GMC fitness-to-practise action.

Trainee progression and workplace-based assessment

UK histopathology training spans five years following foundation training, covering broad subspecialty exposure and culminating in the FRCPath examination — Part 1 (written and OSPE) in year three, Part 2 (clinical and microscopy) in year five. The training programme is set by the RCPath curriculum, with workplace-based assessments (WBAs) generating an evidence portfolio of clinical encounters, case-based discussions, multi-source feedback, and direct observation of practical skills. Educational supervisors and clinical supervisors meet the trainee at defined points each year — formative review at three months, summative review at twelve months — and the annual review of competence progression (ARCP) panel signs off readiness for the next training year.

The training portfolio integrates CPD, audit involvement, MDT participation, slide club engagement, EQA performance, and research output. The supervising consultant carries named responsibility for the trainee's progression, and concerns about competence are addressed through structured remediation plans rather than informal conversation. The trainee transition to consultant practice is supported by a final year focused on independent reporting, MDT leadership, and management exposure — preparing the candidate for the breadth of the consultant role.

International benchmarking and comparators

UK pathology operates within an international framework of professional bodies and standards. The College of American Pathologists (CAP) publishes parallel cancer protocols and operates EQA schemes used internationally. The European Society of Pathology (ESP), the International Academy of Pathology (IAP), and the United States and Canadian Academy of Pathology (USCAP) provide international meeting platforms, training resources, and consensus guidance. The International Collaboration on Cancer Reporting (ICCR) is the principal international body for cancer dataset harmonisation, with the RCPath and CAP as key contributing partners. Specialist societies — for example, the International Society of Urological Pathology (ISUP), the International Society of Dermatopathology (ISDP), the European Association for Haematopathology (EAHP) — produce subspecialty consensus on grading, classification, and reporting.

5.11 Medico-legal aspects

Histopathology reports carry medico-legal weight. The reporting pathologist is the named professional accountable for the diagnosis, and the report may be examined in coroners' inquests, criminal trials, civil negligence claims, and General Medical Council fitness-to-practise hearings. The discipline of clear, honest, and contemporaneous documentation protects both the patient and the pathologist. Retention of slides, blocks, and electronic records is governed by RCPath retention guidance — typically 10 years for routine cases, 30 years for paediatric and forensic cases, lifetime for selected categories.

Expert witness work in histopathology is a recognised consultant activity. The expert witness role differs from the routine reporting role — the expert provides an independent opinion to the court, not to the patient's clinical team, and the duty of the expert is to the court rather than to either party in the dispute. The standards for expert witness practice are set by the Civil Procedure Rules and by the General Medical Council; the candidate is not examined on expert witness work at Part 1 but should know that the role exists and that it carries distinct ethical and procedural obligations.

5.12 Learning from complaints and feedback

Patient complaints reach pathology services through the hospital complaints procedure rather than directly, since pathology rarely has direct patient contact. The complaints that do arise often concern delays, report errors, or communication failures to the patient's clinical team. Each complaint is investigated, the patient receives a written response within the statutory timeframe, and learning is fed back to the department through governance. Clinician feedback — both formal (at MDT, in user surveys) and informal (during slide review, in corridor conversation) — is the more frequent source of operational learning, and a healthy departmental culture welcomes critical feedback as the route to improvement.

5.13 Key points

Chapter 5 — key points

AJCC TNM 8: Current edition for most sites. Prefixes p, c, y (post-neoadjuvant), r (recurrent), a (autopsy). Synoptic block at end of report.

Structured reporting: ICCR sets international core and non-core items; RCPath datasets implement for the UK and are referenced by NICE.

Error classification: Pre-analytical errors dominate (60–70%); analytical 15–25%; post-analytical 5–15%. Clerical errors top the audit lists.

Cases of Note: RCPath grades 1–4 by clinical impact. Recurrent grade 3–4 triggers performance review.

Root cause analysis: Five-whys to systemic cause. Never events (specimen swap, wrong patient) trigger duty of candour and serious incident review.

Turnaround time: Biopsies 7 days, resections 10 days, cytology 3–5 days (UK KPIs at 80% threshold). Continuous audit with monthly review.

Second-opinion practice: Documented external review with written opinion; incorporated or divergence noted in the final report.

5.14 Chapter SBAs

Q5.1. Misidentification of a patient or specimen leading to wrong-patient treatment is a defined event in the NHS never-events framework, with mandatory reporting and investigation obligations. A reporting pathologist signs out a left breast core biopsy with invasive ductal carcinoma. The patient has since undergone scheduled mastectomy. At MDT the following week, slide review reveals that the slide labelled with the patient's identifier is in fact from another patient — a labelling error introduced at the cut-up bench. The original patient's correct slides show only benign fibrocystic change. Which single set of actions represents the appropriate institutional response?

A. Issue a corrected report and inform the surgeon by email.

B. Discuss with the patient at the next follow-up clinic.

C. Trigger a serious incident investigation, apply the duty of candour with full disclosure to the patient and family, and undertake root cause analysis.

D. Document the error in the laboratory log and review at the next governance meeting.

E. Refer the case directly to the General Medical Council for fitness-to-practise review.

Answer: C

This event meets the criteria for a never event — specimen mix-up leading to wrong-patient surgical treatment with severe harm (unnecessary mastectomy). The institutional response is structured. First, urgent verbal communication to the surgical team and to the patient's clinicians. Second, formal serious incident investigation under the NHS England serious incident framework, opening within hours of identification. Third, application of the duty of candour — the patient and (where appropriate) the family are informed openly with apology, explanation, and a planned process. Fourth, root cause analysis to identify the system failures that allowed the labelling error and to design preventive actions. Fifth, learning is fed back into departmental governance and into broader NHS reporting if patterns are identified.

Option A is grossly inadequate — a corrected report by email does not meet the duty of candour and does not trigger the systemic response that a never event requires. Option B delays appropriate communication. Option D treats a serious incident as a minor issue. Option E confuses the institutional response with individual fitness-to-practise referral; GMC referral is considered only when individual conduct or competence is in question, and the appropriate primary response remains the structured serious incident investigation.

Q5.2. Structured reporting using defined core data items supports completeness, audit extraction, and MDT discussion. A pathologist completes a report on a colectomy specimen for invasive adenocarcinoma. Which single item is a core data item required in every RCPath colorectal cancer dataset report?

A. The patient's smoking history.

B. The macroscopic length of the resected colon segment.

C. The lymphovascular invasion status (present, absent, or indeterminate).

D. The patient's body mass index.

E. The operating surgeon's name.

Answer: C

Lymphovascular invasion is a recognised independent prognostic factor in colorectal carcinoma and is included as a core data item in the ICCR and RCPath colorectal cancer datasets. The report records the status as present, absent, or indeterminate, and the finding feeds adjuvant chemotherapy decisions for stage II disease where its presence (along with high-risk features such as perineural invasion, poor differentiation, and inadequate lymph node yield) supports the case for chemotherapy.

Reporting lymphovascular invasion consistently is part of the audit-ready cancer report and is one of the elements assessed in RCPath dataset compliance audits.

Option A is patient information that may sit in the clinical record but is not a pathology dataset item. Option B is a macroscopic descriptor that may appear in the macroscopic section of the report but is not classed as a core dataset item. Option D is not a histopathology data item. Option E is part of the request information rather than a dataset item.

Q5.3. External quality assessment provides cross-institutional benchmarking and is a regulatory requirement for accredited laboratories. A laboratory has failed to return three consecutive RCPath EQA distributions for histopathology and one IQN-Path distribution for HER2 IHC. UKAS surveillance is scheduled in two months. Which single statement best describes the regulatory and operational implications?

A. Continued non-participation is acceptable provided the department documents the reasons.

B. Non-participation in an appropriate EQA scheme is an immediate critical non-conformity that places ISO 15189 accreditation at risk.

C. EQA participation is recommended but not required for accreditation.

D. The laboratory should withdraw from accreditation and operate without ISO 15189 status.

E. The HER2 EQA scheme is voluntary because HER2 testing is not regulated.

Answer: B

Participation in an appropriate external quality assessment scheme is an explicit requirement of ISO 15189 (the laboratory medicine quality standard against which UKAS accredits histopathology services). Persistent non-participation — whether through failure to return distributions or through formal withdrawal — constitutes a critical non-conformity that places the laboratory's accreditation at immediate risk. The expected sequence is a UKAS surveillance visit identifying the non-conformity, a defined improvement plan from the laboratory with timelines, and the possibility of accreditation suspension if the plan is not delivered. EQA non-participation is also an indicator that the laboratory may lack the internal capacity to detect performance drift, raising the broader concern that diagnostic quality may not be assured.

Option A is incorrect because no documentation removes the requirement to participate. Option C confuses recommendation with requirement. Option D is a disproportionate response. Option E is factually wrong — HER2 testing is a regulated companion diagnostic with mandated EQA participation through IQN-Path.

5.15 Chapter EMQ

EMQ 5.1. Error classification and response. For each scenario, select the single most appropriate framework, action, or category from the option list. Each option may be used once, more than once, or not at all.

A. Pre-analytical error

B. Analytical error

C. Post-analytical error

D. Cases of Note grade A (no harm)

E. Cases of Note grade C–E (actual harm)

F. Never event

G. Duty of candour

H. Root cause analysis

I. Significant event analysis

J. Routine departmental audit

(1) A specimen container labelled for Patient A is found to contain tissue removed from Patient B, identified through an unrelated MDT slide review three weeks after surgery. The wrong tissue was reported and treatment has been initiated based on the incorrect diagnosis. **Answer: F**

(2) A floater fragment from a positive lymph node case has contaminated a subsequent benign nodal specimen, identified at sign-out by the reporting pathologist before any report was issued. No harm reached the patient. **Answer: B**

(3) A reporting pathologist accidentally enters the wrong patient identifier on a histopathology report. The error is caught by a checking clerical staff member before the report leaves the laboratory. **Answer: C**

(4) A serious incident has been formally declared after a wrong-patient mastectomy. A structured investigation is convened to identify the underlying system failures and to design preventive actions. **Answer: H**

(5) An MDT review identifies that a missed dysplasia diagnosis from six months earlier resulted in delayed treatment of progression. The patient has been informed and the family is asking for further explanation. **Answer: G**

Chapter 6 — Autopsy practice

The autopsy is the original method of pathology — the systematic examination of a body after death to determine the cause and the contributing circumstances. The technique long predates the microscope and the immunohistochemistry platform, and it remains the single most informative investigation in medicine for explaining unexpected death, validating clinical diagnoses, and providing accountability to families and to the legal system. The FRCPath Part 1 examiners assess the principles of autopsy practice rather than the manual technique — consent and legal authority, the systematic examination, the recognition of pathology, the certification of death, and the communication of findings to families and to the courts. This chapter sets out the framework within which the histopathologist performs and reports autopsy work in UK practice.

6.1 Legal authority and consent

Hospital autopsy and the Human Tissue Act

Hospital (consented) autopsy is undertaken at the request of clinicians and with the consent of the deceased's family. The Human Tissue Act 2004 (HTA, applying to England, Wales, and Northern Ireland; the Human Tissue (Scotland) Act 2006 covers Scotland) governs the storage, use, and disposal of human tissue removed at autopsy. Authorisation under the HTA is the legal foundation for hospital autopsy — the nominated representative (the deceased's spouse, civil partner, parent, or other qualifying relative as defined by the HTA) provides written authorisation in a form that confirms understanding for the post-mortem examination, for retention of tissue and organs, and for any subsequent use (research, education, archiving). The form documents specific elements: the scope of the examination (full or limited), retention of small tissue samples, retention of whole organs (for example, the brain for neuropathological assessment), and the eventual disposal pathway for retained material.

Hospital autopsy rates have declined steeply across the developed world over the past half-century — from over fifty per cent of hospital deaths in the 1960s to under five per cent in many UK institutions in 2024. The reasons are multiple: clinical confidence in imaging and laboratory investigations, the operational and emotional burden on families and clinicians, declining trainee exposure to the technique, and limited resources in mortuary services. The decline has consequences — the autopsy remains the gold standard for diagnostic verification — and several published audit series demonstrate that around ten per cent of autopsies reveal a major unexpected finding that would have changed clinical management had it been known antemortem. The candidate should be aware of this paradox and the broader debate around autopsy revival initiatives.

Coroners' autopsies and the coronial system

Coroners' (or, in Scotland, procurator fiscal) autopsies are undertaken under the legal authority of an independent judicial officer charged with investigating sudden, unexpected, or unexplained deaths. The coroner orders an autopsy when the cause of death is not clear from the clinical history, when the death is potentially due to violence, accident, neglect, or unnatural causes, when the death occurred during or shortly after surgery or other medical intervention, when the death may be subject to industrial disease compensation, or when the deceased had not been seen by a doctor in the immediate period before death. The consent of the family is not required for a coroner's autopsy — the coroner's authority overrides familial wishes — though the family is informed and the timing is communicated.

The coroner is currently appointed under the Coroners and Justice Act 2009, with revised regulations updating earlier nineteenth-century statutes. The coroner's pathologist — a histopathologist or forensic pathologist on the coroner's approved list — performs the autopsy and reports directly to the coroner. The report may be limited to the immediate cause of death or may extend to a broader account of contributing pathology, depending on the coroner's request. Findings inform the coroner's decision on inquest, certification, and any referral to other authorities — police, the Health and Safety Executive, or sector regulators where the death raises wider concerns (police, HSE, regulatory bodies).

Authority and scope at a glance

Hospital autopsy: HTA authorisation by nominated representative. Scope set by consent form.

Coroner's autopsy: coroner's authority overrides family consent; performed on coroner's list of approved pathologists.

Forensic autopsy: specialist forensic pathologist; suspected homicide, suspicious deaths, complex cases.

Scotland: Procurator Fiscal directs medico-legal autopsies; Human Tissue (Scotland) Act 2006.

Refusal: hospital autopsy can be refused by family; coroner's autopsy cannot.

6.2 Mortuary safety and infection control

Mortuary practice carries occupational hazards that the candidate should know in principle. Universal precautions apply — gloves, gowns, face shields, and surgical masks for all autopsies. Containment level 3 specimens demand additional protocols — respirator protection, controlled airflow, restricted access, and decontamination of the workspace after each examination: respiratory protection (FFP3 mask) for tuberculosis, viral haemorrhagic fevers, and SARS-CoV-2 in some institutional protocols. The high-risk specimen list includes hepatitis B and C, HIV, prion disease, tuberculosis, and the viral haemorrhagic fevers. Some institutions decline to perform full autopsies on patients with category 4 pathogens, restricting examination to limited cavity inspection or to imaging-only post-mortem investigation.

Prion disease — Creutzfeldt-Jakob disease, variant CJD, kuru, and other transmissible spongiform encephalopathies — presents the highest-risk scenario in mortuary practice. The prion protein resists conventional decontamination by autoclaving, formaldehyde, and standard chemical disinfection, and a single autopsy on a suspected case requires dedicated single-use equipment, careful technique to minimise aerosolisation, and incineration of the dedicated equipment afterwards. Many UK mortuaries refer suspected prion cases to a designated national centre rather than perform the autopsy locally. The 1990s BSE epidemic and the subsequent variant CJD cases reshaped UK mortuary policy, and the contemporary framework is set by the Advisory Committee on Dangerous Pathogens.

6.3 The autopsy technique

External examination and evisceration

Every autopsy begins with external examination — height, weight, body habitus, identifying features, surgical scars, evidence of injury, evidence of intervention (intravenous lines, endotracheal tube, urinary catheter — each documented for context) (intravenous lines, endotracheal tube, urinary catheter), evidence of decomposition (rigor mortis, livor mortis, hypostasis), and any abnormal findings (rashes, oedema, jaundice, cyanosis). External examination is the first and most important data source in suspicious deaths, and photography of any external finding is routine in coronial and forensic practice.

Evisceration follows a standard sequence. The midline incision extends from chin or upper sternum to symphysis pubis. Skin and subcutaneous tissue are reflected; the rib cage is opened with a saw or rib shears; the anterior thoracic plate is removed. The abdominal cavity is opened and inspected in situ for any free fluid, abnormal masses, or unusual relationships. The Rokitansky (en masse) technique removes all the thoracic and abdominal organs as a single block; the Virchow technique removes each organ separately; the Letulle (modified Rokitansky) technique combines features of both. The choice depends on operator preference, the clinical question, and the technical demands of the case. For most contemporary UK practice, a modified Rokitansky or Letulle approach predominates.

Systematic organ examination

After removal, organs are examined systematically — typically heart, lungs, gastrointestinal tract, liver, biliary tree, pancreas, spleen, urinary tract, reproductive tract, and endocrine glands. Each organ is weighed against published reference ranges, externally examined for surface lesions, and sectioned at standard intervals to display the parenchymal architecture and any focal abnormality. Photography supplements the description for unusual or suspicious findings. Histology samples are taken from any focal lesion and from standard sites where systemic pathology is anticipated — for example, anterior descending coronary artery in cardiac death, lung parenchyma representative of both lung fields in respiratory death, liver wedge in hepatobiliary disease.

The brain is removed after the skull cap is reflected — by either a coronal saw cut around the calvarium or a designated mortuary technique that preserves the dura. Fresh brain is heavy and friable; many laboratories suspend the whole brain in formalin for two to three weeks before sectioning, particularly for neuropathological assessment. Coronal sections then display the cortex, basal ganglia, ventricular system, brain stem, and cerebellum, with sampling for histology based on the macroscopic findings and the clinical question.

6.4 Toxicology and ancillary sampling

Toxicology samples — peripheral blood, vitreous, urine, gastric contents — are collected at the start of the autopsy to minimise post-mortem redistribution and contamination. The standard panel comprises peripheral blood (femoral vein is preferred over central blood because of the redistribution phenomenon, in which drugs leak from gastric and hepatic stores into central blood after death), vitreous humour, urine, and gastric contents. Specimens are stored at minus 20 °C and sent to an accredited forensic toxicology laboratory for screening (immunoassay for the standard drug-of-abuse panel) and confirmation (gas chromatography mass spectrometry, liquid chromatography mass spectrometry).

Microbiology samples are taken when infection is suspected — blood cultures from a peripheral vessel, swabs from the lung surface or other suspected source, cerebrospinal fluid where indicated. Sampling discipline matters because the body becomes colonised rapidly after death, generating a high false-positive rate on culture. Molecular methods (16S ribosomal RNA sequencing, multiplex PCR panels) are increasingly used to characterise post-mortem isolates and to distinguish ante-mortem infection from post-mortem colonisation.

6.5 Post-mortem imaging

Post-mortem imaging — predominantly computed tomography (PMCT) and to a lesser extent magnetic resonance imaging (PMMR) — has emerged over the past two decades as a powerful supplement to invasive autopsy and, in selected cases, as an alternative to it. PMCT is fast and widely available; a single scan generates a complete anatomical dataset that can be reviewed and re-reviewed without time pressure. The indications include identification of foreign bodies and projectiles, recognition of skeletal injuries (particularly subtle fractures), demonstration of free intraperitoneal or intrathoracic gas (gut perforation, vascular gas embolism), and demonstration of haemothorax or haemoperitoneum. PMCT-guided biopsy enables targeted sampling without full evisceration.

PMMR is slower, less widely available, and more sensitive to small post-mortem changes — but is superior to PMCT for soft-tissue pathology, particularly in cardiac and neonatal pathology. Imaging-only post-mortem investigation is offered in some institutions as an alternative to invasive autopsy for families who decline a conventional examination on religious or personal grounds; the diagnostic yield is lower than invasive autopsy but the technique resolves a defined proportion of cases without invasive examination. The decision to substitute imaging for invasive autopsy rests with the coroner where coronial authority applies, and with the family and clinical team for hospital autopsies.

6.6 Body identification and documentation

Confirmation of body identity is the first responsibility at autopsy. The standard sequence is verification of identifying wristbands (where present), checking the body against the mortuary register, and confirming any distinguishing physical features against the patient record. In cases of disputed identity, dental records, fingerprints, surgical scars, and DNA matching are the established techniques — dental records are the workhorse for identification of remains in mass casualty incidents and in advanced decomposition. The pathologist documents the identification process in the autopsy report, particularly when the identity is not immediately confirmed.

Documentation at autopsy follows defined conventions. The autopsy report records the date and place of examination, the names of those present, the identifying details of the deceased, the clinical history, the external examination, the internal examination, the ancillary investigations (toxicology, microbiology, histology), the interpretation, and the cause of death. Photography is integrated throughout — overview shots of the body in situ, close-ups of any external finding, and internal photographs of significant lesions. The photographs form part of the medical record and may be required as evidence at inquest or in subsequent proceedings.

System-by-system examination findings

The candidate should know the dominant macroscopic findings to seek in each system. The cardiovascular examination focuses on coronary artery patency at standardised intervals, myocardial integrity (acute infarction is pale in the first six hours and then becomes increasingly mottled and yellow over days), valve morphology, great vessel integrity (aortic dissection demonstrates an intramural haematoma and intimal tear), and pericardial collections. The respiratory examination assesses pulmonary parenchyma for consolidation, oedema, congestion, embolism (saddle and segmental embolism in the main pulmonary arteries), tumour, and asbestos-related disease. The gastrointestinal examination identifies haemorrhage (intraluminal, intramural, retroperitoneal), perforation, ischaemia, obstruction, and tumour. The hepatobiliary examination assesses parenchymal architecture, biliary patency, cirrhotic morphology, and focal lesions. The genitourinary examination assesses renal cortex thickness, parenchymal lesions, and bladder integrity. The central nervous system assesses ventricular volume, parenchymal integrity, haemorrhage (subarachnoid, intracerebral, subdural, epidural), infarction, herniation, and focal lesions.

6.7 Mortality and morbidity meetings

Mortality and morbidity (M&M) meetings are the clinical governance venue at which deaths are reviewed for learning. The structure varies by department, but the standard pattern presents each death in turn — the clinical history, the cause of death, any autopsy findings, and any quality of care issues that arose during the admission. The pathologist contributes the autopsy findings and the integrated interpretation, supporting the clinical team's discussion of whether the death was avoidable, expected, or revealed any system-level learning. The output of the M&M meeting feeds into the broader clinical governance audit and may trigger root cause analysis where significant learning is identified.

The Learning from Deaths framework, introduced by NHS England in 2017, formalised the requirement for NHS trusts to review every death and to identify problems in care that could be addressed. The framework distinguishes deaths classified as having problems in care (further sub-classified by likelihood that better care could have prevented the death) and feeds annual public reports on mortality review. The autopsy findings — when an autopsy has been performed — are a key input to the review. The decline in autopsy rates has therefore affected the precision of the Learning from Deaths process, generating renewed interest in autopsy revival across UK practice.

6.8 Specific autopsy contexts

Sudden cardiac death

Sudden unexpected cardiac death in adults under fifty — including young athletes and apparently healthy adults — is the commonest scenario triggering coroner's autopsy. The autopsy systematically assesses the major coronary arteries (degree of stenosis, plaque morphology, evidence of thrombosis), the myocardium (regional infarction, scar, fibrosis, focal lesions), the conducting system (sinoatrial node, atrioventricular node where indicated), the cardiac valves, and the great vessels. Hypertrophic cardiomyopathy, dilated cardiomyopathy, arrhythmogenic right ventricular cardiomyopathy, channelopathies (long QT, Brugada, catecholaminergic polymorphic ventricular tachycardia) — these are the differential to consider when no macroscopic explanation is found. Heart sampling for histology is standardised — coronary arteries cross-sectioned at 5 mm intervals, myocardial blocks from each ventricular wall and the conducting system. Genetic testing of myocardial DNA may be undertaken in selected cases with consent of the family, to identify channelopathies and inheritable cardiomyopathies of relevance to surviving relatives.

Perinatal and paediatric autopsy

Perinatal autopsy (stillbirth and neonatal death) is a specialised subdiscipline performed by a paediatric or perinatal pathologist. The autopsy includes external examination with anthropometric measurements — crown-heel and crown-rump length, foot length, head circumference, chest circumference — and placental examination (always — the placenta carries information critical to interpretation of fetal pathology), full evisceration with detailed cardiac and central nervous system examination, photography of any congenital anomalies, and karyotyping or microarray analysis of fetal tissue. The cause of death analysis often defines a primary obstetric or fetal cause and one or more contributing factors. The findings inform parental counselling, support reproductive planning for subsequent pregnancies, and contribute to the maternal-fetal mortality audit.

Sudden infant death syndrome (SIDS) is a coronial responsibility and is investigated under the Joint Agency Response (JAR) protocol in England, with parallel arrangements across the devolved nations. The protocol coordinates police, social services, paediatric, and pathology investigation — its purpose is to exclude inflicted injury, metabolic disorder, and identifiable cardiac, respiratory, or infectious cause. Microbiological, toxicological, metabolic, and genetic investigations supplement the autopsy, and a multidisciplinary case discussion concludes the investigation. Unexplained sudden infant deaths that meet the SIDS criteria are certified accordingly; identified causes are certified by the relevant ICD code.

Post-surgical death

Death within thirty days of surgery is a coronial event in most UK jurisdictions, triggering a coroner's autopsy with particular focus on the operative site and the perioperative pathway. The autopsy examines the operative site for haemorrhage, anastomotic leak, surgical material left in situ, and infection. Systemic complications — pulmonary embolism, myocardial infarction, sepsis, fluid management complications, transfusion reactions, anaesthetic complications — are sought in the relevant organ systems. The findings inform any clinical investigation, the inquest process, and any clinical governance learning at the institution.

Sepsis and infectious death

Autopsy after death attributed to sepsis or other infectious cause aims to identify the source of infection, the extent of organ involvement, and any predisposing factor. Blood cultures are taken from a peripheral vessel before evisceration. The presumed source (chest, abdomen, urinary tract, skin, surgical site) is examined directly with sampling for histology and microbiology. End-organ damage — acute kidney injury, hepatic dysfunction, disseminated intravascular coagulation manifestations, adrenal haemorrhage suggesting Waterhouse-Friderichsen syndrome — is documented. The findings support certification, may identify a preventable infection control failure, and contribute to mortality and morbidity review.

6.9 Death certification and the medical examiner system

In England and Wales the death certification process has changed markedly in the past five years — the introduction of the medical examiner (ME) system, which from 2024 became mandatory for non-coronial deaths in NHS hospitals. The ME is a senior clinician (often a histopathologist or other consultant) who scrutinises the proposed cause of death on the Medical Certificate of Cause of Death (MCCD), engages with the bereaved family, identifies cases requiring referral to the coroner, and confirms the certification before the death is registered. The system aims to improve the accuracy of death certification, support bereaved families, and identify quality of care concerns. Parallel systems operate in Scotland and Northern Ireland with local variations.

The MCCD records the sequence of conditions leading to death — the immediate cause (Part 1a), the antecedent cause (Part 1b), the underlying cause (Part 1c), and significant contributing conditions (Part 2). The discipline of MCCD completion is taught to all UK doctors and is examined in postgraduate certification — the candidate is expected to know the sequence and the rules. Common errors include certifying old age as a cause without supporting underlying pathology, certifying sepsis without naming the source, and conflating the underlying cause with the mode of death (for example, certifying 'cardiac arrest' rather than the underlying ischaemic or cardiomyopathic process).

Cremation forms

Cremation in the United Kingdom requires statutory medical certification — historically two separate medical certificates (the Cremation 4 and Cremation 5 forms), now streamlined to a single Cremation 4 form following changes implemented alongside the medical examiner system. The completing doctor confirms that the cause of death is known, that the death is not subject to coronial investigation, and that there is no medical reason to delay cremation. The medical examiner reviews the certification before cremation can proceed. The forms reflect the historical concern that cremation destroys post-mortem evidence and therefore demands greater certainty about cause of death than burial.

6.10 The inquest

An inquest is the public legal hearing convened by the coroner to determine four specific questions about a death — who the deceased was, when they died, where they died, and how they came by their death. The inquest is investigative rather than adversarial; the coroner asks questions of witnesses, and there are no parties in the conventional sense. Verdicts are recorded in defined categories — natural causes, accident, suicide, unlawful killing, lawful killing, open verdict, and narrative conclusion — each reflecting the coroner's assessment of the circumstances (where the coroner sets out the circumstances in narrative form rather than a single-word verdict).

The pathologist who performed the autopsy is commonly called as a witness at inquest. The witness role demands clear, evidence-based testimony presented in plain language to a non-medical audience that includes the bereaved family. The witness explains the autopsy findings, identifies the cause of death, and answers questions from the coroner, the family or their legal representative, and any other interested party. Maintaining objectivity while expressing genuine empathy for the family — both at once — is the discipline; the witness is there to inform the inquest, not to advocate for any party.

6.11 Communication with families

Bereaved families are at the centre of the autopsy process even when they are not legally required to consent. Communication with the family typically falls to the clinical team who knew the patient — supported by the pathologist for specific queries about the autopsy findings. The discipline of clear, sensitive, jargon-free communication is critical — families want to know what happened, why it happened, and whether anything could have been done differently. The findings are explained without minimising or overstating, and any limitations or uncertainties in the autopsy interpretation are stated openly.

Particular sensitivity attaches to perinatal and paediatric autopsy, to autopsies of patients with mental health crises, and to autopsies on individuals from minority communities where religious and cultural considerations may inform the timing, scope, and conduct of the examination. The pathologist works within these frameworks, declining to perform autopsies that conflict with consent or with the coroner's authority and supporting alternative pathways (limited autopsy, post-mortem imaging) where appropriate.

6.12 Teaching and learning at autopsy

The autopsy is the foundational teaching activity in pathology — direct correlation between gross findings, microscopy, and clinical history is unmatched as a learning experience. Histopathology trainees attend autopsies, observe technique, perform components under supervision, and present cases at departmental mortality and morbidity meetings. The decline in autopsy volume has affected training opportunities, and many UK training programmes have responded by concentrating autopsy training at designated centres with high case volumes. Trainees signed off at FRCPath level are competent to perform routine coronial autopsies under appropriate supervision and to report the findings; forensic autopsy specialisation requires additional specific training and Forensic Pathology certification.

6.13 Key points

Chapter 6 — key points

Hospital autopsy: HTA-authorised by nominated representative. Scope set by the consent form; family can refuse.

Coroner's autopsy: Coroner's authority overrides family consent. Statutory referrals: violent or unnatural death, sudden death of unknown cause, death in custody.

Forensic autopsy: Specialist forensic pathologist; suspected homicide and other suspicious deaths. Chain-of-custody preserved throughout.

Scotland: Procurator Fiscal directs medico-legal autopsies; Human Tissue (Scotland) Act 2006 applies.

Technique: External examination, evisceration, organ block dissection, weights and measurements, histology of targeted blocks, toxicology where indicated.

Special situations: Sudden cardiac death (review conduction system, send tissue for genetic testing); maternal death (placenta retained); paediatric death (referred specialist pathway).

Report: Cause of death in WHO format: 1a immediate, 1b underlying due to 1a, 1c underlying due to 1b; 2 contributory.

6.14 Chapter SBAs

Q6.1. Coronial authority overrides familial consent in defined circumstances under the Coroners and Justice Act 2009 and parallel legislation. A 72-year-old man dies suddenly at home, having seen his general practitioner one week earlier with stable angina. He had been seen by no doctor in the days immediately before death. The family wishes to decline post-mortem examination on religious grounds. Which single statement best describes the appropriate pathway?

A. The autopsy is declined in accordance with the family's wishes.

B. A hospital autopsy is performed with the family's consent under the HTA.

C. The death is referred to the coroner; the coroner has the legal authority to order an autopsy independently of the family's wishes.

D. The general practitioner certifies the death as ischaemic heart disease and no further investigation is required.

E. A forensic autopsy is performed because the death is suspicious.

Answer: C

Sudden, unexpected death of a person who had not been seen by a doctor in the immediate period before death meets the criteria for referral to the coroner. The coroner, exercising independent judicial authority, decides whether autopsy is required to establish the cause of death and, if so, what scope the autopsy should take. The coroner's authority overrides familial wishes — the family is informed but does not have a veto. The discipline of respectful communication with the family, explaining the legal framework and the reasons for the coroner's decision, sits alongside the legal authority and is part of good practice. The autopsy may, in some cases, be undertaken in a limited form (for example, restricted to cavity examination) to accommodate religious or cultural concerns, but the decision rests with the coroner.

Option A is incorrect because the family does not have authority to decline a coroner's autopsy. Option B applies only to hospital autopsies under the HTA, which is not the appropriate pathway when coronial referral is required. Option D bypasses the legal framework — the GP cannot certify a death that meets coronial criteria without referral. Option E confuses coroner's with forensic autopsy; forensic autopsies are reserved for suspected homicide and other suspicious or complex cases, and the scenario describes neither.

Q6.2. Post-mortem drug redistribution from gastric and hepatic stores into central vessels can elevate measured blood concentrations and confound interpretation of toxicology results. A coroner's autopsy is being performed on a patient suspected of overdose. Which single sampling site is the preferred source of blood for toxicology analysis?

A. Right atrium (cardiac blood).

B. Inferior vena cava just below the diaphragm.

C. Femoral vein (peripheral blood).

D. Portal vein.

E. Subclavian vein.

Answer: C

Post-mortem redistribution is the phenomenon by which drugs and metabolites diffuse from tissue reservoirs (the gastric contents, the liver, the lungs) into central blood after death. Central blood (cardiac and great vessel) measurements may therefore overestimate the antemortem blood concentration and confound interpretation. Peripheral blood — most reliably from the femoral vein — is less affected by redistribution and is the preferred source for forensic toxicology. The femoral vein is accessed before evisceration with a clean technique to minimise contamination, and a defined volume is collected into preservative-free and preservative-containing tubes for separate analyses.

Option A (right atrium) is precisely the site most affected by redistribution and is the worst choice for quantitative interpretation. Options B and E are also subject to redistribution from adjacent organs. Option D (portal vein) is the most contaminated source because it drains the gastrointestinal tract directly — the highest-concentration drug reservoir after oral ingestion.

Q6.3. The Medical Certificate of Cause of Death records a defined sequence of conditions leading to death, with discipline expected in distinguishing underlying cause from mode of death. A 78-year-old woman dies in hospital. She had longstanding ischaemic heart disease, a prior myocardial infarction, and developed a chest infection three days before death. Which single sequence is the most appropriate MCCD entry?

A. Part 1a: Cardiac arrest. Part 1b: Old age.

B. Part 1a: Pneumonia. Part 1b: Ischaemic heart disease.

C. Part 1a: Bronchopneumonia. Part 1b: Acute exacerbation of chronic ischaemic heart disease. Part 1c: Coronary artery atherosclerosis.

D. Part 1a: Sepsis. Part 1b: Old age.

E. Part 1a: Multi-organ failure. Part 1b: Frailty.

Answer: C

Good MCCD certification records the sequence of conditions in causal order — the immediate cause that produced death (1a), the antecedent cause that led to the immediate cause (1b), and the underlying cause that initiated the sequence (1c, if applicable). For this patient, bronchopneumonia is the immediate cause, the chronic cardiac disease (acute exacerbation) is the antecedent contributory cause, and coronary artery atherosclerosis is the underlying disease. The certification supports public health analysis and informs the cancer or non-cancer mortality registries.

Option A treats cardiac arrest as a cause when it is in fact a mode of death — the heart stops when any patient dies, and 'cardiac arrest' carries no causative information. 'Old age' is an unhelpful certification in the presence of identifiable contributory disease. Option B reverses the antecedent and underlying logic — pneumonia is the immediate cause, and ischaemic heart disease is the contributing factor, but the underlying coronary atherosclerosis is missing. Option D conflates the mode (sepsis as final pathway) with the underlying cause. Option E uses non-specific terminology that does not support meaningful certification.

6.15 Chapter EMQ

EMQ 6.1. Autopsy pathway and authority. For each scenario, select the single most appropriate pathway or action from the option list. Each option may be used once, more than once, or not at all.

A. Hospital autopsy with HTA authorisation by the nominated representative

B. Coroner's autopsy ordered by the coroner

C. Forensic autopsy by a forensic pathologist

D. Limited autopsy with restricted scope by family agreement

E. Post-mortem imaging only (no invasive autopsy)

F. Refer to a designated prion-disease centre

G. Joint Agency Response (JAR) protocol

H. Medical Certificate of Cause of Death issued without autopsy

I. Refer to the Procurator Fiscal (Scotland)

J. Cremation 4 form completion by medical examiner

(1) A 35-year-old man dies four days after a road traffic collision in which another driver was involved. Police suspect that mechanical failure may have contributed. **Answer: C**

(2) An 80-year-old woman with documented dementia and end-stage congestive cardiac failure dies at home under hospice care. Her general practitioner had visited two days earlier and the cause of death is straightforwardly established. **Answer: H**

(3) A 9-month-old infant is found unresponsive in his cot by his parents and cannot be resuscitated. No injury or illness is documented in the recent history. **Answer: G**

(4) A 60-year-old patient with rapidly progressive dementia, ataxia, and myoclonus has died. Suspected Creutzfeldt-Jakob disease is documented in the clinical notes. **Answer: F**

(5) A 50-year-old man dies suddenly while playing tennis. He had no documented cardiac history and had seen his GP a year earlier with no significant findings. Death occurred in Glasgow. **Answer: I**

Chapter 7 — Cytopathology principles

Cytopathology is the diagnosis of disease from cells rather than from tissue architecture — a discipline founded by George Papanicolaou in the 1940s on cervical smears and now extending across virtually every organ system. The morphological substrate is fundamentally different from histopathology: individual cell features (nucleus, cytoplasm, nucleolar prominence, chromatin pattern) dominate the diagnosis, supported by background features (necrosis, inflammation, mucus, colloid) and limited architectural information from cell clusters. The FRCPath Part 1 examiners assess cytological technique, the major standardised classification systems, and the integration of cytology with histology and ancillary investigations. This chapter covers the principles that recur across organ-specific cytology and introduces the international reporting frameworks that define contemporary practice.

7.1 Sample acquisition and preparation

Fine-needle aspiration

Fine-needle aspiration (FNA) is the foundational technique. A 22- to 25-gauge needle is passed into the lesion under palpation or imaging guidance, suction is applied, and material is drawn into the needle. Multiple passes maximise yield. The aspirated material is expelled onto slides and processed by one of three pathways — direct smear preparation (the classical technique, with a second slide drawn rapidly across the first to spread cells in a monolayer), rinse into liquid-based cytology medium, or cell-block preparation by centrifugation and paraffin processing. Many laboratories use a combined approach with direct smears for rapid assessment and an additional rinse for ancillary studies.

Image guidance has transformed FNA practice. Ultrasound guidance is the routine method for superficial lesions and for accessible deep targets (thyroid, salivary, breast, lymph node, liver, pancreas via endoscopic ultrasound). Computed tomography guidance is preferred for deep retroperitoneal and pulmonary lesions where ultrasound penetration is limited. Endobronchial ultrasound (EBUS) is the standard technique for mediastinal lymph node staging in lung cancer. Endoscopic ultrasound (EUS) with FNA samples pancreatic, gastric submucosal, and peri-oesophageal lesions. Rapid on-site evaluation (ROSE) — a cytopathologist or trained cytotechnologist evaluates the sample at the procedure to confirm adequacy — reduces non-diagnostic rates markedly.

Liquid-based cytology and cell blocks

Liquid-based cytology (LBC) collects the sample into a preservative fluid (ThinPrep methanol-based or SurePath ethanol-based being the dominant commercial systems). The fluid suspends cells, lyses red blood cells, and provides a substrate for automated filtration or sedimentation onto a slide. LBC delivers a clean monolayer free of blood and obscuring material, supports ancillary molecular and immunocytochemical testing on the residual fluid, and is the substrate for HPV testing in cervical screening. The technique has displaced conventional smears for cervical cytology in most modern programmes and is increasingly applied across non-gynaecological cytology.

Cell blocks are paraffin blocks generated from residual cytological material — fluid sediment, FNA washings, or scraped cell pellets — embedded as small tissue samples and processed identically to surgical specimens. The cell block enables immunohistochemistry, in-situ hybridisation, and molecular testing on cytological material, bringing the full ancillary toolkit of histopathology to bear on cells. The cell block is now a standard adjunct to FNA across organs where lineage definition, biomarker testing, or molecular profiling is anticipated — for example, lung adenocarcinoma EBUS samples where TTF-1, napsin A, and PD-L1 IHC plus molecular profiling are routine.

7.2 Staining methods in cytology

Two staining traditions dominate cytology, and each highlights different morphological features. The Papanicolaou stain — haematoxylin, orange G, and EA-50 (eosin azure 50) — provides excellent nuclear detail with crisp chromatin pattern and clear nucleoli, plus differential cytoplasmic staining (orange for keratinised squamous cells, blue-green for non-keratinised). Papanicolaou is the international standard for cervical cytology and the dominant stain for fine-needle aspiration cytology where nuclear features drive the diagnosis. The technique requires fixation in alcohol (95 per cent ethanol) and a multi-step staining sequence that takes around twenty minutes to complete.

The Romanowsky family of stains — Diff-Quik, May-Grunwald-Giemsa, Wright-Giemsa — uses methylene blue and eosin derivatives to produce striking colour contrast. The stains highlight cytoplasmic features (granules, vacuoles, mucin), background material (colloid in thyroid, lymphoglandular bodies in lymph node, mucin in mucinous tumours), and lymphoid cells with great clarity. The trade-off is less detailed nuclear chromatin pattern. Diff-Quik in particular is the rapid stain of choice for ROSE adequacy assessment — its three-minute protocol gives a usable preparation while the patient is still on the procedure table. Many laboratories run paired smears, one fixed for Papanicolaou and one air-dried for Romanowsky, combining the strengths of both traditions.

Pap versus Romanowsky — when to use which

Papanicolaou: nuclear chromatin, nucleoli, squamous keratinisation. Cervical screening, FNA where nuclear detail dominates.

Romanowsky (Diff-Quik, MGG): cytoplasmic detail, granules, mucin, background, lymphoid cells. ROSE adequacy, lymph node cytology, fluid cytology.

Combined approach: paired smears (alcohol-fixed Pap + air-dried Romanowsky) maximise information.

Cell block: paraffin H&E for ancillary IHC, ISH, molecular work.

7.3 Adequacy criteria

A cytology specimen is diagnostically useful only when adequate — sufficient representative cells, well-preserved morphology, and absence of obscuring blood or inflammation. Each major cytology system specifies its own adequacy criteria. Cervical cytology under the Bethesda system requires a minimum number of well-preserved squamous cells (around 5,000 for conventional smears, 8,000 for

LBC), with a transformation zone component (endocervical cells or squamous metaplastic cells) supporting adequate sampling. Thyroid FNA under the Bethesda system for reporting thyroid cytopathology (TBSRTC) requires at least six groups of well-preserved follicular cells, each containing at least ten cells; lesions with abundant colloid alone may be classified as benign without strict cell count if the clinical context supports a colloid nodule.

Inadequate samples are reported as non-diagnostic with explicit guidance on the reason — scant cellularity, obscuring blood, technical artefact, or absence of representative components. The risk of malignancy in non-diagnostic samples is not zero and varies by organ. In thyroid cytology the risk of malignancy in a non-diagnostic FNA is around 5 to 10 per cent; in salivary FNA it is somewhat higher; in pancreatic EUS-FNA the inadequate rate has been reduced by ROSE to under 10 per cent. The reporting pathologist recommends repeat sampling when clinically appropriate, with the timing depending on the lesion and the clinical urgency.

7.4 Major cytology classification systems

Standardised reporting systems improve communication, allow comparison across institutions, and link the cytological diagnosis to an estimated risk of malignancy (ROM) that informs clinical management. Each major system shares a common structure — discrete diagnostic categories, defined adequacy criteria, ROM estimates per category, and recommended management for each category. The FRCPath candidate should know the principal categories of each system, the canonical ROM estimates, and the broad management implications.

The Bethesda System for Reporting Thyroid Cytopathology

TBSRTC, now in its third edition (2023), classifies thyroid FNA into six categories. Bethesda I (non-diagnostic) — repeat FNA recommended; ROM around 13 per cent (range 5 to 20 per cent in published cohorts). Bethesda II (benign) — clinical follow-up; ROM under 4 per cent. Bethesda III (atypia of undetermined significance or follicular lesion of undetermined significance, AUS/FLUS) — repeat FNA or molecular testing; ROM 13 to 30 per cent depending on local cohort. Bethesda IV (follicular neoplasm or suspicious for follicular neoplasm) — surgical lobectomy or molecular testing; ROM 23 to 34 per cent. Bethesda V (suspicious for malignancy) — surgical resection; ROM 67 to 83 per cent. Bethesda VI (malignant) — surgical resection or definitive management; ROM 97 to 99 per cent.

Molecular testing for indeterminate Bethesda III and IV categories has reshaped thyroid management over the past decade. Commercial panels (Afirma gene expression classifier, ThyroSeq, ThyGeNEXT/ThyraMIR) integrate genomic and transcriptomic data to refine the risk estimate, supporting decisions on surgical versus observational management for borderline lesions. UK uptake is variable, and the candidate is not expected to memorise commercial panel performance but should know that molecular adjuncts exist for indeterminate cytology.

The Milan System for Reporting Salivary Gland Cytopathology

The Milan system (2018, with refinements published since) classifies salivary FNA into six categories paralleling the structure of TBSRTC. Milan I (non-diagnostic) — repeat FNA; ROM around 25 per cent reflecting the higher pre-test probability of significant disease in salivary lesions referred for FNA.

Milan II (non-neoplastic) — clinical follow-up; ROM around 10 per cent. Milan III (atypia of undetermined significance) — repeat FNA; ROM around 20 per cent. Milan IVa (benign neoplasm — pleomorphic adenoma, Warthin tumour, basal cell adenoma) — surgical resection or observation depending on lesion; ROM under 5 per cent. Milan IVb (salivary neoplasm of uncertain malignant potential, SUMP) — surgical resection; ROM 35 per cent. Milan V (suspicious for malignancy) — surgical resection; ROM around 60 per cent. Milan VI (malignant) — definitive surgical management; ROM over 90 per cent.

The Paris System for Reporting Urinary Cytology

The Paris System (TPS-Urine, current second edition 2022) classifies urinary cytology into seven categories with focus on high-grade urothelial carcinoma (HGUC) detection rather than low-grade lesions, which the cytology cannot reliably identify. Categories include non-diagnostic, negative for HGUC, atypical urothelial cells (AUC), suspicious for HGUC, HGUC, low-grade urothelial neoplasm (LGUN), and other malignancies (small cell, squamous, adenocarcinoma). The system emphasises specific cytological criteria — increased nucleus-to-cytoplasm ratio above 0.7, hyperchromatic chromatin, and irregular nuclear membrane — to distinguish HGUC from reactive atypia. ROM for the principal categories ranges from very low (negative) to over 90 per cent (HGUC).

The IAC Yokohama System for Reporting Breast Cytopathology

The Yokohama system (2019) classifies breast FNA into five categories: insufficient, benign, atypical (cells lacking definite features of malignancy but warranting further investigation), suspicious for malignancy, and malignant. Each category carries a ROM and a management recommendation. The role of breast FNA has shifted in modern practice — most breast cancer diagnoses are made on core biopsy rather than FNA, with FNA reserved for selected scenarios (cystic lesions, lymph node staging, recurrent disease confirmation). The system retains relevance for these scenarios and for centres that maintain FNA capacity.

The Bethesda System for cervical cytology

The Bethesda System for reporting cervical cytology (TBS-Cerv, latest edition 2014) covers the entire cervical screening workflow. Squamous cell categories run from NILM (negative for intraepithelial lesion or malignancy) through ASC-US (atypical squamous cells of undetermined significance), LSIL (low-grade squamous intraepithelial lesion encompassing CIN1 and HPV cytopathic change), ASC-H (atypical squamous cells, cannot exclude high-grade), HSIL (high-grade squamous intraepithelial lesion encompassing CIN2 and CIN3), and squamous cell carcinoma. Glandular categories run from AGC (atypical glandular cells) through endocervical adenocarcinoma in situ and adenocarcinoma. The system informs management algorithms tied to HPV co-testing — primary HPV testing is now the dominant cervical screening modality in the UK and several other countries, with cytology used as a reflex test on HPV-positive samples.

The WHO Reporting System for Lung Cytopathology

The WHO 2023 Reporting System for Lung Cytopathology — developed jointly by the International Academy of Cytology, the American Society of Cytopathology, and the Papanicolaou Society —

provides a five-tier classification for respiratory cytology including bronchoalveolar lavage, bronchial brushings, bronchial washings, and EBUS-FNA. Categories are non-diagnostic, benign, atypical, suspicious for malignancy, and malignant — each with associated risk of malignancy and recommended management. The system parallels the structure of the thyroid and salivary systems and supports international harmonisation of lung cytology reporting. Ancillary testing on EBUS-FNA samples (TTF-1, p40, napsin A, ALK, ROS1, PD-L1 immunocytochemistry on cell block; molecular profiling on liquid residual or cell block extraction) is the standard adjunct for malignant samples to guide treatment.

7.5 Cervical screening — principles and operational framework

The UK cervical screening programme covers women aged 25 to 64. The screening interval depends on HPV status: HPV-negative individuals are recalled at five-yearly intervals across the full age range (25-49 and 50-64). The five-yearly interval for the 25-49 age group was implemented by NHS England from 1 July 2025 (Scotland and Wales had moved to a five-yearly interval at earlier dates), bringing the entire screening age range to a uniform five-yearly recall for HPV-negative results. Individuals testing HPV-positive at screening, or with a recent history of HPV, are recalled more frequently (typically annually for surveillance) until HPV clearance or dysplasia is detected. The programme moved from cytology-primary to HPV-primary screening in 2019 — samples are first tested for high-risk HPV (the 14 oncogenic types), with reflex cytological assessment on HPV-positive samples and immediate return to routine recall for HPV-negative samples. The transition reduced the cytological workload markedly and concentrated cytological assessment on the population most at risk of dysplasia.

Quality assurance in the screening programme operates at multiple levels — laboratory-level QA (proportion of inadequate samples, throughput, processing turnaround), screener-level QA (annual workload audit, rapid review of negative slides, internal QA exercises), and programme-level audit (coverage, recall rates, biopsy-proven dysplasia detection rates, interval cancer rates). The screening programme is operated within a national governance framework with named regional and national leads and an established communication pathway for incident reporting. Cervical screening errors are among the most documented in healthcare quality literature and have informed the broader development of laboratory error management.

7.6 Automation in cytology

Automated image analysis has been deployed in cervical cytology screening since the late 1990s — initially the AutoPap and PAPNET systems, more recently the Hologic Genius Digital Diagnostics System and the BD FocalPoint slide profiler. The principle is the same in each platform — whole-slide imaging captures the slide, an algorithm identifies the regions most likely to contain abnormal cells, and the screener reviews those regions in priority order. Computer-assisted screening (CAS) improves sensitivity for high-grade dysplasia and reduces the cognitive load of full-field screening. Most UK laboratories now use CAS for primary cervical cytology screening, with manual review of the algorithm-flagged regions.

Automation in non-gynaecological cytology is less established but is expanding. Whole-slide imaging supports remote review, slide sharing for second opinion, and the application of deep learning algorithms for pattern recognition in selected applications (urinary cytology screening for high-grade urothelial carcinoma, thyroid FNA categorisation). The technology is in the validation phase for routine diagnostic use in non-gynaecological settings, and accreditation frameworks are evolving alongside.

7.7 Renal mass cytology

Percutaneous renal mass biopsy and FNA are now established techniques for the characterisation of small renal masses, particularly when active surveillance or ablation is being considered as an alternative to surgery. Cytology distinguishes the major renal cell carcinoma subtypes — clear cell, papillary, chromophobe — and identifies oncocytoma and angiomyolipoma as benign mimics. The cytological features differ between subtypes: clear cell carcinoma shows clear or finely granular cytoplasm with delicate vasculature in the smears; papillary carcinoma shows papillary architecture and foamy macrophages in the background; chromophobe carcinoma shows perinuclear halos and binucleation; oncocytoma shows oxyphilic cytoplasm and round monomorphic nuclei. Cell-block IHC supports lineage definition — CK7 and CA9 for clear cell, AMACR for papillary, KIT and CK7 for chromophobe and oncocytoma differential, HMB-45 and Melan-A for angiomyolipoma.

7.8 Organ-specific FNA cytology

Thyroid FNA

Thyroid FNA is the most extensively standardised cytology service. The cytological features of papillary thyroid carcinoma are diagnostic in classical cases — nuclear enlargement, nuclear grooves, intranuclear pseudo-inclusions, powdery optically-clear chromatin, and three-dimensional architectural fragments with intricate papillary configuration. Cytological diagnosis of papillary carcinoma maps to Bethesda V or VI depending on the strength of the features. The follicular-patterned lesions (follicular adenoma, follicular carcinoma, follicular variant of papillary carcinoma, NIFTP) present the diagnostic limit of cytology — the distinction between adenoma and carcinoma requires histological assessment of capsular and vascular invasion, and cytology can position the lesion as Bethesda III or IV but cannot resolve the categorical question.

Lymph node FNA

Lymph node FNA addresses two principal questions. The first is metastatic carcinoma — relevant in head and neck cancer staging, in unknown primary work-up, and in re-staging of treated disease. Cytological recognition of carcinoma in a lymph node is generally straightforward when classical features are present; lineage assignment uses immunocytochemistry on cell block sections. The second question is primary lymphoma. Cytological diagnosis of lymphoma is limited — classification depends on architecture, immunophenotype, and molecular work that cytology alone cannot deliver. FNA can suggest a lymphoid process and refer for excisional biopsy, or can support diagnosis when combined with flow cytometry on a separate aspirate, with cell block immunohistochemistry, and with molecular clonality analysis. Excisional biopsy remains the gold standard for primary lymphoma diagnosis in the United Kingdom and most international centres.

Pancreatic EUS-FNA

Endoscopic ultrasound-guided FNA of pancreatic lesions distinguishes the major categories — ductal adenocarcinoma, neuroendocrine tumour, intraductal papillary mucinous neoplasm (IPMN), mucinous cystic neoplasm, solid pseudopapillary neoplasm, serous cystadenoma, and pancreatitis. The Papanicolaou Society of Cytopathology guidelines structure the reporting categories and the recommended ancillary testing. Cell block immunocytochemistry differentiates ductal adenocarcinoma (CK7, CK20 variable, CA19-9, MUC1) from neuroendocrine tumour (synaptophysin, chromogranin, INSM1) and from solid pseudopapillary neoplasm (beta-catenin nuclear, CD10, vimentin). Cystic lesions are evaluated with cyst fluid CEA, CA19-9, glucose, and amylase measurements alongside cytological assessment of any aspirate.

Body fluid cytology

Pleural, peritoneal, and pericardial fluid cytology addresses the question of malignancy in serous effusions. Reactive mesothelial cells are abundant in any inflamed serous cavity and constitute the principal cytological pitfall — they form sheets and papillary clusters, show variable nuclear enlargement, and may be mistaken for adenocarcinoma. Discriminating features include the cohesive monolayered architecture of mesothelial cells, the central pale 'window' between adjacent mesothelial cells, and the lack of true gland formation. Immunocytochemistry on cell block sections distinguishes mesothelial cells (calretinin, WT1, D2-40 positive) from carcinoma (BerEP4, MOC-31, CEA, organ-specific markers positive). Malignant mesothelioma is the most challenging differential — cytology alone cannot reliably distinguish reactive mesothelial hyperplasia from mesothelioma, and effusion cytology positive for mesothelioma requires histological correlation.

7.9 Ancillary techniques on cytology material

Immunocytochemistry on cell block sections operates identically to histological IHC and supports lineage definition, biomarker assessment, and predictive testing. Cell block sections are also the substrate for FISH (HER2 amplification, ALK and ROS1 rearrangement in lung), in-situ hybridisation for viral signal (EBER for EBV, high-risk HPV in cervical), and for molecular testing through dedicated extraction protocols. Some platforms enable molecular testing directly on liquid-based cytology residuals without cell block preparation — particularly useful for lung adenocarcinoma EBUS samples and for thyroid molecular profiling.

Flow cytometry on cytological samples is the standard initial workup for suspected lymphoma on FNA — a separate aspirate is collected into RPMI or similar transport medium and run on the flow platform to identify the cell population by surface marker phenotype. The flow result feeds back into the cytological assessment and supports an integrated cytological diagnosis. Excisional biopsy follows when architectural assessment is needed for definitive classification.

7.10 Errors and pitfalls in cytology

Cytological misinterpretation is a recognised source of diagnostic error, with characteristic patterns. False-negative errors arise from sampling failure (the lesion was missed by the needle), from screening error in cervical cytology (the abnormal cells were on the slide but were not identified), and from interpretation error (atypical cells were seen but were misclassified as reactive). False-positive errors arise from over-interpretation of reactive atypia in inflammatory contexts, from confusion of metaplasia with neoplasia, and from contamination by floater cells from a previous case. The discipline of double-screening for cervical cytology and double-reporting for difficult non-gynaecological cases mitigates both error categories, and rapid review of negative slides under defined criteria is a recognised QA technique.

Specific pitfalls include reactive ductal hyperplasia in breast FNA mimicking ductal carcinoma in situ, lymphocytic thyroiditis with Hurthle cell change mimicking follicular neoplasia, reactive mesothelial cells in effusion cytology mimicking metastatic carcinoma, atypical squamous cells of undetermined significance representing post-inflammatory change rather than dysplasia, and benign reactive lymph node features mimicking low-grade lymphoma. Each pitfall is addressed by knowledge of the pattern, by ancillary testing, and by integration of cytological findings with clinical and radiological context.

7.11 Reporting and integration with histology

A cytological report identifies the specimen and the procedure, describes the cytological findings, applies the relevant standardised classification, and provides the diagnosis with risk of malignancy where appropriate. The report explicitly states the management recommendation arising from the result — repeat sampling for non-diagnostic, surgical resection for malignant, observation for benign — referring to local guidelines where relevant. When ancillary testing is performed on cell block or residual fluid, the cytology report integrates those findings into a single coherent diagnostic statement rather than separate parallel reports.

Cytology-histology correlation is a standard QA activity. When a cytological diagnosis is followed by a surgical specimen on the same lesion, the two reports are compared for concordance. Discordance triggers review of both materials, with the outcome documented in the laboratory record. The exercise supports continuous calibration of cytological interpretation against the histological gold standard and identifies patterns of diagnostic difficulty that inform departmental education and protocol development.

7.12 Key points

Chapter 7 — key points

Sample types: Exfoliative (cervix, urine, serous fluids), abrasive (brushings), FNA (palpable or image-guided), ROSE.

Stains: Papanicolaou for nuclear chromatin and squamous keratinisation (alcohol-fixed);

Romanowsky (Diff-Quik, MGG) for cytoplasm, granules, lymphoid background (air-dried).

Cell block: Paraffin H&E plus IHC, ISH, and molecular work. Critical for lung adenocarcinoma biomarker panel.

ROSE: Rapid on-site evaluation confirms adequacy and triages material to cell block, microbiology, flow cytometry, molecular.

Cervical cytology: Bethesda 2014: NILM, ASC-US, LSIL, ASC-H, HSIL, AGC. HPV testing co-tests or triages by local pathway.

Thyroid FNA: Bethesda TBSRTC: I non-diagnostic, II benign, III AUS, IV follicular neoplasm, V suspicious, VI malignant. Risk of malignancy and management mapped to each category.

Fluid cytology: Serous effusions classified by IAC Sydney system. Adenocarcinoma vs mesothelioma vs reactive mesothelium: panel of calretinin, WT1, BAP1, MOC-31, BerEP4.

7.13 Chapter SBAs

Q7.1. Defined cytological categories with associated risks of malignancy guide subsequent management in thyroid cytology. A 45-year-old woman has thyroid FNA of a 2 cm hypoechoic nodule. Cytology shows microfollicular architecture with mild nuclear atypia but no classical papillary features. The lesion is classified as Bethesda IV (follicular neoplasm or suspicious for follicular neoplasm). Which single statement best describes the typical risk of malignancy and the recommended next step?

A. Risk of malignancy under 5 per cent; clinical follow-up only.

B. Risk of malignancy 23 to 34 per cent; surgical lobectomy or molecular testing for further risk stratification.

C. Risk of malignancy over 95 per cent; total thyroidectomy.

D. Risk of malignancy not defined; repeat FNA in six months.

E. Risk of malignancy under 1 per cent; no further investigation.

Answer: B

Bethesda IV (follicular neoplasm or suspicious for follicular neoplasm) carries a risk of malignancy in the range of 23 to 34 per cent according to the third edition of TBSRTC, reflecting the inability of cytology to distinguish follicular adenoma from follicular carcinoma (the distinction requires assessment of capsular and vascular invasion on the resected lesion). The recommended next step is either surgical lobectomy for definitive histological assessment, or molecular testing using a validated commercial panel to refine the risk estimate before deciding on surgery. The choice depends on patient factors, lesion size, ultrasound features, and local pathway availability. The 2023 ATA guidelines and parallel UK guidance support both surgical and molecular triage pathways for Bethesda IV lesions.

Option A understates the ROM and gives an inappropriate management. Option C overstates the ROM — Bethesda VI (malignant) carries an ROM over 95 per cent, not Bethesda IV. Option D is incorrect because Bethesda IV does have a defined ROM range. Option E understates and proposes no investigation, which is inappropriate for a Bethesda IV result.

Q7.2. Distinction of reactive mesothelial cells from metastatic adenocarcinoma in serous effusions depends on a defined immunocytochemistry panel applied to cell block sections. A 70-year-old man presents with a unilateral pleural effusion and prior history of colorectal carcinoma. Pleural fluid cytology shows a population of cohesive cells in three-dimensional clusters with abundant cytoplasm and uniform nuclei. The differential is reactive mesothelial cells versus metastatic adenocarcinoma. Which single panel is the most appropriate first-line approach on the cell block?

A. Pan-cytokeratin alone.

B. Calretinin, WT1, and D2-40 to confirm mesothelial lineage; BerEP4, MOC-31, and CDX2 to support metastatic colorectal carcinoma.

C. Ki-67 alone to assess proliferation.

D. Vimentin alone to demonstrate mesenchymal origin.

E. BRAF V600E IHC to support metastatic disease.

Answer: B

The differential between reactive mesothelial cells and metastatic carcinoma in serous effusions is the canonical cell-block immunocytochemistry question. The recommended panel includes mesothelial markers (calretinin, WT1, D2-40) and carcinoma markers (BerEP4, MOC-31, CEA), with lineage-specific markers added for the suspected primary site (CDX2 and CK20 for colorectal origin in this patient). Mesothelial cells stain positively for calretinin, WT1, and D2-40 and negatively for the carcinoma markers; metastatic adenocarcinoma shows the reverse pattern. The integrated panel produces a definitive lineage assignment in the majority of cases. Malignant mesothelioma — which would also stain positively for mesothelial markers — is the residual concern; cytology alone cannot reliably distinguish reactive mesothelial hyperplasia from mesothelioma, and pleural biopsy is the gold standard if mesothelioma remains in the differential.

Option A is insufficient — pan-cytokeratin stains both mesothelial cells and adenocarcinoma. Option C provides proliferative information but does not address lineage. Option D is inadequate — vimentin is non-specific in this context. Option E focuses on a mutation-specific marker that does not help with the categorical lineage question.

Q7.3. Adequacy of a cytology specimen is defined by the relevant classification system and is the prerequisite for diagnostic interpretation. A thyroid FNA of a 1.5 cm hypoechoic nodule shows only three groups of five well-preserved follicular cells each, with abundant red blood cell background. No colloid is identified. Which single classification and recommendation is the most appropriate?

A. Bethesda II (benign), recommend clinical follow-up.

B. Bethesda III (AUS/FLUS), recommend repeat FNA in 3 months.

C. Bethesda I (non-diagnostic), recommend repeat FNA under ultrasound guidance.

D. Bethesda V (suspicious for malignancy), recommend surgical resection.

E. Bethesda VI (malignant), recommend total thyroidectomy.

Answer: C

TBSRTC adequacy requires at least six groups of well-preserved follicular cells, each containing at least ten cells. The described sample (three groups of five cells each) falls below this threshold and is therefore non-diagnostic — Bethesda I. The recommended next step is repeat FNA, typically under ultrasound guidance to maximise yield from the lesion, often after a delay of three to six months to allow resolution of any haemorrhagic interference at the original biopsy site. Lesions with abundant colloid may be classified as benign without strict cell count criteria, but the described sample lacks colloid and is not eligible for this exception.

Option A is incorrect — the sample does not meet adequacy criteria and cannot be called benign without sufficient cellularity. Options B, D, and E all imply a diagnostic interpretation that the inadequate sample cannot support. The discipline of classifying inadequate samples as Bethesda I rather than overcalling or undercalling them protects the integrity of the system and ensures that the appropriate management (repeat sampling) follows.

7.14 Chapter EMQ

EMQ 7.1. Cytology classification systems. For each scenario, select the single most appropriate classification system from the option list. Each option may be used once, more than once, or not at all.

A. The Bethesda System for reporting thyroid cytopathology (TBSRTC)

B. The Milan System for reporting salivary gland cytopathology

C. The Paris System for reporting urinary cytology

D. The IAC Yokohama System for reporting breast cytopathology

E. The Bethesda System for reporting cervical cytology

F. The Papanicolaou Society of Cytopathology pancreatobiliary system

G. International System for Reporting Serous Fluid Cytopathology

H. WHO Reporting System for Lung Cytopathology

I. WHO Classification of Soft Tissue Tumours

J. ICCR Cancer Datasets

(1) A 50-year-old woman has FNA of a 3 cm parotid gland mass. Cytology shows monomorphic basaloid cells with myxoid stroma; the differential includes pleomorphic adenoma and adenoid cystic carcinoma. **Answer: B**

(2) A 65-year-old man with painless haematuria has a voided urine cytology sample submitted to screen for high-grade urothelial neoplasia. **Answer: C**

(3) A 70-year-old woman has thoracentesis of a unilateral pleural effusion. The cytology shows reactive mesothelial cells and the question is whether malignant cells are present in the fluid. **Answer: G**

(4) A 40-year-old woman has FNA of a 1.8 cm thyroid nodule with hypoechoic features on ultrasound. The cytological assessment will be reported as a Bethesda category. **Answer: A**

(5) A 60-year-old man has EUS-guided FNA of a 2 cm head of pancreas mass. The cytological findings need a standardised reporting framework with risk of malignancy estimates. **Answer: F**

Chapter 8 — Oesophagus

The oesophagus presents the FRCPath Part 1 candidate with a focused syllabus dominated by inflammatory and neoplastic disease. The mucosa transitions from non-keratinising stratified squamous epithelium in the body of the oesophagus to columnar gastric epithelium at the gastro-oesophageal junction (GOJ), and this transition zone is the seat of the most clinically significant oesophageal disease, Barrett's oesophagus and the adenocarcinomas that arise within it. This chapter covers the principal entities encountered in oesophageal biopsy and resection practice — reflux oesophagitis, eosinophilic oesophagitis, infectious oesophagitis, Barrett's oesophagus with dysplasia grading, oesophageal adenocarcinoma, squamous cell carcinoma, and the mesenchymal and neuroendocrine entities — together with the WHO 5th edition classification, the AJCC 8 TNM framework, and the assessment of response to neoadjuvant therapy.

8.1 Anatomy and normal histology

The oesophagus extends from the cricopharyngeal sphincter at C6 to the GOJ at around T10–T11, with a length of approximately 25 cm in the adult. The mucosa is lined by non-keratinising stratified squamous epithelium throughout most of its length: basal cells with a small dark nucleus give rise to maturing squamous cells with increasing cytoplasmic glycogen toward the surface. The lamina propria contains scattered lymphocytes and occasional plasma cells. The muscularis mucosae forms a thin double layer of smooth muscle that separates the lamina propria from the submucosa, and the submucosa contains mucous glands (submucosal seromucous glands characteristic of the oesophagus) along with vessels, nerves, and the submucosal lymphoid tissue. The muscularis propria is striated in the upper third, mixed in the middle third, and smooth in the lower third, a quirk of embryological derivation that occasionally features in examiner discussion.

The gastro-oesophageal junction is defined endoscopically as the upper margin of the gastric folds and histologically as the point where squamous epithelium meets columnar epithelium (the squamocolumnar junction, SCJ). The normal SCJ coincides with the GOJ — when columnar epithelium is found proximal to the GOJ, the lesion is termed Barrett's oesophagus subject to defined diagnostic criteria. A short segment of columnar-lined mucosa less than 1 cm above the GOJ is the so-called 'irregular Z line' and is generally not classified as Barrett's in current UK guidance.

Normal oesophageal histology — key features

Mucosa: non-keratinising stratified squamous epithelium; basal cells small with dark nuclei, maturing toward surface.

Lamina propria: scattered lymphocytes, occasional plasma cells; vascular papillae extend partway into epithelium.

Muscularis mucosae: thin double smooth muscle layer.

Submucosa: submucosal seromucous glands (characteristic of the oesophagus), vessels, nerves.

Muscularis propria: striated upper, mixed middle, smooth lower.

GOJ: upper margin of gastric folds; SCJ coincides with GOJ normally.

8.2 Reflux oesophagitis (GORD)

Gastro-oesophageal reflux disease (GORD) is the commonest oesophageal pathology and the principal source of biopsy material from the lower oesophagus. The histological features of reflux include basal cell hyperplasia (extending more than 15 per cent of epithelial thickness from the basement membrane), elongation of the lamina propria papillae (extending more than two-thirds of the epithelial thickness toward the surface), intraepithelial inflammatory cells (neutrophils and eosinophils, the latter scattered and few in number), spongiosis (intercellular oedema), and sometimes erosion or ulceration with granulation tissue and acute inflammation at the surface.

Eosinophils are present in reflux oesophagitis but are typically scattered, few in number, and not concentrated at the surface or in microabscesses — the threshold widely cited for clinical suspicion of eosinophilic oesophagitis is 15 or more eosinophils per high-power field at peak count, and this number serves as the principal discriminator from reflux. Reactive squamous atypia can be marked in active reflux and care is needed to distinguish it from dysplasia — reactive atypia shows preserved maturation, an inflammatory background, and surface differentiation, whereas dysplasia shows architectural disorder, loss of polarity, and atypia that extends to the surface.

8.3 Eosinophilic oesophagitis

Eosinophilic oesophagitis (EoE) is a chronic immune-mediated inflammatory disease of the oesophagus characterised by intense eosinophilic infiltration and a clinical syndrome of dysphagia, food impaction, and oesophageal stricturing predominantly in children and young adults. The diagnostic histology requires more than 15 eosinophils per high-power field at peak count, typically in the absence of significant changes in the rest of the gastrointestinal tract. Additional supportive features include eosinophilic microabscesses (clusters of more than four eosinophils), surface layering of eosinophils, basal cell hyperplasia, papillary elongation, dilated intercellular spaces, and subepithelial fibrosis. Multiple biopsies from the proximal and distal oesophagus are recommended because the disease can be patchy.

The differential diagnosis includes severe GORD (where eosinophil counts can exceed 15 per HPF in some patients), eosinophilic gastroenteritis (where eosinophil infiltration extends through the stomach and small bowel), parasitic infection, drug hypersensitivity, and connective tissue disease. The clinical context, response to proton-pump inhibitor therapy (PPI-responsive EoE versus PPI-refractory EoE in current terminology), and the distribution of disease are the principal discriminators. The candidate is not expected to memorise the entire ACG-NASPGHAN guideline but should know the 15-eosinophil threshold and the principal differential.

8.4 Infectious oesophagitis

Three infectious agents account for the bulk of oesophageal infection in immunocompromised patients — Candida, herpes simplex virus (HSV), and cytomegalovirus (CMV). Candida oesophagitis shows pseudohyphae and budding yeast within an inflammatory exudate at the surface, typically demonstrated with PAS or Grocott methenamine silver staining. Endoscopy reveals adherent white plaques, and biopsy confirms the diagnosis.

Herpes simplex oesophagitis affects the squamous epithelium with characteristic nuclear inclusions — multinucleated cells with ground-glass nuclei, peripheral chromatin margination, and the classical Cowdry type A intranuclear eosinophilic inclusion. Lesions are typically punched-out ulcers in the upper or middle oesophagus, and the diagnostic cells are found at the edge of the ulcer rather than at its base. Immunohistochemistry for HSV-1 and HSV-2 confirms the diagnosis when morphology is suggestive but inclusions are scarce.

Cytomegalovirus oesophagitis affects endothelial cells, fibroblasts, and stromal cells (not the squamous epithelium) — the diagnostic cells show enlarged nuclei with single eosinophilic nuclear inclusion surrounded by a clear halo (so-called 'owl-eye' nuclei) and basophilic cytoplasmic inclusions. The diagnostic cells are found at the base of the ulcer (the opposite of HSV) and CMV immunohistochemistry is the standard confirmatory test. The distinction matters clinically because the antiviral therapy differs (aciclovir for HSV, ganciclovir for CMV).

Viral oesophagitis at a glance — HSV vs CMV

HSV: squamous epithelium affected; multinucleated cells, ground-glass nuclei, Cowdry A inclusions; cells at edge of ulcer.

CMV: endothelial/fibroblast cells affected; owl-eye nuclear and cytoplasmic inclusions; cells at base of ulcer.

Site discriminator: HSV upper/middle; CMV anywhere but typically with broader systemic CMV disease.

Therapy: HSV → aciclovir; CMV → ganciclovir.

IHC: HSV-1, HSV-2, CMV antibodies routinely available; confirm when morphology suggestive.

8.5 Other forms of oesophagitis

Pill oesophagitis arises from prolonged contact of medication with the oesophageal mucosa — bisphosphonates, doxycycline, potassium chloride, iron salts, NSAIDs, and other agents are the recurring culprits. Endoscopy shows ulceration at sites of pill impaction, often at the level of the aortic arch where the oesophagus is anatomically narrowed. Histology reveals ulceration with granulation tissue and acute inflammation, and crystalline foreign material may be seen within the ulcer base. Radiation oesophagitis follows mediastinal radiotherapy and shows the spectrum of acute mucosal injury (ulceration, atypical fibroblasts in the lamina propria, telangiectatic vessels) progressing to chronic stricturing with submucosal fibrosis.

Lichenoid oesophagitis — a band-like lymphocytic infiltrate at the epithelial-stromal interface with squamous apoptosis and Civatte bodies — has emerged as a recognised entity within the past decade. The differential includes drug-induced injury, autoimmune oesophagitis (lichen planus, paraneoplastic), and graft-versus-host disease in the post-transplant setting. The pattern recognition is important because the systemic associations differ; identification of band-like lichenoid inflammation in oesophageal biopsy prompts review of medication, dermatological history, and immune status.

8.6 Barrett's oesophagus

Definition and diagnostic criteria

Barrett's oesophagus is the replacement of the normal stratified squamous epithelium of the distal oesophagus by columnar epithelium of metaplastic origin. UK practice diverges from US practice on the histological threshold. The British Society of Gastroenterology (BSG) defines Barrett's as endoscopically visible columnar-lined oesophagus extending at least 1 cm above the gastro-oesophageal junction and confirmed histologically as metaplastic columnar mucosa — with or without intestinal metaplasia (goblet cells) (Fitzgerald RC et al., Gut 2014;63:7–42). The American College of Gastroenterology and the American Gastroenterological Association, by contrast, require goblet cells (intestinal metaplasia) for the diagnosis. The WHO 5th edition acknowledges both positions. Candidates for the UK examination should know the BSG threshold and the rationale: the absence of goblet cells on a given biopsy often reflects sampling rather than true absence, and the BSG view is that adequate biopsy of any columnar-lined oesophagus will usually reveal intestinal metaplasia over time.

The clinical context matters. The endoscopist describes the length of columnar-lined oesophagus using the Prague C and M criteria — the circumferential extent (C) and the maximal extent (M) of columnar mucosa above the GOJ. Short-segment Barrett's (less than 3 cm) carries lower risk of progression than long-segment Barrett's (3 cm or more). The diagnosis requires both endoscopic identification of columnar epithelium above the GOJ and histological confirmation of intestinal metaplasia with goblet cells.

Surveillance and risk of progression

Patients with Barrett's enter an endoscopic surveillance programme designed to detect dysplasia and early adenocarcinoma at a curable stage. Surveillance interval depends on segment length, presence of dysplasia, and patient factors. Non-dysplastic short-segment Barrett's is reviewed at 3–5 year intervals, non-dysplastic long-segment at 2–3 year intervals, low-grade dysplasia at 6 month intervals with consideration of endoscopic ablation, and high-grade dysplasia or intramucosal carcinoma prompts endoscopic eradication therapy or surgical resection. Annual cancer risk in non-dysplastic Barrett's is around 0.3 per cent — sizeable population risk but low individual risk, which informs the surveillance economics.

8.7 Dysplasia in Barrett's oesophagus

Grading and terminology

Dysplasia in Barrett's is graded into four categories — negative for dysplasia, indefinite for dysplasia, low-grade dysplasia, and high-grade dysplasia. WHO 5th edition retains this terminology alongside the parallel Vienna Classification (Vienna 4 = HGD, Vienna 5 = invasive carcinoma). Low-grade dysplasia shows nuclear stratification confined to the basal half of the epithelium, nuclear enlargement and hyperchromasia, loss of polarity, and preserved surface maturation. High-grade dysplasia shows nuclear stratification to the surface, marked nuclear pleomorphism, prominent nucleoli, loss of architectural orientation with cribriform or back-to-back glands, and loss of surface maturation.

Indefinite for dysplasia is the diagnostic refuge for biopsies where atypia is present but cannot be confidently distinguished from reactive change in the setting of active inflammation or surface ulceration. The category triggers anti-inflammatory therapy (intensive proton pump inhibitor) and repeat biopsy after a defined interval — typically 3 to 6 months — to clarify the diagnosis. Persistent atypia after intensive therapy raises the index of suspicion for true dysplasia.

Diagnostic adjuncts in dysplasia

Two consultant pathologists confirm a diagnosis of dysplasia in Barrett's in UK practice — the BSG guidance is explicit about double-reporting before patients enter ablation pathways. P53 immunohistochemistry supports the assessment in difficult cases — aberrant p53 expression (either strong diffuse nuclear positivity indicating gain-of-function TP53 mutation, or complete null pattern with retained internal control indicating loss-of-function mutation) supports a diagnosis of dysplasia or early neoplasia, while a heterogeneous wild-type pattern supports a reactive interpretation. Ki-67 expansion (proliferation extending to the surface) supports dysplasia. AMACR can be positive in dysplastic Barrett's but is non-specific. The pathologist integrates these findings with the morphology rather than relying on any single ancillary marker.

Dysplasia in Barrett's — diagnostic discipline

Negative: no nuclear atypia beyond physiological. No surveillance acceleration.

Indefinite: atypia present but inflammation or ulceration limits assessment. PPI + repeat biopsy 3–6 months.

Low-grade: nuclear changes confined to basal half; preserved surface maturation. 6-monthly review or endoscopic ablation.

High-grade: full-thickness atypia, architectural disorder, loss of surface maturation. Endoscopic eradication or surgical resection.

Double-reporting: two consultants confirm dysplasia before ablation. p53 IHC supports difficult cases.

8.8 Oesophageal adenocarcinoma

Oesophageal adenocarcinoma is the dominant malignancy of the distal oesophagus and GOJ in Western populations. The incidence has risen markedly over recent decades — paralleling the rise of obesity and GORD — and adenocarcinoma now exceeds squamous cell carcinoma in most Western series. The majority of adenocarcinomas arise within Barrett's oesophagus, supporting the rationale for Barrett's surveillance. The clinical presentation is typically dysphagia or weight loss in advanced disease; early lesions are detected on surveillance biopsy or as incidental findings during endoscopy for other indications.

Histologically, oesophageal adenocarcinoma shows gland formation with mucin production, variable architectural complexity, and a spectrum of grade from well-differentiated tubular and papillary patterns to poorly-differentiated solid sheets with signet-ring cells. The Siewert classification of GOJ tumours distinguishes Siewert type I (centred 1–5 cm above the GOJ — oesophageal), type II (centred 1 cm above to 2 cm below the GOJ — true GOJ), and type III (centred 2–5 cm below the GOJ — gastric cardia). The classification informs the surgical approach and the staging conventions, with type I and II tumours staged as oesophageal and type III as gastric under AJCC 8.

Molecular features

Oesophageal adenocarcinoma shows high tumour mutational burden, TP53 mutation in over 70 per cent of cases, and frequent amplifications of HER2, EGFR, MET, and other receptor tyrosine kinases. HER2 testing is now standard practice in advanced disease, with positive cases eligible for trastuzumab-based therapy. PD-L1 testing supports immune checkpoint inhibitor selection. The molecular landscape parallels that of gastric adenocarcinoma, and the TCGA molecular classification of upper GI adenocarcinoma defines four subtypes — chromosomal instability (CIN), microsatellite instability (MSI), Epstein-Barr virus-positive, and genomically stable. The CIN subtype dominates oesophageal adenocarcinoma.

8.9 Squamous cell carcinoma

Squamous cell carcinoma of the oesophagus remains the dominant malignancy globally, particularly in regions of high incidence (China, Iran, parts of South America and East Africa). Risk factors include tobacco, alcohol, hot beverage consumption, achalasia, caustic injury, and nutritional deficiencies. The tumour typically arises in the middle third of the oesophagus and presents with dysphagia. Histology shows squamous differentiation with keratinisation, intercellular bridges, and keratin pearls in well-differentiated cases; poorly-differentiated tumours lose these features and may require IHC (p40, p63, CK5/6 positive; TTF-1 negative) for confirmation.

Squamous dysplasia is the precursor lesion and is graded into low-grade and high-grade categories under the WHO 5th edition. Low-grade dysplasia shows basal cell hyperplasia with nuclear atypia confined to the lower half of the epithelium and preserved surface maturation. High-grade dysplasia shows full-thickness atypia, loss of polarity, and absent surface maturation. The transition to invasive squamous cell carcinoma is defined by stromal invasion through the basement membrane. Early invasive lesions confined to the lamina propria (superficial invasive carcinoma) carry distinct staging and management implications.

8.10 TNM staging — AJCC 8 for oesophageal cancer

The AJCC 8 staging system for oesophageal cancer applies separate categorisations for adenocarcinoma and squamous cell carcinoma, reflecting differences in prognosis. The T category records depth of invasion — Tis (carcinoma in situ or high-grade dysplasia), T1a (invasion to lamina propria or muscularis mucosae), T1b (invasion to submucosa), T2 (invasion to muscularis propria), T3 (invasion to adventitia), T4a (invasion of resectable adjacent structures — pleura, pericardium, diaphragm), T4b (invasion of unresectable structures — aorta, vertebral body, trachea). The N category records regional lymph node involvement — N0 (none), N1 (1–2 nodes), N2 (3–6 nodes), N3 (7 or more nodes). M0 versus M1 records distant metastasis.

Stage groupings differ between adenocarcinoma and squamous cell carcinoma and integrate tumour location, grade, and histological type. The candidate is not expected to memorise the complete stage grouping tables but should know the T-category criteria, the lymph node thresholds, and the principle of histology-specific staging. Pathological staging (pTNM) on resected specimens incorporates depth of invasion as assessed on serial sections, with the deepest invasive front determining the pT category. A count of all lymph nodes examined and involved completes the dataset.

8.11 Neoadjuvant therapy response assessment

Many oesophageal cancer patients receive neoadjuvant chemotherapy or chemoradiotherapy before surgical resection (the CROSS regimen of carboplatin-paclitaxel-radiotherapy is the dominant UK protocol). The response is assessed on the resected specimen using a tumour regression grading (TRG) system. The Mandard system grades from TRG1 (complete response — no viable tumour) to TRG5 (no response — no significant therapy effect). The Becker system uses a similar five-tier scale. The College of American Pathologists (CAP) recommends a four-tier grade — 0 (no viable tumour), 1 (single cells or small groups), 2 (residual tumour with stromal response), 3 (extensive residual tumour with minimal response). The RCPath dataset specifies the system to use for UK reporting.

Complete pathological response (no viable tumour at the primary site and no nodal disease) is the most powerful prognostic indicator and is achieved in around 25 to 35 per cent of patients with squamous cell carcinoma and 15 to 25 per cent with adenocarcinoma after CROSS-style therapy. The pathologist samples the post-treatment tumour bed extensively — entire macroscopic tumour and adjacent fibrosis where no tumour is grossly identifiable — to support accurate assessment. The 'y' prefix (ypT, ypN, ypM) denotes post-neoadjuvant staging.

8.12 Endoscopic resection — EMR and ESD specimen handling

Endoscopic mucosal resection (EMR) and endoscopic submucosal dissection (ESD) have transformed the management of early oesophageal neoplasia — high-grade dysplasia, intramucosal carcinoma, and selected superficial submucosal invasive carcinoma — allowing curative resection without surgery in appropriately selected patients. The pathological assessment is detailed and protocol-driven, because the management decision (further endoscopic surveillance versus oesophagectomy versus combination therapy) depends critically on the depth of invasion, the differentiation, the lymphovascular involvement, and the resection margin status.

EMR specimens are typically piecemeal — multiple fragments of mucosa removed via a cap-snare or band-ligation technique. The pathologist orients each fragment, marks the deep and lateral margins with ink, embeds the fragments en face or perpendicular to the mucosal surface, and obtains serial sections through each block. The report records the histological type and grade of each fragment, the depth of invasion (intramucosal versus submucosal, with quantitative depth in micrometres for submucosal invasive lesions), the lymphovascular invasion status, and the resection margins (deep and lateral). ESD specimens are removed en bloc as a single tissue piece, supporting cleaner margin assessment and more accurate staging — the European Society of Gastrointestinal Endoscopy guidelines favour ESD over EMR for lesions larger than 15 mm or those with submucosal invasion suspicion.

T1 sub-staging — the critical decision point

T1 oesophageal cancer is subdivided into T1a (invasion limited to the lamina propria or muscularis mucosae) and T1b (invasion of the submucosa). The distinction drives the management decision. T1a lesions with favourable features (well or moderately differentiated, no lymphovascular invasion, complete resection with clear margins) are typically managed by endoscopic resection alone — the risk of lymph node metastasis is under 5 per cent. T1b lesions carry a markedly higher risk of nodal metastasis (15 to 25 per cent or more), and most patients are offered oesophagectomy with lymphadenectomy. Submucosal invasion is further sub-classified by depth — sm1 (upper third of submucosa, less than 500 micrometres invasion), sm2 (middle third), sm3 (deepest third) — with risk increasing through the sub-stages. Quantitative measurement of submucosal invasion depth in micrometres is a standard reporting item.

T1 oesophageal cancer — depth and management implications

T1a (intramucosal): invasion to lamina propria or muscularis mucosae; nodal risk <5%; endoscopic resection adequate if favourable features.

T1b (submucosal): invasion of submucosa; nodal risk 15–25%+; oesophagectomy typically indicated.

Sub-staging sm1/sm2/sm3: based on depth of submucosal invasion in micrometres; sm1 (<500 μm) lowest risk.

Favourable features: well/moderately differentiated, no lymphovascular invasion, clear margins.

Adverse features: poorly differentiated, lymphovascular invasion, positive margin, deep submucosal invasion.

8.13 Predictive biomarker testing in oesophageal adenocarcinoma

HER2 testing

HER2 testing is now standard practice in metastatic oesophageal and GOJ adenocarcinoma — positive cases are eligible for trastuzumab-based first-line therapy (the ToGA trial) and for second-line trastuzumab deruxtecan. The testing algorithm is ICCR-aligned. IHC scoring uses a four-tier scale — 0 (no membrane staining or staining in less than 10 per cent of tumour cells), 1+ (faint barely perceptible membrane staining in 10 per cent or more), 2+ (weak to moderate complete or basolateral membrane staining in 10 per cent or more), 3+ (strong complete or basolateral membrane staining in 10 per cent or more). The 10 per cent threshold for oesophageal and gastric adenocarcinoma is lower than the breast 10 per cent threshold; biopsy interpretation accepts membrane staining in 5 contiguous cells. IHC 3+ is reported as HER2-positive. IHC 2+ is equivocal and triggers reflex in-situ hybridisation; a HER2:CEP17 ratio of 2.0 or higher (or copy number 6 or more) confirms amplification.

PD-L1 combined positive score

PD-L1 testing in oesophageal adenocarcinoma and squamous cell carcinoma is reported using the Combined Positive Score (CPS) — the number of PD-L1-positive cells (tumour cells, lymphocytes, macrophages) divided by the total number of viable tumour cells, multiplied by 100. CPS thresholds vary by indication and by drug — the KEYNOTE-859 trial established CPS 1 or higher for pembrolizumab in advanced gastric and GOJ adenocarcinoma, while squamous cell carcinoma is treated with checkpoint inhibitors at lower thresholds. The 22C3 PharmDx assay is the principal companion diagnostic. PD-L1 scoring is operator-dependent — UK NEQAS proficiency data show variable inter-laboratory concordance, particularly at low CPS values, supporting regular EQA participation and pathologist training.

8.14 Crypt dysplasia and the Barrett's diagnostic frontier

Crypt dysplasia — dysplasia confined to the basal portion of the crypts without involvement of the surface epithelium — is an emerging morphological pattern recognised within the past decade. The classical surface-based criteria for Barrett's dysplasia do not capture this pattern, and historical interpretation classified crypt dysplasia as 'negative' or 'indefinite'. Current expert practice recognises crypt dysplasia as a real precursor lesion with quantifiable progression risk, and the candidate should be aware of the entity even if its routine recognition is not yet uniform. Distinguishing features include disorganised crypt architecture, basal atypia with loss of surface maturation in cross-sectioned crypts, and aberrant p53 expression confined to the basal cells.

Foveolar-type dysplasia is a non-intestinal variant of Barrett's dysplasia recognised in the WHO 5th edition. The cytological pattern shows abundant pale or mucin-filled apical cytoplasm with nuclear atypia in cells resembling gastric foveolar epithelium rather than intestinal cells. Foveolar dysplasia carries similar progression risk to intestinal-type dysplasia and is graded into low-grade and high-grade categories. Recognition matters because the cytological subtleties differ from the more familiar intestinal pattern, and missed foveolar dysplasia is a recognised source of false-negative biopsy reports. Serrated dysplasia — characterised by serrated architecture with epithelial proliferative changes resembling colonic sessile serrated lesions — is a third pattern, with progression behaviour still being characterised in published series.

8.15 Primary oesophageal melanoma

Primary mucosal melanoma of the oesophagus is rare (under 0.5 per cent of oesophageal malignancies) but is occasionally encountered in surgical pathology. The tumour typically arises in the distal oesophagus, presents as a pigmented or non-pigmented polypoid mass, and shows the morphological features of melanoma — epithelioid or spindle cells with prominent nucleoli, intracellular melanin pigment (in some tumours), and an invasive growth pattern. Immunohistochemistry confirms the lineage — S100, SOX10, HMB-45, Melan-A, MITF positive — and the molecular profile differs from cutaneous melanoma, with NF1 and KIT mutations more common and BRAF V600E less common. Prognosis is poor with high rates of distant metastasis at diagnosis. The diagnostic challenge is distinguishing primary oesophageal mucosal melanoma from metastatic cutaneous melanoma to the oesophagus — the clinical context, the presence or absence of cutaneous primary disease, and the depth of invasion in the oesophageal wall are the discriminators.

8.16 Mesenchymal and neuroendocrine tumours

Mesenchymal tumours of the oesophagus include leiomyoma (the most common), gastrointestinal stromal tumour (GIST, rarer in the oesophagus than in the stomach), and granular cell tumour (a Schwann cell-derived tumour with characteristic granular eosinophilic cytoplasm and S100/SOX10 positivity). Oesophageal GIST shares the molecular biology of gastric GIST — KIT exon 11 mutation most common, exon 9 and PDGFRA less frequent in oesophagus, with imatinib sensitivity correlating with the mutation profile. Leiomyoma is the dominant submucosal lesion and is benign in nature.

Neuroendocrine tumours of the oesophagus are uncommon. The WHO 5th edition classifies them into well-differentiated neuroendocrine tumours (NET grade 1–3 based on mitotic count and Ki-67) and poorly-differentiated neuroendocrine carcinomas (small cell and large cell types). Small cell carcinoma of the oesophagus is histologically and clinically aggressive, often presenting with metastatic disease and managed similarly to small cell carcinoma of lung.

8.17 Reporting and integration

Oesophageal cancer reports follow the RCPath dataset, with required core items including specimen type and procedure, tumour location (in relation to incisors and GOJ), histological type and subtype, histological grade, dimensions, depth of invasion (T category), proximal, distal, and circumferential margin status, lymphovascular invasion, perineural invasion, lymph node count and involvement, response to neoadjuvant therapy (where applicable), and biomarker results (HER2 IHC and ISH for adenocarcinoma, PD-L1 where commissioned). The synoptic block sits at the end of the report and supports MDT presentation and registry submission.

8.18 Key points

Chapter 8 — key points

Normal histology: Non-keratinising stratified squamous; submucosal seromucous glands; muscularis propria striated upper, smooth lower.

Infective oesophagitis: HSV at ulcer edge (multinucleate, Cowdry A); CMV at ulcer base (owl-eye in endothelium/fibroblasts); Candida pseudohyphae on PAS.

Barrett's: Specialised intestinal metaplasia with goblet cells. Surveillance per BSG/NICE; biopsies labelled by level.

Dysplasia: Negative, indefinite, low-grade, high-grade. Two-consultant confirmation before ablation; p53 supports difficult cases.

Oesophageal SCC and adenocarcinoma: Type, grade, depth, lymphovascular invasion, margins. HER2 reflex on adenocarcinoma.

T1 staging: T1a (intramucosal) → endoscopic resection adequate if favourable. T1b (submucosal) → oesophagectomy; sub-stage sm1/sm2/sm3 by depth.

Eosinophilic oesophagitis: ≥15 eosinophils/HPF in peak field; basal zone hyperplasia, surface microabscesses, lamina propria fibrosis.

8.19 Chapter SBAs

Q8.1. Distinction between reactive squamous atypia and dysplasia in oesophageal biopsies is the recurring diagnostic challenge in chronic reflux. A 60-year-old woman with longstanding reflux symptoms has a biopsy from the lower oesophagus showing scattered eosinophils, basal cell hyperplasia, and marked squamous atypia. Surface maturation is preserved. Which single statement best characterises the appropriate interpretation?

A. High-grade dysplasia — recommend endoscopic eradication therapy.

B. Reactive squamous atypia secondary to reflux — recommend intensive PPI and repeat biopsy if symptoms persist.

C. Low-grade dysplasia — recommend 6-monthly surveillance.

D. Invasive squamous cell carcinoma — recommend staging investigations.

E. Eosinophilic oesophagitis — recommend dietary therapy.

Answer: B

The preservation of surface maturation is the single most reliable discriminator between reactive atypia and dysplasia in oesophageal squamous epithelium. Reactive atypia in active reflux can be marked — basal cell hyperplasia, nuclear enlargement, prominent nucleoli, mitotic activity in the lower epithelium — but the atypical cells mature toward the surface, retaining the orderly squamous architecture. True dysplasia shows full-thickness atypia, loss of polarity, and absent surface maturation. The inflammatory background supports a reactive interpretation. The appropriate management is intensive PPI therapy and repeat biopsy if symptoms or endoscopic findings persist; if atypia remains after intensive anti-reflux treatment, the diagnosis warrants reconsideration with possible reclassification.

Option A overcalls — dysplasia would require loss of surface maturation. Option C is similarly overcalled. Option D is not supported by the described findings. Option E confuses two different oesophageal pathologies; eosinophilic oesophagitis requires ≥15 eosinophils per HPF and a distinct clinical context (typically dysphagia in younger patients).

Q8.2. Diagnosis of Barrett's oesophagus by current UK guidance requires both endoscopic and histological criteria. A 55-year-old man undergoes endoscopy for chronic reflux. The endoscopist identifies tongues of salmon-coloured mucosa extending 2 cm above the GOJ. Biopsies show columnar epithelium without goblet cells but with cardia-type mucous glands. Which single statement best describes the diagnosis under current UK BSG guidance?

A. Barrett's oesophagus is established — initiate surveillance.

B. Barrett's oesophagus is not established because UK BSG guidance, like the ACG, mandates demonstration of intestinal metaplasia.

C. Barrett's oesophagus is established only if subsequent biopsy shows goblet cells.

D. The diagnosis cannot be made until p53 IHC is performed.

E. The diagnosis requires HER2 testing on the biopsy.

Answer: A

Current UK BSG guidance (Fitzgerald RC et al., Gut 2014;63:7–42) defines Barrett's oesophagus as endoscopically visible columnar-lined oesophagus extending at least 1 cm above the GOJ with histological confirmation of metaplastic columnar mucosa, with or without intestinal metaplasia. The described tongue of salmon-coloured mucosa extending 2 cm above the GOJ exceeds the 1 cm threshold, and the histology confirms metaplastic columnar mucosa. Under UK BSG criteria the diagnosis is therefore established, regardless of the absence of goblet cells on this biopsy. The BSG position differs from the ACG and AGA position, which requires demonstration of intestinal metaplasia (goblet cells); the WHO 5th edition acknowledges both. The UK rationale rests on the observation that absence of goblet cells often reflects sampling, since intestinal metaplasia is patchy, and that adequate biopsy will usually reveal goblet cells over subsequent endoscopies. Enrolment in Barrett's surveillance is therefore appropriate, with the surveillance interval dictated by segment length and dysplasia status.

Option B reflects the US ACG/AGA position rather than UK BSG and is incorrect for the question stem. Option C is overcautious — UK BSG considers the diagnosis already established, with subsequent biopsies relevant only to dysplasia surveillance. Options D and E describe ancillary tests that do not establish the diagnosis of Barrett's.

Q8.3. Pathological response to neoadjuvant therapy in oesophageal cancer is a powerful prognostic indicator and is captured using a defined grading system. A 65-year-old man with locally advanced adenocarcinoma has completed neoadjuvant chemoradiotherapy and has undergone oesophagectomy. The resection specimen shows extensive fibrosis at the previous tumour site with no viable tumour cells identified on extensive sampling, and all 18 examined lymph nodes are uninvolved. Which single statement best describes the staging and the prognostic implication?

A. ypT0 ypN0 — complete pathological response with the strongest prognostic association.

B. pT0 pN0 — no neoadjuvant prefix is required.

C. ypT1 ypN0 — fibrosis represents residual tumour.

D. Staging not applicable after neoadjuvant therapy.

E. ypTX ypNX — staging cannot be assessed.

Answer: A

Complete pathological response to neoadjuvant therapy is defined as no viable tumour cells at the primary site and no involvement of regional lymph nodes (ypT0 ypN0). The 'y' prefix is required to indicate post-neoadjuvant staging — distinguishing the result from a primary surgical resection with no residual disease. Complete pathological response is the most powerful prognostic indicator in oesophageal cancer after neoadjuvant therapy, with five-year survival around 50 to 70 per cent compared with around 20 to 30 per cent for incomplete responders. The discipline of extensive sampling of the post-treatment tumour bed is essential to support the ypT0 designation; UK practice typically samples the entire macroscopic abnormality plus serial sections through the adjacent oesophagus.

Option B is incorrect because the 'y' prefix is required for neoadjuvant context. Option C misinterprets fibrosis as residual tumour — fibrosis without viable tumour cells is consistent with complete response. Option D is incorrect; staging is the standard reporting framework after neoadjuvant therapy with the 'y' prefix. Option E (ypTX ypNX) describes an unassessable category and does not apply when assessment has been performed.

8.20 Chapter EMQ

EMQ 8.1. Oesophageal pathology — pattern recognition. For each scenario, select the single most appropriate diagnosis from the option list. Each option may be used once, more than once, or not at all.

A. Reflux oesophagitis

B. Eosinophilic oesophagitis

C. Herpes simplex oesophagitis

D. Cytomegalovirus oesophagitis

E. Candida oesophagitis

F. Barrett's oesophagus with low-grade dysplasia

G. Barrett's oesophagus with high-grade dysplasia

H. Oesophageal adenocarcinoma

I. Oesophageal squamous cell carcinoma

J. Granular cell tumour

(1) A 28-year-old man with longstanding dysphagia and intermittent food impaction has biopsies from the proximal and distal oesophagus showing 30+ eosinophils per high-power field with eosinophilic microabscesses and surface layering. **Answer: B**

(2) A 45-year-old patient on chemotherapy presents with odynophagia. Biopsies from the edge of a punched-out ulcer in the upper oesophagus show multinucleated squamous cells with ground-glass nuclei and peripheral chromatin margination. **Answer: C**

(3) A 60-year-old man on dialysis presents with retrosternal pain. Biopsies from the base of a mid-oesophageal ulcer show enlarged cells with single eosinophilic nuclear inclusions surrounded by a clear halo, in cells with the morphological features of endothelial cells rather than squamous epithelium. **Answer: D**

(4) A 55-year-old woman with chronic reflux has a biopsy of a 3 cm tongue of salmon-coloured mucosa above the GOJ. Histology shows columnar epithelium with goblet cells; nuclei are stratified to the basal half of the epithelium with mild nuclear atypia and preserved surface maturation. **Answer: F**

(5) A 70-year-old man has an endoscopic mucosal resection of a 1.5 cm distal oesophageal lesion in a background of long-segment Barrett's. The resection shows complex glandular architecture, full-thickness nuclear atypia, and invasion through the basement membrane into the lamina propria. **Answer: H**

Chapter 9 — Stomach

Gastric pathology underpins a large fraction of routine and on-call histopathological practice. The mucosal biopsy is the workhorse — addressing the questions of inflammation, infection, metaplasia, dysplasia, and early malignancy — and the resection specimen carries the staging and biomarker assessment that drive adjuvant and palliative therapy. The FRCPath Part 1 candidate is expected to know the histology of normal stomach by region, the principal forms of gastritis with their causes and morphological features, the staging frameworks for chronic atrophic gastritis (OLGA and OLGIM), the dysplasia framework, the Lauren and WHO 5th edition classifications of adenocarcinoma, the TCGA molecular framework, and the principal mesenchymal and neuroendocrine entities including gastrointestinal stromal tumour (GIST) and MALT lymphoma. This chapter sets out the discipline against the international classification and reporting frameworks current in 2026.

9.1 Normal gastric histology

The stomach is divided into anatomical and histological regions with distinct mucosal architecture. The cardia is a narrow zone immediately below the gastro-oesophageal junction — lined by mucinous columnar epithelium with simple branched mucous glands. The body (corpus) and fundus carry the acid-secreting oxyntic mucosa, with parietal cells (acid and intrinsic factor production), chief cells (pepsinogen production), and surface foveolar epithelium overlying the glands. The antrum and pylorus show shorter foveolae overlying mucous glands without parietal cells, and gastrin-producing G cells within the antral glands. The pyloric channel transitions into the duodenum at the pylorus.

Identification of the biopsy site by histology is part of routine assessment. Body or fundic biopsies show oxyntic glands with the characteristic foveolar-to-gland ratio of approximately 1:4, the diagnostic glandular preponderance. Antral biopsies show a 1:1 ratio with predominantly mucous glands. The transition between body and antrum is gradual, and biopsies from the lesser curve incisura may show mixed features. Diagnostic and prognostic conclusions depend on knowing the biopsy site, particularly in atrophic gastritis assessment where the staging system separates antral and corpus involvement.

9.2 Helicobacter pylori gastritis

Helicobacter pylori is the principal infective cause of chronic gastritis, of peptic ulcer disease, and of gastric adenocarcinoma in much of the world. The bacterium colonises the mucous layer above the surface epithelium, demonstrated on H&E as small curved bacilli (best seen with toluidine blue, Giemsa, or modified Genta stains; widely available specific immunohistochemistry confirms the diagnosis in ambiguous cases). The mucosa shows chronic inflammation with lymphocytes and plasma cells, active inflammation with neutrophilic infiltrate of glandular epithelium — the activity component of the Sydney classification — and lymphoid follicles in the mucosa or submucosa — particularly in younger patients.

The updated Sydney System grades gastritis on five parameters — chronic inflammation, activity (neutrophils), Helicobacter density, atrophy, and intestinal metaplasia — each scored as none, mild, moderate, or marked. The biopsy protocol samples five sites: two antrum, two body, and one incisura, with separate identification. Cure of Helicobacter infection typically reverses the active component within weeks — but the chronic inflammation, atrophy, and intestinal metaplasia may persist for months to years. The candidate should know the Sydney parameters and the biopsy protocol.

OLGA and OLGIM staging

The Operative Link on Gastritis Assessment (OLGA) and the parallel OLGIM (Operative Link on Gastric Intestinal Metaplasia) provide systems for staging the extent of gastric atrophy and intestinal metaplasia, respectively. Both use a 0–IV stage based on the combined severity of changes in the antrum (including incisura) and body. OLGA III and IV (advanced atrophy) and OLGIM III and IV (advanced intestinal metaplasia) identify patients at markedly elevated risk of gastric adenocarcinoma — and guide the surveillance interval and guide surveillance pathways. The MAPS guidelines (European Society of Gastrointestinal Endoscopy) build on OLGA/OLGIM to recommend three-yearly surveillance for stage III/IV disease.

Sydney classification at a glance

Chronic inflammation: lymphocytes and plasma cells in lamina propria.

Activity: neutrophils infiltrating glandular epithelium — implies active Helicobacter or other process.

Helicobacter density: graded on H&E or with specific stains.

Atrophy: loss of native oxyntic or antral glands.

Intestinal metaplasia: replacement of native glands by intestinal-type epithelium with goblet cells.

Biopsy protocol: five sites — two antrum, two body, one incisura — separately labelled.

9.3 Autoimmune gastritis

Autoimmune gastritis (atrophic gastritis of the corpus type, type A gastritis) results from immune-mediated destruction of parietal cells with sparing of the antrum. The histology shows oxyntic atrophy with loss of parietal cells, pseudopyloric metaplasia (replacement of oxyntic glands by pyloric-type glands), intestinal metaplasia, and chronic inflammation in the body and fundus. The antrum is typically histologically normal or shows only mild changes. Linear and nodular enterochromaffin-like (ECL) cell hyperplasia is a characteristic finding — driven by elevated gastrin from antral G cells in response to achlorhydria. Anti-parietal cell and anti-intrinsic factor antibodies are diagnostic markers in the clinical context.

The clinical syndrome includes pernicious anaemia — vitamin B12 deficiency from intrinsic factor loss — and an increased risk of gastric type 1 neuroendocrine tumours arising from ECL cell hyperplasia, as well as gastric adenocarcinoma. Endoscopic surveillance in established autoimmune atrophic gastritis is offered, with intervals based on the extent of changes and the presence of associated lesions.

9.4 Other forms of gastritis

Reactive (chemical) gastritis — bile reflux, NSAID injury, or alcohol exposure — follows several insults. The histology shows foveolar hyperplasia with corkscrew-shaped pits, vasodilation in the lamina propria, smooth muscle fibres extending into the lamina propria from the muscularis mucosae, and relative paucity of inflammatory cells. The pattern is recognisable and the differential from Helicobacter gastritis is important because management differs (cessation of NSAID or addressing reflux versus eradication therapy). Eosinophilic gastritis is part of the eosinophilic gastrointestinal disease spectrum; lymphocytic gastritis (with marked intraepithelial lymphocytosis) is associated with coeliac disease and Helicobacter; collagenous gastritis is a rare entity with a thickened subepithelial collagen band; granulomatous gastritis raises the differential of Crohn's disease, sarcoidosis, tuberculosis, and other granulomatous infections.

9.5 Gastric polyps

Fundic gland polyps are the commonest gastric polyp in Western practice — usually small, multiple, located in the body and fundus, and histologically composed of dilated cystic oxyntic glands lined by parietal and chief cells. Sporadic fundic gland polyps are strongly associated with proton pump inhibitor use; multiple fundic gland polyps in a young patient or in the antrum raise the suspicion of familial adenomatous polyposis (FAP), and warrant investigation. Dysplasia in fundic gland polyps is uncommon but recognised.

Hyperplastic polyps are inflammatory polyps with elongated tortuous hyperplastic foveolae, oedematous and inflamed lamina propria, and often arise in a background of chronic gastritis. Adenomatous polyps (intestinal-type and gastric foveolar-type) show low or high-grade dysplasia and carry a measurable risk of progression to adenocarcinoma; excision is recommended. Pyloric gland adenoma is a less common but increasingly recognised entity composed of compact pyloric-type glands with low or high-grade dysplasia, with an elevated risk of high-grade dysplasia and invasive carcinoma compared to other gastric adenoma subtypes. Foveolar-type and gastric-type adenomas have characteristic mucin patterns — MUC5AC and MUC6 positive, MUC2 negative — that distinguish them from intestinal-type adenomas.

9.6 Dysplasia and early gastric cancer

Gastric dysplasia is graded into low-grade and high-grade categories, paralleling Barrett's dysplasia. The Vienna Classification (a Western-Eastern consensus reaching its 2002 revision) provides a five-category framework — Category 1 (negative for dysplasia), 2 (indefinite), 3 (low-grade), 4 (high-grade), 5 (invasive). The Japanese classification has historically incorporated 'non-invasive carcinoma' (Vienna 4.2) and 'intramucosal carcinoma' (Vienna 4.4) as separate diagnostic categories with treatment implications, reflecting different morphological thresholds in different traditions.

Western and Japanese pathologists have reconciled most aspects of the disagreement, and the Vienna framework is the accepted bridge.

Early gastric cancer is defined as adenocarcinoma confined to the mucosa or submucosa, regardless of lymph node involvement. The macroscopic classification (the Paris classification of superficial lesions) groups early lesions into type 0-I (protruded), 0-IIa (slightly elevated), 0-IIb (flat), 0-IIc (slightly depressed), and 0-III (excavated). The macroscopic type predicts the histological type and the likelihood of submucosal invasion, supporting decisions about endoscopic versus surgical resection. T1a (mucosal) lesions with favourable features (well or moderately differentiated, no lymphovascular invasion, less than 2 cm) qualify for endoscopic submucosal dissection in many UK and international guidelines.

9.7 Gastric adenocarcinoma

Lauren classification

The Lauren classification (1965) divides gastric adenocarcinoma into intestinal type, diffuse type, and mixed type. The intestinal type forms glands and tubular structures, shows cohesive growth, and is typically associated with chronic Helicobacter infection, intestinal metaplasia, and stepwise progression through atrophic gastritis and dysplasia. The clinical pattern is more common in older patients, in men, in lower socioeconomic groups, and in certain geographical regions (East Asia, parts of Eastern Europe and Latin America). The diffuse type shows poorly cohesive cells infiltrating singly or in small clusters, often with signet ring morphology (intracytoplasmic mucin displacing the nucleus to the cell margin), and carries a worse prognosis stage-for-stage than intestinal type. The diffuse type more commonly affects younger patients and women, and underlies most cases of hereditary diffuse gastric cancer (CDH1 germline mutation).

WHO 5th edition classification

The WHO 5th edition (2019) classifies gastric adenocarcinoma into five major subtypes: tubular, papillary, mucinous, poorly cohesive (including signet ring carcinoma), and mixed. Additional rare variants include hepatoid adenocarcinoma (with AFP production and morphology resembling hepatocellular carcinoma), micropapillary, lymphoepithelioma-like (Epstein-Barr virus-associated, with prominent lymphocytic stroma and good prognosis), and adenocarcinoma with enteroblastic differentiation. The classification aligns broadly with Lauren — tubular and papillary correspond to the intestinal Lauren type, poorly cohesive to the diffuse Lauren type, and mixed to the Lauren mixed type.

TCGA molecular classification

The Cancer Genome Atlas (TCGA) gastric adenocarcinoma analysis defined four molecular subtypes that complement the morphological classifications. Chromosomal instability (CIN) tumours show extensive aneuploidy and amplification of receptor tyrosine kinases — HER2, EGFR, MET; they correspond morphologically to intestinal-type Lauren tumours of the GOJ and proximal stomach. Microsatellite instability (MSI) tumours show MMR deficiency, high mutational burden, and are predictive of immune checkpoint inhibitor response; they are commoner in older patients and in the antrum. Epstein-Barr virus-positive tumours show CpG island methylation, PIK3CA mutation, and PD-L1 amplification, and correspond morphologically to lymphoepithelioma-like carcinoma. Genomically stable tumours predominantly correspond to the diffuse Lauren type and are enriched for CDH1 and RHOA mutations. The classification is research-grade in 2026 — clinical molecular testing in the UK is restricted to HER2, MMR, EBER, and PD-L1 in most NHS pathways.

Gastric adenocarcinoma — classifications overview

Lauren: intestinal (cohesive, glands, Helicobacter-associated); diffuse (poorly cohesive, signet ring, CDH1).

WHO 5: tubular, papillary, mucinous, poorly cohesive, mixed + rare variants (hepatoid, EBV-LELC, micropapillary).

TCGA: CIN (HER2+), MSI (MMR-deficient), EBV-positive, genomically stable.

HDGC: germline CDH1 mutation — bilateral diffuse gastric and lobular breast cancer risk.

9.8 Hereditary diffuse gastric cancer

Hereditary diffuse gastric cancer (HDGC) is the autosomal dominant syndrome caused by germline CDH1 mutation (and a smaller proportion by CTNNA1 mutation), characterised by very high lifetime risk of diffuse-type gastric adenocarcinoma (around 70 per cent in men, 55 per cent in women) and lobular breast carcinoma in women (around 40 per cent). The International Gastric Cancer Linkage Consortium (IGCLC) criteria identify families for genetic testing — two or more cases of gastric cancer in first or second-degree relatives with one diffuse type at any age, or one diffuse gastric cancer under age 40, or a personal or family history of diffuse gastric and lobular breast cancer. Carriers are offered prophylactic total gastrectomy — or intensive endoscopic surveillance — depending on clinical circumstance. Prophylactic gastrectomy specimens characteristically show multiple small foci (often hundreds) of intramucosal signet ring carcinoma scattered throughout the stomach, with normal background mucosa — the pathologist samples the entire stomach to document the burden of disease.

9.9 HER2 and predictive biomarker testing

HER2 testing in gastric and GOJ adenocarcinoma follows the same dual IHC and ISH algorithm as in oesophageal adenocarcinoma. IHC 0 and 1+ are negative; 3+ is positive; 2+ is equivocal and triggers reflex ISH. The 10 per cent threshold (with biopsy 5-cell rule) differs from breast cancer scoring. HER2-positive disease is eligible for first-line trastuzumab plus chemotherapy (the ToGA regimen) and for second-line trastuzumab deruxtecan. The intratumoural heterogeneity of HER2 expression in gastric cancer is greater than in breast — supporting interpretation of the basolateral staining pattern and the use of multiple biopsy or block sampling.

MMR IHC is increasingly tested at diagnosis on every gastric adenocarcinoma — supporting MSI-driven immune checkpoint inhibitor selection in metastatic disease and identifying potential Lynch syndrome cases for clinical genetics referral. EBV testing (EBER ISH) is performed selectively, particularly in tumours with lymphoepithelioma-like morphology where the result drives understanding of biological behaviour. PD-L1 testing using CPS scoring informs immune checkpoint inhibitor eligibility. Claudin 18.2 is an emerging biomarker — the antibody zolbetuximab targets claudin 18.2-expressing tumours and has shown survival benefit in trials — with companion diagnostic IHC assays now being deployed.

9.10 Gastrointestinal stromal tumour

GIST is the most common mesenchymal tumour of the GI tract, with the stomach being the commonest site (around 60 per cent). The tumour arises from interstitial cells of Cajal or their precursors and is defined by KIT (CD117) immunoreactivity in most cases, with DOG1 and CD34 supporting the diagnosis. Spindle cell GIST (around 70 per cent) shows fascicles of uniform spindle cells with eosinophilic cytoplasm; epithelioid GIST (around 20 per cent) shows polygonal cells with clear or eosinophilic cytoplasm — mixed types account for the remainder. Approximately 80 per cent of gastric GISTs harbour KIT mutations (most commonly exon 11), 10 per cent harbour PDGFRA mutations (commonly D842V in the gastric epithelioid type), and 10 per cent are wild-type for KIT and PDGFRA. The wild-type group includes SDH-deficient GIST (germline or somatic SDH-subunit mutation; SDHB IHC loss; younger patients; multifocal disease; epithelioid morphology), NF1-associated GIST (often small bowel; multifocal), and BRAF-mutant GIST (rare).

Risk stratification — Miettinen-Lasota

Risk of malignant behaviour in GIST is stratified by tumour size, mitotic count, and primary site (the Miettinen-Lasota / AFIP 2006 system). Gastric GISTs have the lowest baseline risk for a given size and mitotic count compared with small bowel and other sites, reflecting different biological behaviour. The system divides cases into very low, low, intermediate, and high risk categories based on the combination of size (under 2 cm, 2 to 5 cm, 5 to 10 cm, over 10 cm) and mitotic count (under 5 per 5 mm squared, 5 or more per 5 mm squared). Imatinib adjuvant therapy is offered to high-risk cases — treatment selection informed by mutation profile (imatinib-sensitive mutations versus imatinib-insensitive PDGFRA D842V or wild-type cases).

9.11 Gastric neuroendocrine tumours

Gastric neuroendocrine tumours (NETs) are classified by clinical context into three types. Type 1 NETs arise in chronic atrophic gastritis — typically autoimmune — on a background of ECL cell hyperplasia driven by hypergastrinaemia from achlorhydria; they are usually small (under 2 cm), multifocal, indolent, and managed by endoscopic resection with surveillance. Type 2 NETs arise in Zollinger-Ellison syndrome (gastrinoma-driven hypergastrinaemia, often MEN1-associated); they share morphology with type 1 but the clinical management addresses the underlying gastrinoma. Type 3 NETs arise sporadically without hypergastrinaemia, are typically solitary and larger at presentation, and behave more aggressively with higher metastatic potential — surgical resection with lymphadenectomy is standard.

Grading uses the WHO 5th edition NET grade based on mitotic count and Ki-67 — NET grade 1 (mitoses under 2 per 2 mm squared, Ki-67 under 3 per cent), NET grade 2 (mitoses 2-20 or Ki-67 3-20 per cent), NET grade 3 (mitoses over 20 per 2 mm squared or Ki-67 over 20 per cent with well-differentiated morphology). Poorly-differentiated neuroendocrine carcinoma (small cell or large cell type, with Ki-67 typically over 50-60 per cent) is a separate category with worse prognosis and different management.

9.12 Gastric MALT lymphoma

Mucosa-associated lymphoid tissue (MALT) lymphoma — extranodal marginal zone lymphoma of MALT type — is the principal primary lymphoma of the stomach. The tumour is driven in around 90 per cent of cases by chronic Helicobacter pylori infection, with neoplastic small lymphoid cells (marginal zone phenotype) infiltrating the lamina propria with characteristic lymphoepithelial lesions (clusters of neoplastic lymphocytes infiltrating gland epithelium). Eradication of Helicobacter induces lymphoma regression in around 70-80 per cent of localised cases — particularly those with the t(11;18) BIRC3-MALT1 translocation absent. The t(11;18)-positive cases are less likely to respond to Helicobacter eradication alone and may require oncological therapy.

9.13 TNM staging and reporting

Gastric cancer staging under AJCC 8 records T (tumour depth: Tis, T1a/T1b, T2, T3, T4a, T4b), N (number of involved regional lymph nodes: N0, N1 [1-2], N2 [3-6], N3a [7-15], N3b [16+]), and M (distant metastasis). Lymph node count expectations differ from oesophageal staging — at least 15 lymph nodes should be recovered for accurate pN assessment, with submission of all peri-gastric nodes and named station lymph nodes — D1 plus D2 dissection provides the standard yield in oncological gastrectomy.

Reporting datasets follow the RCPath gastric cancer template, with core items covering specimen type, tumour location, Lauren and WHO subtype, grade, dimensions, depth of invasion, margins (proximal, distal, omental, radial), serosal involvement, lymphovascular and perineural invasion, lymph node count and involvement, response to neoadjuvant therapy where applicable, and biomarker results (HER2, MMR, EBER where commissioned, PD-L1 where requested). The synoptic block supports MDT presentation and registry submission.

9.14 Key points

Chapter 9 — key points

Sydney biopsy protocol: Five sites — two antrum, two body, one incisura — separately labelled. Chronic inflammation, activity, Helicobacter, atrophy, intestinal metaplasia each graded.

Helicobacter detection: H&E, modified Giemsa, Warthin-Starry, or immunohistochemistry. Eradication confirmed at 6 weeks post-therapy.

Lauren classification: Intestinal (cohesive, glands, Helicobacter-driven) vs diffuse (poorly cohesive, signet ring, CDH1-associated).

WHO 5e: Tubular, papillary, mucinous, poorly cohesive, mixed, plus rare variants (hepatoid, EBV-LELC, micropapillary).

TCGA molecular: Chromosomal instability (HER2+), MSI (MMR-deficient), EBV-positive, genomically stable.

HDGC: Germline CDH1 — bilateral diffuse gastric and lobular breast cancer risk. Prophylactic gastrectomy considered; pathologist samples entire stomach in mapped grid.

Gastric MALT: Helicobacter eradication first-line. t(11;18) MALT1::API2 predicts non-response to eradication and need for chemotherapy.

9.15 Chapter SBAs

Q9.1. Distinction between sporadic fundic gland polyposis and inherited polyposis syndromes is clinically critical because the surveillance and treatment pathways differ markedly. A 30-year-old woman has multiple fundic gland polyps identified during gastroscopy for dyspepsia. She has no known family history of cancer. Which single feature would most strongly raise suspicion of familial adenomatous polyposis (FAP)?

A. Identification of low-grade dysplasia within one of the polyps.

B. Polyps localised to the gastric body and fundus.

C. Polyps less than 5 mm in diameter.

D. Multiple polyps including some located in the antrum.

E. Negative Helicobacter pylori status.

Answer: A

Sporadic fundic gland polyps in young patients without PPI exposure, and particularly fundic gland polyps with any degree of dysplasia, raise suspicion of familial adenomatous polyposis (FAP). FAP patients characteristically develop multiple fundic gland polyps with a higher frequency of dysplasia than sporadic cases, and the presence of dysplasia in any fundic gland polyp in a young patient should prompt referral to clinical genetics for APC germline testing. The other typical features of FAP-associated gastric polyposis include greater polyp density, larger numbers (often hundreds), and association with duodenal adenomas. The differential of FAP also includes attenuated FAP, MUTYH-associated polyposis, and gastric adenocarcinoma and proximal polyposis of the stomach (GAPPS) — a more recently described entity caused by APC promoter 1B point mutations.

Option B describes the typical location of sporadic fundic gland polyps and is not discriminatory. Option C describes typical sporadic morphology. Option D is the opposite — polyps localised to the antrum are typically hyperplastic or adenomatous rather than fundic gland polyps, and antral fundic gland polyps are not characteristic of FAP. Option E is unhelpful because fundic gland polyps are not typically associated with active Helicobacter infection.

Q9.2. Risk-of-malignant-behaviour stratification in gastrointestinal stromal tumour (GIST) depends on tumour size, mitotic count, and anatomical site. A 5 cm gastric GIST in a 60-year-old patient shows 8 mitoses per 5 mm squared on extensive sampling. KIT exon 11 mutation is confirmed. Which single statement best describes the risk category and the management implication?

A. Very low risk — observation only.

B. High risk — adjuvant imatinib for at least three years is supported by current guidance.

C. Low risk — surgical resection only without adjuvant therapy.

D. Intermediate risk — adjuvant imatinib for one year is supported.

E. Risk cannot be stratified without molecular profiling.

Answer: B

Under the Miettinen-Lasota / AFIP 2006 risk system, a gastric GIST measuring 5 to 10 cm with mitotic count above 5 per 5 mm squared falls into the high-risk category — irrespective of whether the upper or lower part of the size range applies. High-risk GIST is associated with high recurrence rates after surgical resection alone, and adjuvant imatinib for at least three years (the SSGXVIII/AIO trial supports this duration) is the standard of care for KIT-sensitive mutations. KIT exon 11 mutations respond well to imatinib, supporting the use of adjuvant therapy. The treatment decision is also informed by the genotype — PDGFRA D842V mutations are imatinib-resistant and are not candidates for adjuvant imatinib.

Option A understates the risk markedly. Option C also understates. Option D fits an intermediate-risk profile but the mitotic count above 5 per 5 mm squared with size in this range places the lesion in the high-risk category. Option E is incorrect because risk stratification can be performed from morphology alone (size and mitotic count); molecular profile informs treatment selection rather than risk stratification.

Q9.3. Gastric MALT lymphoma is the principal primary gastric lymphoma and responds to Helicobacter eradication in a defined proportion of cases. A 65-year-old man has gastric biopsies showing a dense lymphoid infiltrate with characteristic lymphoepithelial lesions. Immunohistochemistry confirms a marginal zone B-cell phenotype, and Helicobacter pylori is identified on the same biopsy. Which single factor most strongly predicts non-response to Helicobacter eradication alone?

A. Patient age over 60.

B. Antral as opposed to corpus location.

C. Presence of the t(11;18)(q21;q21) BIRC3-MALT1 translocation.

D. Helicobacter eradication has not been attempted in this patient.

E. Tumour size less than 2 cm on endoscopic ultrasound.

Answer: C

Around 90 per cent of gastric MALT lymphomas are Helicobacter-driven, and 70 to 80 per cent of localised cases respond to eradication therapy with histological regression. The principal predictor of non-response is the t(11;18)(q21;q21) BIRC3-MALT1 translocation — present in around 25 per cent of cases overall and markedly more common in non-responders. The translocation is detected by FISH using break-apart probes. t(11;18)-positive cases typically require oncological therapy (rituximab, chemotherapy, or radiotherapy) in addition to or instead of eradication. Other adverse predictors include deep mural invasion on endoscopic ultrasound and absence of detectable Helicobacter infection at presentation.

Options A, B, and E are not strong predictors of response or non-response. Option D is not a predictor — it describes a starting point rather than a biological characteristic of the tumour.

9.16 Chapter EMQ

EMQ 9.1. Gastric pathology — diagnosis. For each scenario, select the single most appropriate diagnosis from the option list. Each option may be used once, more than once, or not at all.

A. Helicobacter pylori-associated chronic active gastritis

B. Autoimmune (corpus type A) atrophic gastritis

C. Reactive (chemical) gastritis

D. Eosinophilic gastritis

E. Hyperplastic polyp

F. Fundic gland polyp

G. Pyloric gland adenoma

H. Intestinal-type gastric adenocarcinoma

I. Diffuse-type gastric adenocarcinoma with signet ring features

J. Type 1 gastric neuroendocrine tumour

(1) A 55-year-old woman has gastric body biopsies showing oxyntic atrophy, pseudopyloric metaplasia, linear ECL cell hyperplasia, and chronic inflammation. Antral biopsies are histologically normal. Anti-parietal cell antibodies are positive. **Answer: B**

(2) A 70-year-old man with chronic NSAID use has antral biopsies showing foveolar hyperplasia with corkscrew-shaped pits, vasodilation, and smooth muscle fibres extending into the lamina propria, with relatively few inflammatory cells. **Answer: C**

(3) A 35-year-old woman with Helicobacter-associated atrophic gastritis has a 6 mm polyp in the gastric body. The polyp shows dilated cystic oxyntic glands lined by parietal and chief cells. **Answer: F**

(4) A 42-year-old woman has gastric body biopsies showing scattered cells with intracytoplasmic mucin displacing the nucleus to the cell margin, infiltrating singly through the lamina propria. The cohesive glands are absent. The patient's mother and sister had gastric cancer in their forties. **Answer: I**

(5) A 78-year-old man with longstanding autoimmune atrophic gastritis has a 1.2 cm polypoid lesion in the gastric body. Biopsy shows a well-differentiated neuroendocrine tumour with Ki-67 of 2 per cent. **Answer: J**

Chapter 10 — Small bowel and appendix

Small bowel pathology occupies a defined and well-bounded section of the syllabus. The mucosal biopsy work is dominated by coeliac disease and its differential, by Crohn's disease and the broader inflammatory bowel disease spectrum, and by infectious enteritides. The resection specimens carry ischaemia, obstruction, perforation, and the spectrum of small bowel neoplasia — adenocarcinoma, neuroendocrine tumours, lymphomas, and rare entities. The appendix has its own focused syllabus dominated by acute appendicitis and its variants, the mucinous neoplasm spectrum (LAMN, HAMN, mucinous adenocarcinoma), goblet cell adenocarcinoma, and the neuroendocrine tumour group. This chapter sets out the principal entities, the WHO 5th edition classification of small bowel and appendiceal tumours, and the staging conventions for invasive disease.

10.1 Normal small bowel histology

The small bowel comprises duodenum, jejunum, and ileum, each with broadly similar histological organisation and characteristic regional features. The mucosa shows villous architecture — finger-like projections of lamina propria covered by absorptive enterocytes with apical brush border, goblet cells, and scattered neuroendocrine cells. The lamina propria contains lymphocytes, plasma cells, eosinophils, mast cells, and macrophages within a loose connective tissue framework. The crypts of Lieberkuhn extend down to the muscularis mucosae and contain Paneth cells (with prominent apical eosinophilic granules) at the crypt base. The submucosa contains Brunner's glands in the duodenum (mucous glands secreting bicarbonate-rich alkaline mucus, a characteristic regional feature) and Peyer's patches (large lymphoid aggregates) in the terminal ileum. The muscularis propria has inner circular and outer longitudinal layers separated by the myenteric plexus.

Villous-to-crypt ratio is the principal measure of mucosal architecture, normally 3:1 to 5:1 with longer villi in the proximal duodenum and shorter villi distally. The intraepithelial lymphocyte (IEL) count is normally less than 25 lymphocytes per 100 enterocytes in adults; counts above 25 raise the question of coeliac disease or related lymphocytic enteropathy. The Brunner's glands extending into the submucosa identify the biopsy as duodenal in origin.

10.2 Coeliac disease

Coeliac disease is the immune-mediated enteropathy triggered by dietary gluten in genetically susceptible individuals (HLA-DQ2 and DQ8 haplotypes). The histological hallmarks are intraepithelial lymphocytosis, crypt hyperplasia with crypt elongation, and villous atrophy of variable severity. The Marsh classification (refined by Oberhuber and others) grades the changes from Marsh 0 (normal architecture) through Marsh 1 (intraepithelial lymphocytosis only), Marsh 2 (intraepithelial lymphocytosis with crypt hyperplasia), and Marsh 3 (villous atrophy graded as 3a partial, 3b subtotal, 3c total). The biopsy site is critical — duodenal bulb and second part biopsies (at least four biopsies, of which at least one from the bulb) maximise diagnostic yield because changes are often patchy and proximal-predominant.

Serological correlation — anti-tissue transglutaminase IgA (tTG-IgA) antibodies and anti-endomysial IgA — supports the histological diagnosis and is essential for case interpretation. Seronegative villous atrophy raises a wide differential including drug-induced enteropathy (olmesartan, methotrexate), tropical sprue, common variable immunodeficiency, autoimmune enteropathy, Whipple disease, eosinophilic enteritis, peptic duodenitis, and giardiasis. Refractory coeliac disease (persistent villous atrophy despite strict gluten-free diet) is sub-classified by intraepithelial lymphocyte phenotype — type I shows polyclonal T-cells, type II shows aberrant clonal T-cells with loss of CD8 surface expression and is the precursor to enteropathy-associated T-cell lymphoma (EATL).

Coeliac disease essentials

HLA: DQ2 (95%) and DQ8 (most of remainder) — genetic susceptibility.

Marsh classification: 0 normal; 1 IEL only; 2 IEL + crypt hyperplasia; 3a–c villous atrophy partial/subtotal/total.

Biopsy: ≥4 duodenal biopsies including ≥1 from the bulb; changes patchy and proximal-predominant.

IEL threshold: >25 per 100 enterocytes raises diagnostic suspicion.

Seronegative villous atrophy: drug (olmesartan), tropical sprue, CVID, autoimmune enteropathy, Whipple, eosinophilic, giardiasis.

Refractory type II: aberrant T-cell clone; EATL precursor.

10.3 Crohn's disease and inflammatory bowel disease

Crohn's disease is the chronic granulomatous inflammatory bowel disease (IBD) that may affect any part of the gastrointestinal tract from mouth to anus. The classical small bowel involvement is in the terminal ileum, with ileal stricturing, mucosal ulceration, transmural inflammation, and skip lesions interspersed with normal mucosa. The histological hallmarks include non-caseating granulomas (present in around 40 per cent of cases when surgical resections are sampled extensively, fewer in mucosal biopsies), transmural inflammation, fissuring ulceration, lymphoid aggregates extending through the bowel wall, neural hypertrophy, and pyloric metaplasia of the small bowel epithelium (an architectural marker of chronic injury). Fat wrapping (creeping fat) around the involved bowel is a macroscopic feature characteristic of Crohn's disease.

The differential of granulomatous inflammation in the small bowel includes tuberculosis (caseating granulomas typically present, with acid-fast bacilli demonstrable by Ziehl-Neelsen or by molecular methods), yersiniosis (resembles Crohn's but with appropriate microbiology), sarcoidosis (multisystem), foreign body reaction, and rare entities (chronic granulomatous disease of childhood). Distinguishing Crohn's from intestinal tuberculosis is particularly important in regions with high TB prevalence and in patients with relevant risk factors — caseation, larger granulomas with confluent pattern, and demonstration of acid-fast bacilli support TB. Indeterminate cases warrant clinical and microbiological correlation before commitment to immunosuppressive therapy.

10.4 Acute and chronic ischaemia

Acute mesenteric ischaemia presents in elderly patients with sudden severe abdominal pain disproportionate to physical findings. Resection specimens show transmural haemorrhagic infarction with surface fibrinopurulent exudate and friable necrotic bowel wall. The histology shows coagulative necrosis of the mucosa extending into the deeper layers, with vascular thrombosis in larger vessels of the mesentery. The causes include embolism (often from atrial fibrillation), thrombosis on atherosclerotic vessel disease, low-flow non-occlusive ischaemia, and venous thrombosis. Determining the cause from the resection specimen is sometimes possible — atheroma at the SMA origin, fresh thrombus in larger arteries, or organising venous thrombus.

Chronic ischaemia produces a different histological pattern: mucosal atrophy with reduced villous height, submucosal fibrosis, hyalinisation of lamina propria, and pseudomembrane formation in severe cases. The clinical context (post-prandial pain, weight loss, mesenteric vascular disease) supports the diagnosis. Localised ischaemic injury — for example following intussusception or strangulation in a hernia — shows segmental changes corresponding to the affected loop.

10.5 Small bowel neoplasia

Adenocarcinoma

Small bowel adenocarcinoma is rare (around 3 per cent of GI cancers) but is the second commonest small bowel neoplasm after neuroendocrine tumours. The duodenum is the commonest site, particularly the periampullary region. The tumour typically arises from adenoma — sporadic, FAP-associated, MUTYH-associated polyposis, Peutz-Jeghers, or Lynch syndrome. Lynch syndrome accounts for around 5 per cent of small bowel adenocarcinomas and is the indication for routine MMR IHC testing on every small bowel adenocarcinoma. The histology mirrors colorectal adenocarcinoma — glandular architecture with variable mucin, ranging from well to poorly differentiated. Staging follows AJCC 8 for small bowel cancer with site-specific T categories.

Small bowel neuroendocrine tumours

Small bowel neuroendocrine tumours arise most commonly in the terminal ileum, often as multiple lesions, and characteristically secrete serotonin causing the carcinoid syndrome (flushing, diarrhoea, right-heart valve disease) when liver metastases are present. The tumours are well-differentiated, with insular or trabecular architecture, uniform cells with stippled chromatin, and characteristic immunoreactivity for synaptophysin, chromogranin, and INSM1. CDX2 is positive (the tumour is enteric in origin). Grade is determined by Ki-67 and mitotic count under the WHO 5th edition framework — grade 1 (Ki-67 under 3 per cent), grade 2 (3-20 per cent), grade 3 (over 20 per cent with well-differentiated morphology). Multifocality, mesenteric desmoplasia (with fibrosis encasing mesenteric vessels), and liver metastases are characteristic features.

Lymphoma

The small bowel is the commonest extranodal site for non-Hodgkin lymphoma in the GI tract. The principal entities include diffuse large B-cell lymphoma (the most common), MALT lymphoma (small bowel involvement uncommon), follicular lymphoma (often duodenal, indolent), mantle cell lymphoma (multiple lymphomatous polyposis pattern), and enteropathy-associated T-cell lymphoma (EATL — associated with refractory coeliac disease type II, aggressive). The diagnostic approach combines morphology, immunophenotyping (flow cytometry on fresh tissue and IHC on FFPE), molecular clonality (IGH and TCR rearrangement studies), and FISH for diagnostic translocations. Excisional or generous endoscopic biopsy is preferred to support classification.

10.6 The appendix — acute appendicitis

Acute appendicitis is the commonest emergency abdominal surgical specimen, and the appendicectomy specimen requires structured macroscopic and microscopic assessment. The macroscopic features include erythema, fibrinopurulent exudate on the serosa, dilatation, perforation, faecolith impaction in the lumen, and any masses or wall thickening. Microscopic examination samples the tip, mid-portion, and base, with at least one block to demonstrate the muscularis propria and the resection margin. The histology of acute appendicitis shows transmural neutrophilic infiltration, mucosal ulceration, surface fibrinopurulent exudate, and vascular thrombosis in advanced cases. Perforated appendicitis adds the additional findings of full-thickness inflammation extending to and through the serosa.

Specific appendicular entities to recognise include enterobius vermicularis (pinworm — visible parasites within the lumen, usually incidental), schistosomiasis (eggs with characteristic spines in the wall in endemic regions), tuberculosis (granulomatous inflammation, the appendix may be involved in disseminated abdominal TB), endometriosis (endometrial glands and stroma in the appendiceal wall), and diverticular disease (acquired diverticula with inflammation). The acute appendicitis differential always includes considering whether the inflammation has masked an underlying neoplasm — and every appendix specimen is sampled to address that question.

10.7 Appendiceal mucinous neoplasms

The classification of appendiceal mucinous neoplasms was reorganised with the WHO 5th edition (2019) and the PSOGI (Peritoneal Surface Oncology Group International) consensus. The diagnostic categories now are mucinous adenoma (confined to the lumen with no invasion of the wall, true neoplasm with low-grade dysplasia), low-grade appendiceal mucinous neoplasm (LAMN — with replacement of mucosa by villous or flat low-grade neoplastic epithelium and pushing-margin extension into the wall with diverticulum-like outpouchings; no infiltrative invasion), high-grade appendiceal mucinous neoplasm (HAMN — same architectural pattern as LAMN but high-grade cytological atypia), mucinous adenocarcinoma (true infiltrative invasion of the wall, may be well, moderate, or poorly differentiated, with or without signet ring cells), and goblet cell adenocarcinoma (formerly called goblet cell carcinoid — see below).

LAMN with acellular mucin breaching the serosa — but without epithelial cells outside the appendix — is classified as pT4a under AJCC 8 staging, reflecting the recognised potential for development of pseudomyxoma peritonei from the rupture of mucinous epithelium and its extension to the peritoneal cavity. LAMN with neoplastic epithelium outside the appendix on the serosa is pT4a but with worse prognostic implications. Pseudomyxoma peritonei is staged separately and graded by cellularity and grade of epithelium — low-grade mucinous carcinoma peritonei (acellular or paucicellular low-grade) is the classical complication of LAMN, while high-grade mucinous carcinoma peritonei follows HAMN and mucinous adenocarcinoma.

Appendiceal mucinous neoplasia — WHO 5 / PSOGI

Mucinous adenoma: luminal neoplasm with low-grade dysplasia; no wall invasion.

LAMN: low-grade pushing-margin pattern with wall outpouchings; no infiltrative invasion.

HAMN: LAMN architecture with high-grade cytology.

Mucinous adenocarcinoma: true infiltrative invasion; well/moderate/poor differentiation; with or without signet ring.

Goblet cell adenocarcinoma: dual mucinous and neuroendocrine differentiation; graded 1–3.

pT4a with mucin: acellular peritoneal mucin from LAMN — pseudomyxoma risk.

10.8 Goblet cell adenocarcinoma and appendiceal NETs

Goblet cell adenocarcinoma (the renamed entity formerly called goblet cell carcinoid) is unique to the appendix and shows simultaneous mucinous and neuroendocrine differentiation. The tumour comprises tubules and clusters of goblet-like cells (with intracytoplasmic mucin) admixed with neuroendocrine cells, infiltrating the wall in a distinctive concentric annular pattern. The Tang classification (refined by Yozu and the WHO 5th edition) grades the tumour into three tiers based on architectural distortion, single-cell pattern, and signet-ring features — grade 1 (well-differentiated goblet cell pattern predominant), grade 2 (around 50 per cent showing signet ring or single cell infiltration), grade 3 (predominant signet ring or undifferentiated pattern). The grade strongly predicts prognosis.

Appendiceal neuroendocrine tumours (NETs) are usually small (under 1 cm), located at the tip, and discovered incidentally in appendicectomy specimens for presumed appendicitis. The tumours are well-differentiated with insular and trabecular architecture, uniform cells, and characteristic IHC (synaptophysin, chromogranin, INSM1, CDX2). Surgical management depends on size (under 1 cm — appendicectomy adequate; 1 to 2 cm — depends on grade, location, and lymphovascular invasion; over 2 cm — right hemicolectomy generally indicated). Grading uses the WHO 5th edition NET grade based on mitotic count and Ki-67.

10.9 Reporting and staging

Small bowel and appendiceal cancer reports follow the RCPath and ICCR datasets. Core items include specimen type, tumour location (with anatomical reference), histological type and grade, dimensions, depth of invasion, margins, lymphovascular invasion, perineural invasion, lymph node count and status, MMR status (mandatory for adenocarcinoma to identify Lynch syndrome candidates), and any treatment effect. Pseudomyxoma peritonei findings are reported separately when the appendix is the presumed primary, including grade and extent. The synoptic block follows the structured reporting convention.

10.10 Key points

Chapter 10 — key points

Coeliac disease: HLA-DQ2 (95%) or DQ8. Marsh 0–3 (normal → IEL → crypt hyperplasia → villous atrophy). ≥4 duodenal biopsies including bulb; IEL threshold >25/100 enterocytes.

Seronegative villous atrophy: Drug (olmesartan), tropical sprue, CVID, autoimmune enteropathy, Whipple, eosinophilic enteritis, giardiasis.

Inflammatory bowel disease: Ileitis assessment; granulomas favour Crohn's (30% biopsies, 60% resections).

Appendiceal mucinous neoplasia: Mucinous adenoma → LAMN → HAMN → mucinous adenocarcinoma. WHO 5/PSOGI nomenclature; pT4a acellular peritoneal mucin signals pseudomyxoma risk.

Goblet cell adenocarcinoma: Dual mucinous and neuroendocrine differentiation; graded 1–3.

Small bowel NETs: Most common in ileum; chromogranin and synaptophysin positive; Ki-67 grades G1/G2/G3.

Vasculopathy and ischaemia: Mesenteric artery occlusion, vasculitis, radiation enteritis — recognise by transmural ischaemic pattern.

10.11 Chapter SBAs

Q10.1. Distinction between intestinal tuberculosis and Crohn's disease in the terminal ileum is critical because the management is fundamentally different. A 45-year-old patient with weight loss and abdominal pain has a right hemicolectomy for terminal ileal stricture. The histology shows transmural inflammation with non-caseating granulomas, lymphoid aggregates, and fat wrapping. Which single feature, if present, would most strongly favour intestinal tuberculosis rather than Crohn's disease?

A. Presence of multiple non-caseating granulomas.

B. Fat wrapping of the involved bowel.

C. Caseating granulomas with confluent pattern and Ziehl-Neelsen-positive acid-fast bacilli.

D. Skip lesions interspersed with normal mucosa.

E. Pyloric metaplasia in the small bowel epithelium.

Answer: C

Caseating granulomas with confluent pattern and demonstrable acid-fast bacilli are the principal histological discriminator between intestinal tuberculosis and Crohn's disease. Crohn's granulomas are characteristically non-caseating, small, and scattered; TB granulomas are typically larger, often confluent, frequently caseating, and may show acid-fast bacilli on Ziehl-Neelsen staining or by molecular methods (PCR for Mycobacterium tuberculosis complex). The distinction matters because

Crohn's is treated with immunosuppression while TB requires antimicrobial therapy — and starting immunosuppression in unrecognised intestinal TB risks dissemination. Clinical context (geographical risk, contact history, chest findings, HIV status) and microbiological investigations support the diagnosis.

Option A is non-discriminatory because both Crohn's and TB show granulomas (Crohn's: non-caseating; TB: caseating). Option B (fat wrapping) is characteristic of Crohn's, not TB. Option D (skip lesions) is also more characteristic of Crohn's. Option E (pyloric metaplasia) indicates chronic injury and is seen in Crohn's; it is not a feature of TB.

Q10.2. Refractory coeliac disease type II is the recognised precursor of enteropathy-associated T-cell lymphoma, and its identification carries important prognostic and surveillance implications. A 60-year-old man with long-standing histologically-confirmed coeliac disease has been on a strict gluten-free diet for two years but continues to have persistent villous atrophy on duodenal biopsy. Intraepithelial T cells show aberrant surface phenotype with loss of CD8 expression and demonstrate clonal T-cell receptor rearrangement on molecular testing. Which single statement best describes the diagnosis and the management implication?

A. Coeliac disease with poor dietary adherence — repeat dietary counselling.

B. Refractory coeliac disease type II with high risk of progression to EATL.

C. Common variable immunodeficiency mimicking coeliac.

D. Tropical sprue.

E. Drug-induced enteropathy.

Answer: B

Persistent villous atrophy despite documented strict gluten-free diet defines refractory coeliac disease. The phenotype of the intraepithelial lymphocytes determines the sub-classification — type I (polyclonal T cells with normal surface CD3, CD8, TCR alpha/beta expression) is less aggressive and may respond to additional dietary and pharmacological intervention. Type II (aberrant clonal T cells with loss of CD8 surface expression, sometimes loss of TCR surface expression, and demonstrable TCR clonality) carries a high risk of progression to enteropathy-associated T-cell lymphoma (EATL) — up to 50 per cent over 5 years in published series. Management of type II disease includes specialist coeliac centre referral, consideration of treatment with cladribine or autologous stem cell transplantation, and intensive surveillance for lymphoma development.

Options A, C, D, and E all describe alternative diagnoses that the clinical, histological, and immunophenotypic findings exclude. The clonal aberrant T-cell phenotype with surface CD8 loss is the defining feature.

Q10.3. Classification of appendiceal mucinous lesions was reorganised with the WHO 5th edition (2019) and PSOGI consensus, and accurate categorisation drives the management. An appendicectomy specimen shows villous neoplastic epithelium with low-grade cytological atypia replacing the mucosa, with pushing-margin extension into the wall forming diverticulum-like outpouchings of mucin into the wall. No infiltrative invasion is identified. Acellular mucin extends through the serosa onto the peritoneal surface. Which single diagnosis and stage is most appropriate under current WHO 5 / PSOGI classification?

A. Mucinous adenoma, pT0.

B. Low-grade appendiceal mucinous neoplasm (LAMN), pT4a.

C. High-grade appendiceal mucinous neoplasm (HAMN), pT3.

D. Mucinous adenocarcinoma, pT4a.

E. Goblet cell adenocarcinoma, pT2.

Answer: B

The described morphology — pushing-margin extension of low-grade neoplastic epithelium into the wall with diverticulum-like outpouchings, no infiltrative invasion, with acellular mucin breaching the serosa — defines low-grade appendiceal mucinous neoplasm (LAMN). The peritoneal extension of acellular mucin alone (without epithelial cells) is staged as pT4a under AJCC 8 staging conventions and is associated with the risk of pseudomyxoma peritonei. Cellular peritoneal mucin (with neoplastic epithelial cells beyond the appendix) would carry a worse prognosis. The clinical management includes consideration of cytoreductive surgery and hyperthermic intraperitoneal chemotherapy (HIPEC) in specialist centres if pseudomyxoma develops.

Option A (mucinous adenoma) is excluded by the wall involvement. Option C (HAMN) is excluded by the low-grade cytology. Option D (mucinous adenocarcinoma) is excluded by the absence of infiltrative invasion. Option E (goblet cell adenocarcinoma) describes a different entity with dual mucinous-neuroendocrine differentiation.

10.12 Chapter EMQ

EMQ 10.1. Small bowel and appendiceal pathology — diagnosis. For each scenario, select the single most appropriate diagnosis from the option list. Each option may be used once, more than once, or not at all.

A. Coeliac disease (Marsh 3b)

B. Crohn's disease

C. Intestinal tuberculosis

D. Refractory coeliac disease type II

E. Small bowel adenocarcinoma

F. Small bowel neuroendocrine tumour

G. Enteropathy-associated T-cell lymphoma

H. Acute appendicitis (uncomplicated)

I. Low-grade appendiceal mucinous neoplasm (LAMN)

J. Goblet cell adenocarcinoma

(1) A 25-year-old woman with chronic diarrhoea has duodenal biopsies showing subtotal villous atrophy, crypt hyperplasia, and intraepithelial lymphocytosis of 80 per 100 enterocytes. Anti-tTG IgA is positive at 10× upper limit of normal. **Answer: A**

(2) A 50-year-old patient with previous coeliac disease and strict gluten-free diet for 5 years has persistent villous atrophy. Intraepithelial T cells show loss of CD8 expression with clonal TCR rearrangement. **Answer: D**

(3) A 65-year-old man has a 6 cm well-differentiated tumour at the ileocaecal junction with insular and trabecular architecture, uniform cells with stippled chromatin, synaptophysin and chromogranin positivity, and intense mesenteric desmoplasia. **Answer: F**

(4) An appendicectomy specimen from an 80-year-old shows a 3 cm tumour with tubules and clusters of goblet-like cells admixed with neuroendocrine cells, infiltrating the wall in a concentric annular pattern. **Answer: J**

(5) An appendicectomy from a 40-year-old shows a dilated lumen with villous low-grade neoplastic epithelium and pushing-margin extension of mucin-filled outpouchings through the wall. No infiltrative invasion is identified. Acellular mucin extends onto the serosa. **Answer: I**

Chapter 11 — Colon, rectum, and anus

Colorectal pathology is the largest single workstream in most general histopathology departments. Mucosal biopsy work is dominated by inflammatory bowel disease, infectious and ischaemic colitis, and bowel cancer screening polyp surveillance. Resection specimens carry colorectal cancer staging, MMR testing, biomarker assessment, neoadjuvant response, and structured ICCR/RCPath reporting. The anus carries its own focused syllabus dominated by anal intraepithelial neoplasia, anal squamous cell carcinoma (HPV-associated), Paget disease, and inflammatory disorders of the perianal skin. This chapter sets out the principal entities, staging and dataset conventions, and the molecular framework that drives contemporary management.

11.1 Normal colorectal histology

Colorectal mucosa shows orderly tubular crypts perpendicular to the muscularis mucosae — uniform in length, with a single basal layer of nuclei and intervening lamina propria of normal cellularity. Surface columnar epithelium and abundant goblet cells overlie the crypts. The lamina propria contains lymphocytes, plasma cells (with a normal density gradient from upper to lower), eosinophils, mast cells, and macrophages. The muscularis mucosae is a thin double smooth muscle layer; the submucosa contains vessels, nerves, and lymphoid aggregates. The muscularis propria has inner circular and outer longitudinal layers — the latter aggregated into three taeniae coli in the colon and forming a continuous layer in the rectum and appendix.

Architectural features assessed in IBD biopsy include crypt density, crypt distortion (branching, dilatation, dropout), surface integrity, basal plasma cell infiltrate, lamina propria cellularity gradient, and Paneth cell metaplasia distal to the hepatic flexure — an architectural marker of chronic injury, since Paneth cells are normally restricted to the right colon and progressively less common moving distally.

11.2 Ulcerative colitis

Ulcerative colitis (UC) is the chronic relapsing inflammatory disease of the colorectum characterised by continuous mucosal inflammation extending proximally from the rectum — the rectum is almost always involved. Histological hallmarks include crypt distortion (the most reliable architectural feature of chronicity), crypt dropout with reduced density, basal plasmacytosis, surface villiform change, Paneth cell metaplasia distal to the hepatic flexure, and during active disease — neutrophilic cryptitis with crypt abscesses and surface ulceration. The disease is mucosal and submucosal; transmural inflammation raises the question of severe acute UC complicated by toxic megacolon, or alternative diagnosis.

Surveillance for colorectal cancer in long-standing UC is a defined endoscopic and histological pathway. Random biopsies at intervals through the colon plus targeted biopsies of abnormal mucosa are reviewed for dysplasia. Dysplasia is graded low-grade or high-grade, and is further classified by visibility — visible (raised or polypoid dysplasia, increasingly resectable by endoscopic submucosal dissection) versus invisible (flat dysplasia identified only on random biopsy). The SCENIC consensus and BSG guidelines structure the management algorithm.

11.3 Crohn's colitis

Crohn's colitis shares many architectural features with UC but is distinguished by characteristic features. The colitis is patchy with intervening normal mucosa (skip lesions), aphthous ulcers overlie lymphoid aggregates, transmural inflammation produces deep fissuring ulcers and lymphoid aggregates extending through the wall, non-caseating granulomas are present in around 30 per cent of biopsies and 60 per cent of resections (when sampled extensively), and the rectum is often spared. Perianal disease (fistulae, abscesses, skin tags) is characteristic of Crohn's and rare in UC. The terminal ileum may be involved as true ileal disease — distinct from the rare backwash ileitis seen in UC pancolitis.

UC vs Crohn's colitis at a glance

Distribution: UC continuous from rectum; Crohn's patchy with skip lesions, rectum often spared.

Depth: UC mucosal/submucosal; Crohn's transmural with fissuring ulcers.

Granulomas: UC absent (cryptolytic only); Crohn's non-caseating 30% biopsies, 60% resections.

Perianal: UC rare; Crohn's characteristic.

Ileum: UC backwash rare; Crohn's true ileal involvement common.

11.4 Other forms of colitis

Infectious colitis is a frequent differential of acute colitis on biopsy. Bacterial infection (Campylobacter, Salmonella, Shigella, enterohaemorrhagic E. coli) produces acute self-limited colitis with neutrophilic infiltration, preserved architecture, and absence of basal plasmacytosis — distinguishing features from acute-on-chronic IBD. Clostridioides difficile pseudomembranous colitis shows characteristic surface pseudomembranes — fibrin, mucin, neutrophils, and necrotic debris in the volcano-like lesion. CMV colitis affects immunocompromised patients with owl-eye inclusions in endothelial cells. Schistosomiasis (eggs with characteristic spines in the lamina propria, granulomatous response) and tuberculosis (caseating granulomas) are important regional considerations.

Microscopic colitis is a clinical syndrome of chronic watery diarrhoea with normal-appearing mucosa at endoscopy. Two histological patterns predominate. Lymphocytic colitis shows intraepithelial lymphocytosis — over 20 per 100 surface enterocytes — with chronic inflammation in the lamina propria and intact architecture. Collagenous colitis shows a thickened subepithelial collagen band (over 10 micrometres on H&E or trichrome stain) with strands of collagen extending into the lamina propria and entrapping capillaries. Ischaemic colitis shows characteristic features at the splenic flexure or sigmoid (watershed areas) with surface ulceration, lamina propria hyalinisation, withered crypts, and pseudomembrane formation in severe cases.

11.5 Colorectal polyps

Adenomatous polyps

Conventional adenomas comprise tubular, tubulovillous, and villous architectures with low or high-grade dysplasia. Tubular architecture predominates in small polyps; villous architecture becomes prominent in larger lesions; tubulovillous occupies the middle ground. High-grade dysplasia shows full-thickness atypia, architectural complexity (cribriform glands, back-to-back arrangement), and loss of polarity. Intramucosal carcinoma — invasion through the basement membrane but confined to the lamina propria — does not metastasise in colorectal practice because the lamina propria lacks lymphatics, and is therefore not classified as invasive carcinoma in current colorectal staging; the lesion is reported as 'intramucosal carcinoma' or as 'high-grade dysplasia' depending on local convention, with the same management.

Serrated lesions

The serrated pathway is now recognised as a parallel mechanism of colorectal carcinogenesis distinct from the conventional adenoma-carcinoma sequence. Hyperplastic polyps are the indolent end of the spectrum — characteristic serrated luminal architecture, no dysplasia, minimal cancer risk. Sessile serrated lesions (SSL, formerly sessile serrated adenoma) show distorted serrated architecture extending to the crypt base with boot-shaped or L-shaped basal crypts, lateral spread along the muscularis mucosae, dilated crypts at the base, and absence of dysplasia in the typical lesion. SSL is the precursor of around 20-30 per cent of colorectal cancers — particularly right-sided, MSI-high, BRAF-mutant cancers. SSL with dysplasia carries elevated short-term cancer risk. Traditional serrated adenomas (TSA) are rarer, characterised by ectopic crypt foci, eosinophilic cytoplasm, and pointed nuclei.

Hereditary polyposis syndromes

Familial adenomatous polyposis (FAP, germline APC mutation) presents with hundreds to thousands of colorectal adenomas in adolescence and adult life. Attenuated FAP shows fewer polyps and later onset. MUTYH-associated polyposis (biallelic MUTYH germline mutation) presents similarly to attenuated FAP. Lynch syndrome (germline mutation in MLH1, MSH2, MSH6, PMS2, or EPCAM deletion) presents with colorectal and endometrial cancer at relatively young ages with characteristic MMR-deficient tumours; polyps are not numerous but cancers arise from a smaller number of adenomas. Peutz-Jeghers syndrome (germline STK11 mutation) presents with mucocutaneous pigmentation and characteristic Peutz-Jeghers polyps with branching smooth muscle. Juvenile polyposis (germline SMAD4 or BMPR1A) and Cowden syndrome (germline PTEN) are the other principal hereditary polyposis syndromes.

11.6 Colorectal adenocarcinoma

Histology and grading

Colorectal adenocarcinoma is the dominant invasive tumour. WHO 5th edition subtypes include adenocarcinoma not otherwise specified (the dominant pattern), mucinous adenocarcinoma (over 50 per cent mucin), signet ring carcinoma, medullary carcinoma (associated with MMR deficiency — sheets of tumour cells with prominent lymphocytic infiltrate, often well-prognosed), serrated adenocarcinoma, micropapillary, and undifferentiated carcinoma. Grading is by gland formation — well-differentiated (over 95 per cent glands), moderately differentiated (50-95 per cent), poorly differentiated (under 50 per cent). Under WHO 5th edition, medullary carcinoma is designated as low-grade despite its poorly differentiated architecture, reflecting the recognised better prognosis of this MMR-deficient subtype; conventional MMR-deficient adenocarcinomas (non-medullary) are still graded by gland formation in the standard way.

Molecular subtypes

The consensus molecular subtypes (CMS) framework defines four subtypes. CMS1 (MSI immune): MMR-deficient, BRAF-mutant, hypermutated, right-sided, prominent immune infiltration, good prognosis after immunotherapy. CMS2 (canonical): WNT and MYC pathway activation, copy-number high, left-sided, the classical adenoma-carcinoma sequence. CMS3 (metabolic): KRAS-mutant, mixed genomic features, metabolic dysregulation. CMS4 (mesenchymal): TGF-beta activation, stromal infiltration, angiogenesis, poor prognosis. In clinical practice, workup includes MMR IHC (or MSI testing) on every colorectal cancer to identify Lynch candidates and inform immunotherapy eligibility, KRAS/NRAS/BRAF mutation analysis to inform anti-EGFR antibody eligibility in metastatic disease, and increasingly HER2 testing and broader NGS profiling in selected metastatic cases.

MMR IHC and Lynch syndrome triage

MMR IHC tests for loss of expression of MLH1, MSH2, MSH6, and PMS2. The dominant patterns are paired loss of MLH1 and PMS2 (most often sporadic via MLH1 promoter hypermethylation; check BRAF V600E IHC and MLH1 methylation as covered in Chapter 3 to triage Lynch versus sporadic) or paired loss of MSH2 and MSH6 (typically germline, refer to genetics). Isolated loss of MSH6 or PMS2 occurs and usually indicates germline mutation in the respective gene. The combined two-step algorithm — BRAF or methylation testing where MLH1/PMS2 are lost — identifies the Lynch candidates for clinical genetics referral.

11.7 TNM staging and CRC reporting

AJCC 8 staging for colorectal cancer records T (Tis, T1 — submucosal, T2 — muscularis propria, T3 — through muscularis propria into pericolorectal tissue, T4a — through serosa, T4b — invading adjacent organs), N (N0; N1a 1 node; N1b 2-3 nodes; N1c tumour deposits without nodal involvement; N2a 4-6 nodes; N2b 7+ nodes), and M (M0; M1a single organ; M1b multiple organs; M1c peritoneal). A minimum of 12 lymph nodes is the standard target for adequate staging, with submission of all pericolic lymph nodes from the specimen.

Reporting follows the RCPath dataset. Core items include specimen type, tumour location (with distance from key landmarks for rectal tumours), histological type and grade, dimensions, depth of invasion, margins (proximal, distal, circumferential — the latter particularly critical for rectal cancer where positive CRM under 1 mm predicts local recurrence), serosal involvement and perforation, lymphovascular invasion, perineural invasion, tumour budding (graded by intensity), lymph node count and status, response to neoadjuvant therapy where applicable, and biomarker results (MMR for all cases; KRAS/NRAS/BRAF for metastatic; HER2 for metastatic per pathway). The synoptic block supports MDT presentation and registry submission.

11.8 Rectal cancer and neoadjuvant therapy

Rectal cancer occupies a special place in the colorectal staging framework — the surgical pathway differs (total mesorectal excision, TME, often preceded by neoadjuvant chemoradiotherapy or short-course radiotherapy). Pathological assessment of the TME specimen records the completeness of the mesorectal resection plane (Quirke grading: good/Quirke 3, moderate/Quirke 2, poor/Quirke 1). The circumferential resection margin (CRM) is measured in millimetres from the deepest invasive front to the inked radial margin — CRM positive (1 mm or less) is the strongest predictor of local recurrence.

Tumour regression grading after neoadjuvant therapy uses the modified Ryan / CAP four-tier system in current UK practice: 0 (complete response, no viable tumour), 1 (near-complete, single cells or small groups), 2 (residual tumour with stromal response), 3 (extensive residual tumour, minimal response). Complete pathological response (ypT0 ypN0) is achieved in 15-25 per cent of patients after standard neoadjuvant chemoradiotherapy and has good long-term outcomes; the 'watch and wait' strategy — offering radiological surveillance instead of resection to clinical complete responders — is now an established option in many centres.

11.9 Anal pathology

The anal canal extends from the dentate (pectinate) line proximally to the anal verge distally, with a transition zone between columnar rectal epithelium proximal to the dentate line and squamous epithelium distally. The histology of the transition zone may show a mixed pattern of columnar, transitional, and squamous epithelium. The anal pathology syllabus is dominated by HPV-associated squamous neoplasia — anal intraepithelial neoplasia (AIN) graded into low-grade (AIN1, condylomatous change) and high-grade (AIN2 and AIN3, the latter sometimes called severe dysplasia or squamous carcinoma in situ), and anal squamous cell carcinoma. The vast majority (over 90 per cent) of anal squamous carcinomas are HPV-associated, with HPV16 as the dominant subtype. Risk groups include immunocompromised patients (HIV-positive, transplant recipients) and men who have sex with men.

Other anal entities include perianal Paget disease — intraepithelial adenocarcinoma (extramammary Paget) with characteristic large pale tumour cells, mucinous cytoplasm, CK7 positive, CK20 negative for primary perianal Paget; CK7+/CK20+ pattern raises the possibility of secondary involvement from underlying GI tumour. Perianal Bowen disease (anal squamous carcinoma in situ on perianal skin), basal cell carcinoma of the perianal skin, melanoma (rare but with characteristic poor prognosis), anorectal lymphoma, and fistulae and abscesses (frequently associated with Crohn's disease) complete the syllabus.

11.10 Reporting and integration

Colorectal cancer reports follow the RCPath dataset with structured synoptic block. The reporting MDT includes the named surgeon, oncologist, radiologist, and pathologist, with dataset items presented systematically. Treatment-relevant findings include MMR status (for immunotherapy eligibility), molecular profile (KRAS, NRAS, BRAF for metastatic anti-EGFR decisions), tumour budding intensity, and CRM status for rectal cancers. Anal cancer reports follow parallel structure with anatomical specifics (distance from anal verge, dentate line position) and HPV-related findings.

11.11 Key points

Chapter 11 — key points

Adenomas: Tubular, tubulovillous, villous; conventional vs serrated lineage. SSL with cytological dysplasia → urgent endoscopic clearance.

CRC reporting: Site, type, grade, size, TNM 8, lymphovascular and perineural invasion, margins (proximal, distal, circumferential), tumour budding, regression score post-neoadjuvant.

Lymph node yield: ≥12 nodes for adequate staging; below threshold reported with reason.

MMR IHC and Lynch: Reflex on all newly diagnosed CRC (NICE). MLH1/PMS2 loss → BRAF V600E IHC or MLH1 methylation; MSH2/MSH6 loss → clinical genetics.

Molecular: KRAS, NRAS, BRAF for metastatic disease; RAS-wildtype eligible for anti-EGFR; BRAF V600E predicts poor prognosis.

IBD-associated dysplasia: Flat or lesional; low- or high-grade. Two-consultant confirmation; chromoendoscopy-guided sampling.

Anal pathology: Anal SCC (HPV-driven, p16 block-positive); anal melanoma; anal Paget's (primary vs secondary).

11.12 Chapter SBAs

Q11.1. Distinction between ulcerative colitis and Crohn's colitis is the recurring diagnostic question on colonic biopsy. A 28-year-old man has multiple colonic biopsies. The terminal ileum shows aphthous ulcers overlying lymphoid aggregates and a single small non-caseating granuloma. The ascending colon shows patchy chronic inflammation with skip lesions of normal mucosa. The rectum is histologically normal. Which single diagnosis is most consistent?

A. Ulcerative colitis affecting the right colon.

B. Crohn's colitis with ileal involvement.

C. Infectious colitis.

D. Microscopic colitis.

E. Diverticular colitis.

Answer: B

The combination of patchy skip lesions with intervening normal mucosa, rectal sparing, terminal ileal involvement with aphthous ulcers over lymphoid aggregates, and a non-caseating granuloma is characteristic of Crohn's colitis. Ulcerative colitis is characteristically continuous from the rectum, mucosal and submucosal in depth (not transmural), and granuloma-free except for cryptolytic granulomas at sites of ruptured crypts. The terminal ileal involvement in Crohn's is true ileal disease, whereas backwash ileitis (rare in UC) involves a short segment of distal ileum due to incompetent ileocaecal valve in pancolitis.

Option A is incorrect because UC is characteristically continuous from the rectum; the described rectal sparing excludes it. Option C (infectious colitis) typically shows preserved crypt architecture with neutrophilic infiltration and would not produce granulomas. Option D (microscopic colitis) shows normal endoscopic appearance with specific histological patterns (lymphocytic or collagenous) that the described biopsies do not match. Option E (diverticular colitis) is segmental disease related to diverticulae and does not fit the distribution described.

Q11.2. MMR IHC pattern interpretation drives Lynch syndrome triage in colorectal cancer. A 50-year-old man has a right-sided colonic adenocarcinoma with MMR IHC showing loss of MLH1 and PMS2 and retained MSH2 and MSH6. BRAF V600E IHC (VE1 clone) is negative. Which single next test is the most appropriate?

A. Repeat MMR IHC on a different block.

B. Refer directly to clinical genetics for Lynch syndrome assessment.

C. MLH1 promoter methylation analysis.

D. Whole-genome sequencing of the tumour.

E. Microsatellite instability testing on a different platform.

Answer: C

The MMR IHC pattern (paired MLH1 and PMS2 loss) is the commonest pattern and most often reflects sporadic disease driven by MLH1 promoter hypermethylation. BRAF V600E mutation is the first triage test — when present, it strongly supports sporadic disease and reduces the priority of genetics referral. When BRAF V600E is absent (as in this case), the next discriminator between sporadic and germline disease is direct MLH1 promoter methylation analysis. A methylated promoter supports sporadic disease; an unmethylated promoter strongly supports germline MLH1 mutation and triggers clinical genetics referral for confirmatory germline testing. The two-step algorithm (BRAF first, then methylation if BRAF wild-type) is widely encoded in national guidance.

Option A is unnecessary — the IHC pattern is clear. Option B is the action that follows an unmethylated promoter result; it is premature here. Option D is disproportionate at this stage. Option E does not discriminate sporadic from germline disease.

Q11.3. Circumferential resection margin (CRM) status is the strongest predictor of local recurrence in rectal cancer. A total mesorectal excision specimen shows an invasive adenocarcinoma extending through the muscularis propria into the perirectal fat. The deepest invasive front is 0.8 mm from the inked radial margin. Quirke grading of the mesorectal resection plane is good. Which single statement best describes the CRM status and the prognostic implication?

A. CRM negative; expected low local recurrence rate.

B. CRM positive (≤1 mm); strongest predictor of local recurrence.

C. CRM cannot be assessed; specimen inadequate.

D. CRM positive but Quirke 3 grading mitigates the prognostic implication.

E. CRM status is not relevant for rectal cancer.

Answer: B

The circumferential resection margin (CRM) is the radial margin of a rectal cancer resection — the closest distance from the deepest invasive tumour front to the inked surface of the mesorectum or perirectal fat. CRM positive is defined as 1 mm or less in the RCPath and ICCR datasets. A CRM of 0.8 mm therefore meets the positive threshold. CRM positivity is the single strongest pathological predictor of local recurrence in rectal cancer, with relative risk multiple-fold higher than CRM-negative cases. Good Quirke grading (Quirke 3) indicates that the surgeon achieved the optimal anatomical resection plane and does not mitigate the prognostic impact of CRM positivity once that margin is reached.

Option A is incorrect because 0.8 mm is below the 1 mm threshold. Option C is incorrect — the assessment has been made. Option D incorrectly suggests Quirke grade mitigates CRM impact. Option E is incorrect — CRM is the central reporting item for rectal cancer.

11.13 Chapter EMQ

EMQ 11.1. Colorectal and anal pathology. For each scenario, select the single most appropriate diagnosis from the option list. Each option may be used once, more than once, or not at all.

A. Ulcerative colitis

B. Crohn's colitis

C. Pseudomembranous colitis

D. Lymphocytic colitis

E. Collagenous colitis

F. Tubular adenoma with low-grade dysplasia

G. Sessile serrated lesion

H. Colorectal adenocarcinoma (MMR-deficient)

I. Anal intraepithelial neoplasia (AIN 3)

J. Perianal Paget disease (primary)

(1) A 35-year-old woman has continuous mucosal inflammation extending from the rectum to the splenic flexure. Crypt distortion with crypt dropout and basal plasmacytosis are prominent. No granulomas are present. The terminal ileum is histologically normal. **Answer: A**

(2) A 65-year-old woman with watery diarrhoea has colonic biopsies with normal endoscopic appearance. Histology shows intraepithelial lymphocytosis exceeding 25 per 100 surface enterocytes with chronic lamina propria inflammation. The crypt architecture is intact. **Answer: D**

(3) A 78-year-old man has a 4 cm flat lesion in the ascending colon. Histology shows serrated architecture extending to the crypt base with boot-shaped basal crypts, lateral spread along the muscularis mucosae, and no dysplasia. **Answer: G**

(4) A 45-year-old patient has a right-sided colonic adenocarcinoma. MMR IHC shows loss of MLH1 and PMS2. BRAF V600E is positive. MLH1 promoter is hypermethylated. **Answer: H**

(5) A 50-year-old HIV-positive man has perianal biopsies showing full-thickness squamous dysplasia with loss of polarity. p16 immunohistochemistry is diffusely positive. **Answer: I**

Chapter 12 — Liver

Liver pathology occupies a large fraction of histopathology workload across both biopsy and resection material. The needle biopsy covers a wide differential — viral hepatitis, autoimmune hepatitis, fatty liver disease, drug-induced liver injury, cholestatic disease, vascular pathology, storage disorders, and transplant pathology. The resection specimen brings hepatocellular adenoma, hepatocellular carcinoma, intrahepatic cholangiocarcinoma, and metastatic disease. The FRCPath Part 1 candidate is expected to interpret the patterns of hepatic injury, recognise the principal entities, and apply the staging frameworks and ancillary techniques that drive diagnosis and management. This chapter sets out the syllabus against the WHO 5th edition classification and current UK reporting standards.

12.1 Normal hepatic architecture

The liver is organised into hepatic lobules — hexagonal arrangements of hepatocyte cords radiating from the central vein toward portal tracts at the periphery. Portal tracts contain three structures (the portal triad): a branch of the portal vein, a branch of the hepatic artery, and an interlobular bile duct. The hepatocytes are organised in plates one to two cells thick, separated by sinusoids lined by fenestrated endothelium and Kupffer cells. The space of Disse, between the sinusoidal endothelium and the hepatocytes, contains hepatic stellate cells (Ito cells) — the principal source of collagen in fibrosis. Reticulin fibres form the framework — reticulin stain demonstrates the orderly cell-plate architecture, and disruption is a key feature of malignancy and regenerative nodules.

Functional zonation divides each acinus into three zones based on distance from the portal tract and exposure to oxygen and nutrients. Zone 1 (periportal, closest to the portal tract) is most exposed to oxygen and toxins; zone 3 (centrilobular, around the central vein) is the most metabolically active and most vulnerable to ischaemic and toxic injury. The zonation determines the distribution of many hepatic injuries — paracetamol toxicity is centrilobular (zone 3) because of CYP450 metabolism; passive congestion is centrilobular; viral hepatitis affects all zones; alcoholic hepatitis is typically centrilobular; haemochromatosis deposits iron periportally first; copper deposition in Wilson's disease is periportal.

12.2 Acute hepatitis

Acute hepatitis on biopsy shows lobular inflammation with hepatocyte ballooning, apoptosis (acidophil bodies — round eosinophilic structures derived from apoptotic hepatocytes), spotty necrosis, and a portal lymphocytic infiltrate. The pattern is shared across viral, autoimmune, drug-induced, and ischaemic causes — the clinical context, serology, and drug history drive the differential. Hepatitis A and E classically produce predominantly portal inflammation with plasma cells. Hepatitis B can present with characteristic 'ground-glass' hepatocytes (chronic carrier state — HBsAg-positive cells with finely granular eosinophilic cytoplasm). Hepatitis C acute infection is often subclinical; the chronic form is more often biopsied.

Drug-induced liver injury (DILI) accounts for a large proportion of acute hepatitis presentations. The pattern is variable — hepatocellular (resembling viral hepatitis), cholestatic (canalicular cholestasis without significant inflammation), mixed, granulomatous (a defined set of drugs including allopurinol, sulphonamides, methyldopa), and microvesicular steatosis (tetracycline, valproate, NRTI antiretrovirals). The clinical history of recent drug exposure and the exclusion of viral aetiology by serology are the principal diagnostic tools.

12.3 Chronic hepatitis

Chronic hepatitis is defined by persistent hepatic inflammation lasting more than six months. The histological pattern shows portal lymphocytic infiltration, with the inflammatory activity assessed by the extent of interface hepatitis (the spillover of lymphocytes from the portal tract into the adjacent lobular parenchyma, with hepatocyte damage at the interface). Fibrosis develops over time and is staged separately from the inflammatory grade. Two grading and staging systems are widely used — the Ishak system (more granular, with 18-point grading and 6-point staging) and the METAVIR system (simpler four-point grading and four-point staging, predominantly used for hepatitis C). The candidate should know the principle of separately reporting grade (inflammation) and stage (fibrosis), and the four-point METAVIR system in common use.

Hepatitis B and C

Chronic hepatitis B is identified by HBsAg and HBcAg immunohistochemistry on biopsy — ground-glass hepatocytes (HBsAg-positive) reflect chronic carriage; HBcAg expression in nuclei (with cytoplasmic spillover) indicates active viral replication. Hepatitis B antiviral therapy (tenofovir, entecavir) is the standard of care for actively replicating disease. Hepatitis C virus infection is the commonest indication for liver transplantation in many Western countries until the advent of direct-acting antiviral therapy (DAAs) — sustained virological response rates above 95 per cent with current 8 to 12 week DAA regimens have transformed the disease landscape and reduced new HCC incidence.

Autoimmune hepatitis

Autoimmune hepatitis (AIH) classically shows portal and interface inflammation with prominent plasma cell infiltrate, lobular hepatitis, and rosette formation of hepatocytes. Anti-nuclear antibodies (ANA), anti-smooth muscle antibodies (SMA), anti-soluble liver antigen (SLA), anti-liver-kidney microsomal antibody (LKM), and elevated serum IgG support the diagnosis in the clinical context. The simplified IAIHG diagnostic criteria integrate histological features with serological and biochemical findings. Treatment with corticosteroids and azathioprine produces remission in most cases; flares on treatment withdrawal are characteristic, and many patients require lifelong therapy.

12.4 Fatty liver disease

Metabolic dysfunction-associated steatotic liver disease (MASLD) — the renamed entity formerly called non-alcoholic fatty liver disease (NAFLD) — is now the commonest cause of chronic liver disease in many Western populations, driven by obesity, type 2 diabetes, and metabolic syndrome. The histological spectrum runs from simple steatosis (macrovesicular fat in over 5 per cent of hepatocytes, predominantly centrilobular) through metabolic dysfunction-associated steatohepatitis (MASH, formerly NASH) — adding hepatocyte ballooning, lobular inflammation, and Mallory-Denk bodies — to fibrosis (perisinusoidal or 'chicken-wire' pattern characteristically zone 3) and ultimately cirrhosis. The NAS (NAFLD activity score) grades steatosis, lobular inflammation, and ballooning each on defined scales, with fibrosis staged separately on a 5-point scale (F0 to F4 cirrhosis).

Alcoholic liver disease produces a histologically similar pattern — steatosis, steatohepatitis (with neutrophilic infiltration more prominent than in MASH), Mallory-Denk bodies, pericellular fibrosis, and cirrhosis. The histological distinction between alcoholic and metabolic steatohepatitis is unreliable on biopsy alone, and the clinical context (alcohol consumption, metabolic syndrome features) drives interpretation. Some published systems integrate the two under the umbrella term 'metabolic dysfunction and alcohol-associated steatotic liver disease' (MetALD) when both factors contribute.

12.5 Cirrhosis

Cirrhosis is the end-stage architectural disorganisation of the liver, characterised by diffuse fibrosis with parenchymal regeneration into nodules separated by fibrous septa. The macroscopic appearance is divided into micronodular (nodules under 3 mm — typical of alcoholic liver disease) and macronodular (nodules over 3 mm — typical of post-viral and post-necrotic cirrhosis), with mixed patterns common. The histology shows variable nodule size, broad fibrous septa with chronic inflammation, distorted vascular architecture, and the underlying aetiology may be inferred from specific features — iron deposition (haemochromatosis), copper accumulation (Wilson's disease), characteristic granulomas (primary biliary cholangitis), bile duct injury (sclerosing cholangitis).

Cirrhosis — common aetiologies and clues

Alcohol: micronodular, Mallory bodies, neutrophilic steatohepatitis, pericellular fibrosis.

MASLD/MASH: steatosis, ballooning, chicken-wire fibrosis, metabolic clinical context.

HBV: ground-glass hepatocytes, HBsAg/HBcAg IHC positive.

HCV: interface hepatitis, portal lymphoid aggregates, steatosis (especially genotype 3).

AIH: plasma cell-rich interface hepatitis, rosettes, ANA/SMA serology.

PBC: florid duct lesion, ductopenia, AMA serology.

PSC: onion-skin periductal fibrosis, MRCP beaded appearance.

Haemochromatosis: periportal iron in hepatocytes (Perls stain), HFE mutation.

Wilson's: periportal copper (rhodanine), ATP7B mutation, low caeruloplasmin.

12.6 Storage and metabolic disease

Hereditary haemochromatosis is the autosomal recessive iron storage disease driven by HFE gene mutation (most commonly C282Y homozygosity). The histology shows iron deposition primarily in hepatocytes — staining with Perls Prussian blue — initially periportal and extending across the lobule with progression. Hepatocellular iron predominates over Kupffer cell iron — the reverse pattern (Kupffer cell iron predominant) suggests secondary iron overload from transfusions or haemolysis. Hepatic iron index (iron concentration per gram dry weight divided by patient age) supports the diagnosis biochemically.

Wilson's disease is the autosomal recessive copper transport defect driven by ATP7B mutation. The histology is variable — fatty change, hepatitis pattern, cirrhosis — and copper deposition is demonstrated by rhodanine or orcein staining, although staining is often patchy and falsely negative. Quantitative hepatic copper estimation on dry tissue (over 250 micrograms per gram dry weight) is more reliable. Low serum caeruloplasmin and elevated urinary copper support the diagnosis biochemically, with confirmatory genetic testing. Alpha-1 antitrypsin deficiency shows characteristic PAS-positive diastase-resistant globules in periportal hepatocytes, with the PiZZ phenotype most commonly producing clinical disease.

12.7 Cholestatic liver disease

Primary biliary cholangitis (PBC, formerly primary biliary cirrhosis) is the autoimmune cholestatic disease of small intrahepatic bile ducts. The histology shows the florid duct lesion — granulomatous destruction of small interlobular bile ducts, with portal lymphocytic and plasma cell infiltrate, periductal granulomas, and progressive ductopenia. Bile duct injury progresses to ductopenia, with secondary biliary cirrhosis and copper deposition in periportal hepatocytes. Anti-mitochondrial antibody (AMA) is the serological hallmark. Ursodeoxycholic acid is the first-line therapy.

Primary sclerosing cholangitis (PSC) is the cholestatic disease of medium and large intrahepatic and extrahepatic bile ducts. The histology shows characteristic onion-skin periductal fibrosis around interlobular bile ducts, with chronic inflammation and progressive ductopenia. The disease is strongly associated with inflammatory bowel disease (around 80 per cent of PSC patients have IBD, predominantly UC). PSC carries elevated risks of cholangiocarcinoma (annual incidence around 1.5 per cent) and colorectal cancer in the IBD-affected cohort. Endoscopic surveillance is offered for both complications.

12.8 Hepatocellular adenoma

Hepatocellular adenomas (HCAs) are uncommon benign tumours predominantly affecting young women on oral contraceptive use. The contemporary molecular classification recognises four subtypes with distinct morphology and clinical behaviour. HNF1A-inactivated HCA (around 35 per cent) shows steatotic morphology, loss of liver fatty acid binding protein (LFABP) on IHC, and benign behaviour. Inflammatory HCA (around 40 per cent) shows inflammatory infiltrate, sinusoidal dilatation, ductular reaction, and positive serum amyloid A (SAA) or C-reactive protein (CRP) IHC; these often carry STAT3-activating mutations or IL6ST mutations. Beta-catenin-mutated HCA (around 10 per cent) shows nuclear beta-catenin positivity and diffuse glutamine synthetase staining; these are associated with elevated HCC progression risk and are typically resected. Unclassified HCA (remainder) lacks specific markers. Telangiectatic HCA is now classified as a variant of inflammatory

HCA. The candidate should know the four subtypes, the characteristic IHC, and the differing management implications.

12.9 Hepatocellular carcinoma

Hepatocellular carcinoma (HCC) is the dominant primary liver malignancy and the third commonest cause of cancer death globally. Most HCC arises on a background of cirrhosis from chronic hepatitis B, hepatitis C, MASH, or alcoholic liver disease. The morphology is variable — trabecular (most common, with thickened liver-cell plates), pseudoacinar, solid, scirrhous, fibrolamellar (a distinct entity in young patients without cirrhosis, characterised by oncocytic eosinophilic cells with prominent fibrous lamellae and DNAJB1-PRKACA fusion), and mixed hepatocellular-cholangiocarcinoma. Grading uses the WHO 5th edition four-tier system based on nuclear features and cytoplasmic differentiation. Reticulin loss (demonstrated on reticulin stain) is the architectural feature distinguishing HCC from adenoma and from regenerative nodules. Specific IHC panels (HepPar-1, arginase-1, glypican-3, AFP) support the diagnosis when morphology is equivocal.

HCC staging and management follow the BCLC (Barcelona Clinic Liver Cancer) framework integrating tumour stage with liver function (Child-Pugh) and performance status. Small HCC (under 2 cm) on cirrhosis is managed by ablation or transplantation; intermediate-stage disease by transarterial chemoembolisation or selective internal radiotherapy; advanced disease by systemic therapy (atezolizumab plus bevacizumab is now first-line; sorafenib and lenvatinib as alternatives). Pathological staging follows AJCC 8 with T categories based on tumour number, size, and vascular invasion. PD-L1 testing is emerging in selected systemic therapy decisions.

12.10 Intrahepatic cholangiocarcinoma and other tumours

Intrahepatic cholangiocarcinoma (iCCA) is the second commonest primary liver malignancy. The histology shows variable glandular architecture with mucin production, infiltrative growth pattern, and dense desmoplastic stromal reaction. The molecular landscape is increasingly characterised — FGFR2 fusions (around 15 per cent of iCCA, with FGFR inhibitors as approved therapy), IDH1 and IDH2 mutations (around 20 per cent, with ivosidenib for IDH1-mutant disease), BAP1 mutations, KRAS, BRAF, and HER2 amplification. Routine molecular profiling is now standard for advanced iCCA. IHC panel for diagnosis includes CK7, CK19 (both positive in iCCA), HepPar-1 (negative), arginase-1 (negative), and a variety of organ-of-origin markers when metastasis is considered.

Hepatoblastoma is the commonest paediatric primary liver tumour, occurring in children under 5 years. The WHO 5th edition recognises epithelial (fetal, embryonal, macrotrabecular, small cell undifferentiated), mixed epithelial and mesenchymal, and teratoid subtypes. Beta-catenin mutations (CTNNB1) drive most cases. Treatment combines chemotherapy and surgery with excellent long-term survival in most stages. Metastatic disease to the liver is the most common malignancy encountered overall — colorectal (the dominant source, with CDX2 and CK20 positivity), pancreaticobiliary, breast, gastric, lung, and melanoma frequently involve the liver, and the IHC panel for liver mass biopsy supports primary tumour identification when the morphological features are equivocal.

12.11 Liver transplantation pathology

Liver transplant biopsies address recurrent disease, rejection, and other complications. Acute T-cell-mediated rejection shows the diagnostic triad of mixed portal inflammation, bile duct injury (lymphocytic cholangitis), and endothelialitis (lymphocytes adherent to and beneath the endothelium of portal and central veins) — assessed using the Banff schema with a Rejection Activity Index (RAI) for severity. Antibody-mediated rejection is recognised by C4d deposition in microvasculature, donor-specific antibody (DSA) detection, and characteristic morphological features. Chronic rejection shows ductopenia (loss of more than 50 per cent of interlobular bile ducts) with foam cell arteriopathy in larger vessels. Recurrent viral hepatitis, recurrent autoimmune disease, recurrent PSC, and recurrent HCC are the principal recurrent diseases. Drug-induced injury from immunosuppressives is a regular consideration.

12.12 Reporting and key points

Liver biopsy reports follow structured templates with separate grade and stage assessment in chronic hepatitis, semiquantitative iron and copper assessment with appropriate staining, and explicit comment on the architecture of the specimen — needle biopsy adequacy is defined by at least 6 to 11 portal tracts and length 1.5 to 2 cm. Resection specimens follow the RCPath HCC, iCCA, and metastasis datasets with structured synoptic reporting including margin status, vascular invasion, lymph node involvement (where present), and biomarker results.

Chapter 12 — key points

Medical liver panel: Masson trichrome (fibrosis), reticulin (architecture), PAS-D (alpha-1 antitrypsin), Perls (iron), orcein or Victoria blue (copper-associated, HBsAg).

Chronic hepatitis: Grade and stage (Ishak or METAVIR). Aetiology: viral, autoimmune, metabolic (MASH), drug-induced.

Steatohepatitis (MASH): Steatosis + ballooning + lobular inflammation ± Mallory-Denk bodies. NAS or SAF score for activity; fibrosis staged separately.

Autoimmune liver disease: AIH (plasma cells, interface hepatitis, rosettes); PBC (florid duct lesion, ductopenia); PSC (onion-skin periductal fibrosis, ducts may be absent in late disease).

Hepatocellular carcinoma: Trabecular thickening >2 cells, reticulin loss. Glypican-3, HSP70, glutamine synthetase triple positive supports HCC.

Cholangiocarcinoma: Intrahepatic (HCC mimic) vs perihilar (Klatskin) vs distal. CK7+/CK20± immunoprofile; molecular: FGFR2 fusions, IDH1/2.

Transplant biopsy: Banff schema; T-cell-mediated rejection (portal inflammation + cholangitis + endothelialitis); AMR (C4d, DSA); chronic rejection (ductopenia, foam cell arteriopathy).

12.13 Chapter SBAs

Q12.1. Hepatocellular adenomas are classified into molecular subtypes with distinct morphology, immunohistochemistry, and clinical behaviour. A 28-year-old woman on long-term oral contraceptive use has a 4 cm hepatic mass resected. The histology shows hepatocellular adenoma with diffuse glutamine synthetase positivity and nuclear beta-catenin staining. Which single statement best describes the implication of these findings?

A. HNF1A-inactivated adenoma — benign behaviour, no further intervention required.

B. Inflammatory adenoma — surveillance recommended.

C. Beta-catenin-mutated adenoma — elevated risk of progression to HCC; resection is generally indicated.

D. Unclassified adenoma — no specific implications.

E. Focal nodular hyperplasia — not a true neoplasm.

Answer: C

Nuclear beta-catenin staining and diffuse glutamine synthetase positivity define the beta-catenin-mutated subtype of hepatocellular adenoma. These tumours carry CTNNB1 (beta-catenin) activating mutations that drive WNT pathway signalling and confer an elevated risk of progression to hepatocellular carcinoma — published series suggest progression rates markedly higher than other HCA subtypes. Surgical resection is generally indicated for beta-catenin-mutated adenomas of any size, in contrast to other subtypes where size threshold and clinical context determine management. The four-subtype molecular classification (HNF1A-inactivated, inflammatory, beta-catenin-mutated, unclassified) is now standard in HCA reporting and informs management decisions.

Option A describes HNF1A-inactivated subtype, characterised by steatotic morphology and loss of LFABP; the IHC pattern described does not fit. Option B describes inflammatory subtype with SAA and CRP positivity, not the described findings. Option D underestimates the risk. Option E describes a different entity entirely — FNH shows central scar and characteristic mapping of glutamine synthetase but not nuclear beta-catenin.

Q12.2. Liver transplant biopsies often present the diagnostic question of acute T-cell-mediated rejection versus other complications. A liver transplant recipient is biopsied 10 days post-transplant for elevated liver enzymes. The biopsy shows mixed portal inflammation with lymphocytes, eosinophils, and plasma cells; lymphocytic injury of small interlobular bile ducts; and lymphocytes adherent to and beneath the endothelium of portal and central veins. Which single diagnosis is most likely?

A. Recurrent hepatitis C.

B. Acute T-cell-mediated rejection.

C. Antibody-mediated rejection.

D. Chronic rejection.

E. Drug-induced liver injury.

Answer: B

The diagnostic triad for acute T-cell-mediated rejection of liver allograft comprises mixed portal inflammation (lymphocytes, eosinophils, plasma cells), bile duct injury (lymphocytic cholangitis affecting small interlobular bile ducts with epithelial injury), and endothelialitis (lymphocytes adherent to and beneath the endothelium of portal and central veins). All three features are present in the described biopsy. The Banff schema grades the severity using the Rejection Activity Index (RAI), scoring each component on a 0-3 scale to produce a composite score that guides management (typically intensification of immunosuppression with bolus corticosteroids).

Option A (recurrent HCV) typically shows portal lymphoid aggregates with interface hepatitis, not the triad of features described. Option C (AMR) requires C4d deposition in microvasculature and donor-specific antibodies, with different morphological features. Option D (chronic rejection) shows ductopenia and foam cell arteriopathy rather than the described acute features. Option E (DILI) typically shows hepatocellular or cholestatic injury patterns without the endothelialitis described.

Q12.3. Pattern of iron deposition in the liver supports the differential between primary and secondary iron overload. A 50-year-old man has a liver biopsy showing extensive iron deposition. The iron is predominantly within hepatocytes, with periportal predominance early in the lobule and minimal Kupffer cell involvement. Which single statement best describes the most likely diagnosis?

A. Secondary iron overload from blood transfusions.

B. Hereditary haemochromatosis (HFE-associated).

C. Acute haemolytic anaemia.

D. African iron overload syndrome.

E. Iron deposition unrelated to systemic iron status.

Answer: B

Hereditary haemochromatosis is characterised by iron deposition predominantly in hepatocytes, with a periportal-to-centrilobular gradient (deposition starts periportally and extends with progression). Kupffer cell iron is typically minimal in early disease, with significant Kupffer cell involvement appearing only in advanced cases. The pattern is driven by the underlying HFE mutation (most commonly C282Y homozygosity) leading to increased intestinal iron absorption and hepatocellular accumulation. The hepatocellular-predominant pattern is the discriminator from secondary iron overload, in which Kupffer cell iron predominates because the iron arrives in macrophage form from extravascular haemolysis or transfusion-derived senescent red cells.

Option A typically shows Kupffer cell-predominant iron from transfusion source. Option C (acute haemolytic anaemia) produces Kupffer cell iron from haemoglobin breakdown rather than hepatocellular accumulation. Option D (African iron overload) has its own pattern with mixed hepatocellular and Kupffer cell involvement. Option E is unlikely given the described extensive iron deposition.

12.14 Chapter EMQ

EMQ 12.1. Liver pathology — diagnosis. For each scenario, select the single most appropriate diagnosis from the option list. Each option may be used once, more than once, or not at all.

A. Acute hepatitis A

B. Chronic hepatitis B

C. Chronic hepatitis C

D. Autoimmune hepatitis

E. Metabolic dysfunction-associated steatohepatitis (MASH)

F. Primary biliary cholangitis

G. Primary sclerosing cholangitis

H. Hereditary haemochromatosis

I. Hepatocellular carcinoma

J. Intrahepatic cholangiocarcinoma

(1) A 60-year-old woman with pruritus has a liver biopsy showing granulomatous destruction of small interlobular bile ducts with portal lymphoplasmacytic infiltrate and ductopenia. AMA is positive at 1:640. **Answer: F**

(2) A 30-year-old woman with elevated transaminases has a liver biopsy showing portal and interface inflammation with prominent plasma cell infiltrate, rosette formation, and lobular hepatitis. ANA and SMA are positive; IgG is elevated. **Answer: D**

(3) A 55-year-old man with ulcerative colitis has a liver biopsy showing periductal concentric onion-skin fibrosis around interlobular bile ducts with chronic inflammation and progressive ductopenia. **Answer: G**

(4) A 45-year-old patient on chronic HBV therapy has a liver biopsy. Hepatocytes show finely granular eosinophilic cytoplasm with ground-glass appearance. HBsAg immunohistochemistry is diffusely positive. **Answer: B**

(5) A 65-year-old man with metabolic syndrome has a liver biopsy showing macrovesicular steatosis in 40% of hepatocytes, centrilobular hepatocyte ballooning, lobular inflammation, and pericellular fibrosis in zone 3. **Answer: E**

Chapter 13 — Biliary tree and gallbladder

Biliary pathology spans the gallbladder and the extrahepatic and intrahepatic bile ducts, with a focused syllabus dominated by inflammatory disease, intraepithelial neoplasia, papillary tumours, and adenocarcinoma. Routine practice is built around the cholecystectomy specimen — gallstone disease and chronic cholecystitis being the dominant findings — supplemented by biliary resections (bile duct resection, Whipple procedure with bile duct sampling, segmental hepatic resection for hilar cholangiocarcinoma) and by biliary brushings and biopsies obtained at endoscopic retrograde cholangiography. The FRCPath Part 1 candidate is expected to know the principal inflammatory entities, the dysplasia-carcinoma sequence in the gallbladder, the WHO 5th edition classification of bile duct neoplasms, and the AJCC 8 staging conventions for both gallbladder and bile duct cancer.

13.1 Normal histology

The gallbladder wall comprises mucosa (a single layer of tall columnar epithelium overlying a delicate lamina propria), muscularis (smooth muscle without a distinct muscularis mucosae, a key anatomical difference from other tubular GI organs that drives staging), perimuscular connective tissue, and serosa (covering the peritoneal aspect; the hepatic-side wall is in direct contact with hepatic parenchyma without a serosal covering). The absence of a true muscularis mucosae has implications for invasion assessment — once tumour breaches the basement membrane it directly enters the lamina propria. Staging is based on depth into the muscle and beyond rather than mucosal versus submucosal as in stomach or colon.

The bile ducts are lined by simple cuboidal to columnar epithelium with mucinous goblet-like cells in larger ducts. Subepithelial periductal glands (Beale glands in the extrahepatic ducts; peribiliary glands in larger intrahepatic ducts) are mucous glands that contribute to physiological bile production and represent a recognised site for tumour origin. The fibroconnective wall of the bile duct contains smooth muscle bundles, particularly in the distal common bile duct and the ampulla of Vater. The ampullary region (the confluence of bile and pancreatic ducts at the duodenum) is a distinct anatomical and pathological site, covered separately under pancreatic and ampullary disease.

13.2 Cholecystitis

Acute cholecystitis follows obstruction of the cystic duct by a stone (calculous cholecystitis, the dominant form) or rarely without stones (acalculous cholecystitis, seen in critically-ill patients). The histology shows acute neutrophilic inflammation with mucosal erosion or ulceration, oedema and haemorrhage of the wall, and serosal fibrinous exudate. Severe disease produces gangrenous changes (transmural haemorrhagic necrosis) or perforation. Acalculous cholecystitis is associated with critical illness, ICU stay, and total parenteral nutrition; the morphology resembles calculous acute cholecystitis but without an identifiable obstructing stone.

Chronic cholecystitis is the commonest finding in cholecystectomy specimens, reflecting longstanding intermittent obstruction or chronic irritation by stones. The histology shows mucosal atrophy with reduced epithelial height, lymphocytic and plasma cell infiltrate in the lamina propria, muscular hypertrophy, and Rokitansky-Aschoff sinuses (mucosal outpouchings through the muscularis caused by repeated luminal pressure). Pyloric metaplasia (mucinous glands resembling antral mucosa) and intestinal metaplasia (with goblet cells and Paneth cell-like cells) develop with progression of chronic injury and represent precursor changes to dysplasia.

Xanthogranulomatous cholecystitis is a distinctive variant with mass-forming inflammation that can mimic gallbladder carcinoma macroscopically and clinically. The histology shows sheets of foamy macrophages (xanthoma cells) with fibrosis and chronic inflammation, often with cholesterol clefts and brown pigment. Recognition is important because the lesion is benign and the clinical and intraoperative appearance can prompt unnecessarily extensive surgery. Frozen-section examination is occasionally requested intraoperatively to distinguish the two entities.

13.3 Gallbladder dysplasia and intracholecystic papillary neoplasm

Dysplasia in the gallbladder arises on a background of chronic cholecystitis with metaplastic change. Low-grade dysplasia (BilIN-1 and BilIN-2 in some classifications, or simply low-grade) shows nuclear stratification confined to the basal half of the epithelium with preserved surface maturation. High-grade dysplasia (BilIN-3, formerly carcinoma in situ) shows full-thickness atypia, loss of polarity, architectural complexity, and is the immediate precursor to invasive adenocarcinoma. Flat (non-papillary) dysplasia is the common pattern in chronic cholecystitis; papillary dysplasia exists but is uncommon.

Intracholecystic papillary neoplasm (ICPN, WHO 5th edition) is the gallbladder counterpart of IPMN of the pancreas and IPNB of the bile duct — a polypoid or papillary intraluminal neoplasm with variable cytological grade. ICPN is subdivided by histological type (intestinal, gastric foveolar, pyloric, biliary) and by grade (low-grade, high-grade). Invasive carcinoma may arise within ICPN, and the proportion of the lesion that is invasive versus in-situ informs staging and prognosis. Recognition of ICPN at cholecystectomy carries a different prognostic implication from flat dysplasia or in-situ carcinoma — the disease has a recognised better prognosis for the in-situ component, although the invasive component when present follows standard adenocarcinoma staging.

Gallbladder precursor lesions at a glance

Pyloric metaplasia: antral-type mucinous glands; chronic inflammation marker.

Intestinal metaplasia: goblet cells, Paneth-like cells; further chronic injury.

BilIN-1/2 (low-grade dysplasia): basal nuclear stratification, preserved surface.

BilIN-3 (high-grade dysplasia): full-thickness atypia, immediate precursor of invasive carcinoma.

ICPN: papillary intraluminal neoplasm; intestinal/gastric/pyloric/biliary types; variable grade.

Adenoma: polypoid lesion with low or high-grade dysplasia, less common pathway.

13.4 Gallbladder polyps

Cholesterol polyps are the commonest gallbladder polyp, identified incidentally on imaging or at cholecystectomy. They are pseudopolyps composed of foamy histiocytes containing cholesterol within the lamina propria, with no neoplastic component — these are reactive changes secondary to cholesterolosis. Cholesterolosis (strawberry gallbladder) — when present diffusely — shows yellow flecks of cholesterol-laden macrophages in the gallbladder mucosa on macroscopic examination. The findings are clinically inconsequential and carry no cancer risk.

Adenomatous polyps are true neoplasms, less common than cholesterol polyps and carrying low-grade or high-grade dysplasia. They are classified by histological type — intestinal-type adenomas (resembling colorectal adenomas), pyloric-gland adenomas (with compact pyloric-type glands), and biliary-type adenomas. Polyps over 1 cm or with growth on serial imaging carry sufficient cancer risk to warrant cholecystectomy. Hyalinising cholecystitis with calcification of the wall ('porcelain gallbladder') is recognised as carrying a small elevated cancer risk historically and is generally an indication for cholecystectomy, although the magnitude of the risk is now considered lower than originally feared.

13.5 Gallbladder carcinoma

Gallbladder adenocarcinoma is the commonest biliary tract malignancy. Risk factors include longstanding cholelithiasis, chronic cholecystitis with metaplasia and dysplasia, ICPN, porcelain gallbladder, primary sclerosing cholangitis, anomalous pancreaticobiliary junction, and certain geographical/ethnic clusters (parts of South America and South Asia). The histology shows variable patterns — typical adenocarcinoma (tubular, papillary, mucinous), adenosquamous carcinoma, squamous cell carcinoma, undifferentiated carcinoma, neuroendocrine carcinoma. Incidental gallbladder cancer (discovered post-cholecystectomy for presumed benign disease) accounts for a large fraction of cases in regions with high cholecystectomy volume.

AJCC 8 staging records T (Tis; T1a — lamina propria; T1b — muscle layer; T2a peritoneal side / T2b hepatic side, both reflecting depth into perimuscular connective tissue with the location-specific distinction reflecting differing prognosis; T3 — through serosa or into hepatic parenchyma or adjacent organ; T4 — main portal vein or hepatic artery, or two or more extrahepatic organs/structures), N (number of involved regional nodes), and M. The peritoneal-side versus hepatic-side T2 distinction (T2a versus T2b) reflects the different anatomical relationship of these surfaces and is unique to gallbladder staging. The reporting follows the RCPath dataset with structured synoptic block.

13.6 Cholangiocarcinoma — extrahepatic

Extrahepatic cholangiocarcinoma comprises perihilar (Klatskin) tumours at the bifurcation of the right and left hepatic ducts (the commonest subtype, around 60 per cent of extrahepatic CCA), and distal cholangiocarcinoma in the distal common bile duct (around 20-30 per cent). The histology shows adenocarcinoma with variable architecture — well-differentiated tubular and papillary patterns in some, poorly differentiated infiltrative patterns in others. Dense desmoplastic stromal reaction is characteristic, and the tumour often shows perineural and lymphovascular invasion. Bismuth-Corlette classification subdivides perihilar tumours by the extent of involvement of the hepatic duct bifurcation (type I — below confluence, type II — at confluence, type IIIa/IIIb — extending into right or left hepatic duct, type IV — extending into both).

Molecular profiling is increasingly relevant. Hilar and distal cholangiocarcinoma overlap with pancreatic ductal adenocarcinoma in their molecular drivers (KRAS, TP53, SMAD4, CDKN2A mutations dominant). FGFR2 fusions, IDH1/2 mutations, and HER2 amplification are more common in intrahepatic disease but occur in extrahepatic cases as well, and routine molecular testing is becoming standard for advanced biliary tract cancer to inform targeted therapy selection. IHC for diagnosis includes CK7, CK19, MUC1, CDX2 (variable), and a panel for distinguishing primary biliary from metastatic disease.

13.7 Intraductal papillary neoplasms of the bile duct

Intraductal papillary neoplasm of the bile duct (IPNB, WHO 5th edition) is a papillary intraductal neoplasm with characteristic mucin production, ranging from low-grade through high-grade dysplasia to invasive adenocarcinoma. The lesion is the biliary counterpart of IPMN of the pancreas and shares similar morphological and behavioural features. Subtyping uses the same four histological categories — intestinal, gastric foveolar, pyloric, and biliary — with characteristic mucin profiles (MUC2 for intestinal, MUC5AC for gastric, MUC6 for pyloric, MUC1 for biliary). The lesion may produce voluminous mucin (mucobilia) leading to biliary obstruction. Surgical resection is the standard treatment, with prognosis depending on grade and the presence of invasive carcinoma. Biliary cystic neoplasms (mucinous cystic neoplasm of the bile duct, BCT/MCN-B) form a separate WHO 5th edition entity characterised by ovarian-type stroma — analogous to the pancreatic MCN.

13.8 Reporting and key points

Cholecystectomy specimens are sampled systematically — the gallbladder is opened longitudinally, examined for stones (which are described and weighed), the wall is sampled at fundus, body, and neck, and any mucosal lesion or thickening is sampled completely. The incidental gallbladder cancer discovered at routine cholecystectomy is the principal cause of difficult re-staging and decision-making about completion oncological resection — sampling discipline at the original specimen drives the accuracy of T-staging and margin assessment. Resection specimens for biliary tract cancer follow the RCPath dataset with structured synoptic reporting and including all key margin assessments (proximal hepatic duct, distal common bile duct, radial margins, hepatic parenchymal margin where applicable).

Chapter 13 — key points

Gallbladder cholecystitis: Acute (neutrophilic, transmural), chronic (Rokitansky-Aschoff sinuses, lymphoplasmacytic). Xanthogranulomatous mimics carcinoma macroscopically.

Gallbladder carcinoma: Often incidental in cholecystectomy. AJCC TNM 8 — pT1a confined to lamina propria; pT1b muscularis; pT2 perimuscular connective tissue without serosa.

Sampling: Open along the long axis; entire mucosa embedded if any thickening or polyp; cystic duct margin separately.

Primary sclerosing cholangitis: Onion-skin periductal fibrosis; ducts may be replaced by fibrous scar in late disease. Associated with IBD and elevated cholangiocarcinoma risk.

IgG4-related sclerosing cholangitis: Storiform fibrosis, obliterative phlebitis, IgG4+/IgG+ plasma cell ratio >40%; mimics cholangiocarcinoma clinically.

Choledochal cysts: Five Todani types; lifelong carcinoma risk; resection standard.

13.9 Chapter SBAs

Q13.1. Distinction between xanthogranulomatous cholecystitis and gallbladder carcinoma is critical because the management differs markedly. A 65-year-old man undergoes cholecystectomy for clinical suspicion of gallbladder mass on imaging. The macroscopic specimen shows wall thickening to 2 cm with yellow nodules. Histology reveals sheets of foamy macrophages with cholesterol clefts, brown pigment, and chronic inflammation, without atypical epithelial cells or invasion. Which single statement best characterises the diagnosis?

A. Xanthogranulomatous cholecystitis — benign inflammatory entity; no further surgery required.

B. Mucinous adenocarcinoma with extensive mucin extravasation.

C. Carcinoid tumour with stromal response.

D. Adenosquamous carcinoma in chronic cholecystitis.

E. Lymphoma of the gallbladder.

Answer: A

Xanthogranulomatous cholecystitis is a distinctive benign inflammatory variant with mass-forming wall thickening. The diagnostic features are sheets of foamy macrophages (xanthoma cells) with cholesterol clefts, brown pigment (haemosiderin and ceroid), and chronic inflammation, without atypical epithelial cells or invasive component. The macroscopic and clinical appearance can mimic carcinoma, prompting concern for malignancy at imaging and at the operating table — which is why frozen-section examination is occasionally requested. Recognition of the histology is important because the lesion is benign and does not require completion oncological surgery — cholecystectomy alone is sufficient. The clinical context (longstanding cholelithiasis, chronic biliary symptoms) supports the diagnosis.

Option B (mucinous adenocarcinoma) would show neoplastic glands and atypical epithelial cells producing mucin, absent in the described biopsy. Option C (carcinoid tumour) would show neuroendocrine cells with characteristic IHC. Option D would show malignant glandular and squamous components. Option E (lymphoma) would show neoplastic lymphoid cells with specific immunophenotype.

Q13.2. Anatomical position-specific staging is unique to gallbladder cancer in the AJCC 8 framework. A cholecystectomy specimen for incidental gallbladder cancer shows an adenocarcinoma invading through the muscle layer into perimuscular connective tissue. The deepest invasive front is on the peritoneal aspect of the gallbladder without involvement of the hepatic parenchymal interface. Which single T category is most appropriate under AJCC 8?

A. T1b — invasion limited to muscle layer.

B. T2a — invasion into perimuscular connective tissue on peritoneal side without serosal extension.

C. T2b — invasion into perimuscular connective tissue on hepatic side.

D. T3 — invasion through serosa.

E. T4 — invasion of main portal vein.

Answer: B

AJCC 8 staging for gallbladder cancer introduced a location-specific T2 subdivision based on whether the deepest invasive front is on the peritoneal side (T2a) or the hepatic side (T2b) of the gallbladder. The distinction reflects the different anatomical relationship — peritoneal-side tumours are covered by serosa, while hepatic-side tumours are in direct contact with hepatic parenchyma without an intervening serosal barrier — and correlates with markedly different prognosis (hepatic-side T2b cases have worse outcomes than peritoneal-side T2a). The described tumour invades into perimuscular connective tissue on the peritoneal aspect without serosal breach and is therefore T2a.

Option A is incorrect because invasion extends beyond the muscle. Option C describes the hepatic-side equivalent which the stem excludes. Option D requires breach of the serosa. Option E describes T4 disease with vascular invasion, not present in the stem.

Q13.3. Intracholecystic papillary neoplasm (ICPN) is the WHO 5th edition entity for papillary intraluminal gallbladder lesions, with variable invasive component. A 70-year-old woman has a cholecystectomy showing a polypoid intraluminal lesion with papillary architecture. Histology shows tall columnar epithelium with intestinal-type goblet cells and high-grade nuclear atypia, without identified invasive component on extensive sampling. Which single statement best describes the diagnosis and the implication?

A. Intestinal-type ICPN with high-grade dysplasia and no invasive component identified — better prognosis than flat in-situ disease.

B. Invasive adenocarcinoma — staged as T1a.

C. Flat high-grade dysplasia (BilIN-3) — equivalent prognosis to ICPN.

D. Cholesterol polyp — clinically inconsequential.

E. Mucinous cystic neoplasm of the gallbladder.

Answer: A

ICPN (intracholecystic papillary neoplasm) is the gallbladder counterpart of IPMN of the pancreas, characterised by a polypoid or papillary intraluminal growth pattern with variable cytological grade. The intestinal-type ICPN shows tall columnar epithelium with goblet cells, MUC2 positivity, and CDX2 positivity. ICPN with high-grade dysplasia and no invasive component carries a recognised better prognosis than flat in-situ disease (BilIN-3) — published series suggest five-year survival approaching 90 per cent for in-situ ICPN compared to lower figures for flat high-grade dysplasia. When invasive carcinoma arises within ICPN, the prognosis follows standard adenocarcinoma staging.

Option B is incorrect because no invasive component is identified. Option C is factually incorrect — ICPN has a better prognosis than flat in-situ disease. Option D would be a non-neoplastic pseudopolyp without dysplastic epithelium. Option E describes a different cystic entity with ovarian-type stroma, not applicable to the described lesion.

13.10 Chapter EMQ

EMQ 13.1. Biliary tract pathology. For each scenario, select the single most appropriate diagnosis from the option list. Each option may be used once, more than once, or not at all.

A. Acute calculous cholecystitis

B. Chronic cholecystitis with pyloric metaplasia

C. Xanthogranulomatous cholecystitis

D. Cholesterol polyp

E. Adenomatous polyp

F. Intracholecystic papillary neoplasm (ICPN)

G. Gallbladder adenocarcinoma

H. Perihilar (Klatskin) cholangiocarcinoma

I. Intraductal papillary neoplasm of bile duct (IPNB)

J. Mucinous cystic neoplasm of the bile duct

(1) A 55-year-old woman undergoes cholecystectomy for gallstone disease. The cholecystectomy shows a 4 mm yellow nodule on the gallbladder mucosa, with histology revealing foamy histiocytes containing cholesterol within the lamina propria; the epithelium is intact and unremarkable. **Answer: D**

(2) A 70-year-old patient undergoes hepatic resection for jaundice. The resection shows a sclerotic mass at the bifurcation of the right and left hepatic ducts (Bismuth type II). Histology reveals well-differentiated tubular adenocarcinoma with desmoplastic stroma and perineural invasion. **Answer: H**

(3) A 65-year-old man has a cholecystectomy. Macroscopically the gallbladder shows multiple 1 cm intraluminal polypoid lesions. Histology reveals papillary fronds lined by intestinal-type columnar epithelium with goblet cells, high-grade nuclear atypia, but no invasion. **Answer: F**

(4) A 75-year-old man undergoes liver resection for an intraductal mucinous lesion. The lesion arises within an intrahepatic bile duct and produces voluminous mucin with biliary obstruction. Histology shows papillary intraductal neoplasm with high-grade dysplasia, MUC5AC positive and MUC2 negative. **Answer: I**

(5) A 50-year-old patient undergoes cholecystectomy for clinically suspected carcinoma. Macroscopically the gallbladder shows wall thickening to 2 cm with yellow nodules. Histology shows sheets of foamy macrophages with cholesterol clefts, brown pigment, fibrosis, and chronic inflammation without atypical epithelial cells. **Answer: C**

Chapter 14 — Pancreas

Pancreatic pathology spans inflammatory disease, cystic neoplasms, ductal adenocarcinoma, neuroendocrine tumours, acinar cell carcinoma, and ampullary tumours, , with each entity driving distinct surgical and oncological management. The fine-needle aspirate from endoscopic ultrasound is the principal biopsy substrate for solid and cystic lesions, supplemented by core biopsy in selected cases. The resection specimens — pancreaticoduodenectomy (Whipple) for periampullary disease, distal pancreatectomy for body and tail lesions, total pancreatectomy for diffuse disease — carry the staging and reporting workload. The FRCPath Part 1 candidate is expected to know the principal entities, the WHO 5th edition classification, the molecular framework, and the AJCC 8 staging conventions for pancreatic and ampullary disease.

14.1 Normal histology

The pancreas comprises exocrine and endocrine compartments in defined anatomical relationship. The exocrine pancreas — approximately 95 per cent of the gland, consists of acini lined by pyramidal cells with abundant apical eosinophilic zymogen granules and basally-located basophilic cytoplasm rich in rough endoplasmic reticulum. The acini drain into a branching duct system — intercalated ducts, intralobular ducts, interlobular ducts, and the main pancreatic duct — lined by cuboidal to columnar epithelium with progressive size increase toward the main duct. The endocrine pancreas comprises the islets of Langerhans — scattered nests of endocrine cells (beta cells producing insulin, alpha cells producing glucagon, delta cells producing somatostatin, PP cells producing pancreatic polypeptide) distributed throughout the gland with regional variation in cell composition.

14.2 Pancreatitis

Acute pancreatitis presents with sudden severe epigastric pain and elevated serum lipase or amylase. The histological hallmark in fatal cases is acinar necrosis with surrounding inflammation, fat necrosis with saponification of pancreatic and peripancreatic adipose tissue, haemorrhage, and vascular thrombosis. The aetiology is dominated by gallstone disease (around 40 per cent) and alcohol (around 30 per cent), with other causes including hypertriglyceridaemia, drugs, autoimmune disease, infection (mumps, Coxsackie), iatrogenic post-ERCP, anatomical variants (pancreas divisum), and idiopathic. Severity grading by the Atlanta classification (revised 2012) integrates clinical and radiological findings with the presence of necrosis and organ failure.

Chronic pancreatitis shows progressive parenchymal atrophy with replacement by fibrosis, ductal dilatation with intraductal calcifications and protein plugs, lobular atrophy with preserved islets (the islets are characteristically the last component to be lost), chronic inflammation, and variable neural prominence and perineural inflammation. Aetiologies include chronic alcohol use (the dominant cause in Western populations), genetic disorders (PRSS1, SPINK1, CFTR mutations in hereditary pancreatitis), tropical pancreatitis (in regions of South and Southeast Asia), and autoimmune pancreatitis.

Autoimmune pancreatitis is sub-classified into type 1 (IgG4-related disease — part of the systemic IgG4-related spectrum) and type 2 (idiopathic duct-centric, associated with inflammatory bowel disease). Type 1 shows lymphoplasmacytic sclerosing pancreatitis with IgG4-positive plasma cells (over 10 per high-power field), storiform fibrosis, and obliterative phlebitis, often with elevated serum IgG4. Type 2 shows granulocytic epithelial lesions in ducts and is more often resectable as a focal mass mimicking carcinoma. Recognition is important because the disease responds dramatically to corticosteroids in contrast to malignancy.

14.3 Cystic neoplasms

Pancreatic cysts span a wide spectrum from non-neoplastic pseudocysts (post-pancreatitis collections lined by inflammatory tissue, not true epithelium) through serous cystadenomas to true mucinous neoplasms with malignant potential. The diagnostic question on EUS-FNA cytology and cyst fluid analysis is the distinction between mucinous and non-mucinous cysts because mucinous cysts (MCN and IPMN) carry malignant potential warranting consideration of resection.

Serous cystadenoma

Serous cystadenoma is a benign neoplasm composed of multiple small cysts (microcystic pattern, often with a central stellate scar on imaging) lined by cuboidal epithelium with clear cytoplasm (glycogen-rich, PAS-positive diastase-sensitive). The lesions occur most commonly in older women in the pancreatic body or tail and have negligible malignant potential. Recognition is important because mistaken classification as a mucinous lesion leads to unnecessary surgery in benign disease.

Mucinous cystic neoplasm

Mucinous cystic neoplasm (MCN) is a true neoplasm with characteristic ovarian-type stroma — the feature that defines the entity. MCN occurs almost exclusively in women (typically 40-50 years old) in the pancreatic body or tail. The cyst is lined by tall columnar mucinous epithelium with variable cytological grade (low-grade, high-grade, invasive). The ovarian-type stroma — composed of spindle cells with elongated nuclei resembling ovarian cortex, ER and PR positive on IHC, sometimes with luteinised cells — supports the diagnosis and distinguishes MCN from other mucinous cystic lesions. The natural history shows risk of progression to invasive carcinoma, supporting resection.

Intraductal papillary mucinous neoplasm

Intraductal papillary mucinous neoplasm (IPMN) arises within the pancreatic ductal system and is classified by anatomical involvement into main-duct, branch-duct, and mixed types. Main-duct IPMN carries higher malignant potential than branch-duct disease. Histological subtypes (paralleling the gallbladder and bile duct papillary neoplasms) include intestinal (MUC2 positive, intestinal goblet cells, often main-duct), gastric foveolar (MUC5AC positive, usually branch-duct, lowest grade), pancreatobiliary (MUC1 positive, more aggressive), and oncocytic (formerly intraductal oncocytic papillary neoplasm, IOPN, now in WHO 5 as a separate entity but historically grouped with IPMN). Each subtype has characteristic mucin profile and behaviour. The Sendai and Fukuoka guidelines structure the imaging and biomarker pathway for IPMN management, with high-risk features driving consideration of resection.

Solid pseudopapillary neoplasm

Solid pseudopapillary neoplasm (SPN) is the rare pancreatic tumour of low malignant potential characterised by predominantly young women (typically 20-30 years old) and a characteristic morphological pattern. The tumour shows solid and pseudopapillary architecture with discohesive cells around fibrovascular cores (pseudopapillae form by degeneration of tumour cells), uniform monomorphic cells, abundant pale to eosinophilic cytoplasm, intracellular and extracellular hyaline globules, and intracytoplasmic vacuolation. The defining molecular driver is CTNNB1 mutation with nuclear beta-catenin accumulation — diffuse nuclear beta-catenin staining is the diagnostic IHC. Other characteristic markers include nuclear cyclin D1, CD10, and abnormal E-cadherin staining (loss of membrane staining with nuclear or cytoplasmic relocalisation).

14.4 Pancreatic ductal adenocarcinoma

Pancreatic ductal adenocarcinoma (PDAC) is the dominant pancreatic malignancy and one of the most lethal solid tumours. The presentation is late in most cases — only 15-20 per cent of patients have resectable disease at diagnosis. Histology shows infiltrative ductal proliferation with desmoplastic stromal reaction, perineural and lymphovascular invasion, and characteristic architectural features including incomplete glandular formation, mucin production, and pleomorphic nuclei often arranged with a single large prominent nucleolus. Subtypes include conventional PDAC (the dominant pattern), undifferentiated carcinoma, undifferentiated carcinoma with osteoclast-like giant cells, colloid (mucinous noncystic) carcinoma, signet ring carcinoma, adenosquamous carcinoma, and rare medullary carcinoma associated with MSI.

Precursor lesions

Pancreatic intraepithelial neoplasia (PanIN) is the principal microscopic precursor of PDAC. The lesion is graded into low-grade and high-grade categories under the WHO 5th edition (replacing the previous three-tier system). Low-grade PanIN shows flat, papillary, or micropapillary architecture with mucinous columnar epithelium and mild to moderate cytological atypia. High-grade PanIN shows full-thickness cytological atypia, loss of polarity, and architectural complexity (cribriforming, budding) — the immediate precursor of invasive disease. PanIN typically occurs in pancreatic ducts smaller than 5 mm; mucinous lesions in larger ducts are reclassified as IPMN.

Molecular profile

PDAC carries a defined set of recurrent molecular alterations driving the disease. KRAS mutation is present in over 90 per cent of cases (most commonly G12D, G12V, G12R) — the founder event in the PanIN-to-PDAC sequence. TP53 mutation is present in around 70 per cent of cases. SMAD4 (DPC4) inactivation occurs in around 50 per cent and is associated with shorter survival and distant metastasis pattern (SMAD4 loss demonstrable by IHC). CDKN2A (p16) inactivation is present in around 90 per cent. Less common but actionable alterations include BRCA1, BRCA2, PALB2 mutations (5-10 per cent — eligible for PARP inhibitor in BRCA-mutant disease), NTRK fusions (rare), and MMR deficiency (under 5 per cent, eligible for immunotherapy). Routine molecular testing in advanced disease covers KRAS, TP53, SMAD4, and the BRCA pathway, with extended panels supporting clinical trial eligibility.

Pancreatic ductal adenocarcinoma — molecular landscape

KRAS: over 90% — founder event; G12D, G12V, G12R most common.

TP53: around 70% — late event in progression.

SMAD4 (DPC4): around 50% — IHC loss demonstrable; associated with metastatic pattern.

CDKN2A: around 90% — p16 inactivation.

BRCA1/2, PALB2: 5-10% — PARP inhibitor eligibility (olaparib).

MSI: under 5% — immunotherapy eligibility.

NTRK fusion: rare — larotrectinib eligibility.

14.5 Pancreatic neuroendocrine tumours

Pancreatic neuroendocrine tumours (PanNETs) range from indolent well-differentiated tumours to aggressive poorly-differentiated neuroendocrine carcinomas. The WHO 5th edition framework grades well-differentiated NETs into three categories based on Ki-67 proliferation and mitotic count — NET grade 1 (Ki-67 under 3 per cent, mitoses under 2 per 2 mm squared), NET grade 2 (Ki-67 3-20 per cent or mitoses 2-20), NET grade 3 (Ki-67 over 20 per cent or mitoses over 20 with well-differentiated morphology). Poorly differentiated neuroendocrine carcinoma (small cell or large cell, Ki-67 typically over 50-60 per cent) is the separate aggressive category with different biology and management.

Functional PanNETs produce hormone-related clinical syndromes — insulinoma (hypoglycaemia, the commonest functional PanNET, usually benign, often small), gastrinoma (Zollinger-Ellison syndrome with peptic ulceration; pancreas or duodenum, often MEN1-associated), glucagonoma (necrolytic migratory erythema, weight loss), VIPoma (Verner-Morrison syndrome with watery diarrhoea, hypokalaemia, achlorhydria), somatostatinoma (diabetes, cholelithiasis, steatorrhoea). Non-functional PanNETs are more common and present as masses without hormone-related symptoms. IHC characterises the tumour — synaptophysin, chromogranin, INSM1 positive across the group; specific hormone IHC supports functional designation. MEN1 syndrome (multiple endocrine neoplasia type 1, germline MEN1 mutation) drives a subset of cases with parallel pituitary and parathyroid involvement.

14.6 Acinar cell carcinoma and ampullary disease

Acinar cell carcinoma is a rare pancreatic malignancy with distinctive morphology — solid and trabecular architecture, monomorphic cells with apical eosinophilic granules (zymogen granules), and single prominent nucleoli. The tumour shows IHC positivity for trypsin, chymotrypsin, and BCL10 — markers absent in PDAC and NET. The tumour may produce lipase hypersecretion syndrome in selected cases (subcutaneous fat necrosis, eosinophilia, polyarthralgia from circulating lipase). The behaviour is intermediate between PDAC and PanNET, with longer survival than PDAC at equivalent stage.

Ampullary carcinomas — arising at the ampulla of Vater where the bile and pancreatic ducts converge into the duodenum — are categorised into two principal types based on the dominant histological pattern. Intestinal-type ampullary carcinoma resembles colorectal adenocarcinoma with glandular architecture, CDX2 and CK20 positive, and tends to have better prognosis than pancreaticobiliary type. Pancreaticobiliary-type ampullary carcinoma resembles pancreatic and biliary ductal carcinoma morphologically and immunohistochemically (CK7, MUC1 positive). Distinguishing between the types matters because the molecular profile, treatment response, and prognosis differ. Intestinal-type cases more often have KRAS mutations and respond better to fluoropyrimidine-based chemotherapy.

14.7 TNM staging and reporting

AJCC 8 staging for pancreatic cancer records T (Tis; T1 — tumour 2 cm or less, with T1a under 0.5 cm, T1b 0.5-1 cm, T1c 1-2 cm; T2 — 2-4 cm; T3 — over 4 cm; T4 — involvement of coeliac axis, superior mesenteric artery, or common hepatic artery — unresectable disease), N (N0; N1 — 1-3 nodes; N2 — 4 or more nodes), and M. The 8th edition removed the previous extrapancreatic extension as a T-defining criterion in favour of size-based criteria.

Reporting follows the RCPath dataset. Core items include specimen type and procedure (Whipple, distal, total), tumour site (head, body, tail, ampullary), histological type and grade, tumour size, multifocality, margin status with detailed margin assessment (pancreatic neck, common bile duct, uncinate / superior mesenteric vein groove margin, posterior / retroperitoneal margin), lymphovascular invasion, perineural invasion (a characteristic feature of pancreatic adenocarcinoma — perineural invasion is identified in over 80 per cent of cases), lymph node count and status, response to neoadjuvant therapy where applicable, and biomarker results where commissioned (MMR, BRCA pathway analysis on resected specimens, KRAS mutation analysis for selected molecular targeting decisions).

14.8 Reporting and key points

Chapter 14 — key points

Ductal adenocarcinoma (PDAC): Most common; perineural invasion characteristic; KRAS, TP53, SMAD4, CDKN2A. Reporting: tumour origin, size, grade, depth, all margins (especially uncinate/posterior), nodes, perineural and lymphovascular invasion.

Margin convention: R0 if >1 mm from any margin (revised UK/RCPath definition); R1 if ≤1 mm. UK practice scrutinises uncinate margin closely.

PanIN: Low-grade and high-grade lesions; high-grade (formerly PanIN-3) is carcinoma in situ.

IPMN: Main-duct (high-risk), branch-duct (lower risk), mixed. Gastric, intestinal, pancreatobiliary, oncocytic subtypes. Worrisome and high-risk stigmata drive resection.

MCN: Ovarian-type stroma diagnostic. Almost exclusively women; tail and body. KRAS and TP53 in invasive component.

Pancreatic NETs: Functioning (insulinoma, gastrinoma) and non-functioning. Grade by mitotic count and Ki-67 (G1 <3%, G2 3–20%, G3 >20%); NEC (small cell or large cell) is separate.

Acinar cell and solid pseudopapillary: Acinar: lipase positive, monomorphic acinar arrangement. SPN: young women, nuclear beta-catenin, CD10 and progesterone receptor positive.

14.9 Chapter SBAs

Q14.1. Distinction between mucinous cystic neoplasm (MCN) and branch-duct intraductal papillary mucinous neoplasm (IPMN) is critical because the management pathways differ, although both are mucinous and have malignant potential. A 45-year-old woman has a 4 cm cystic lesion in the pancreatic tail. Histology shows tall columnar mucinous epithelium with low-grade dysplasia. The underlying stroma comprises spindle cells with elongated nuclei resembling ovarian cortex, with ER and PR positivity on IHC. Which single feature is the defining discriminator of MCN from IPMN?

A. Anatomical location in the pancreatic tail.

B. Presence of low-grade dysplasia.

C. Female sex of the patient.

D. Ovarian-type stroma with ER and PR positivity.

E. Mucinous columnar epithelium.

Answer: D

The defining feature of mucinous cystic neoplasm (MCN) is the presence of ovarian-type stroma — composed of spindle cells with elongated nuclei resembling ovarian cortex, with ER and PR positivity on IHC, sometimes with luteinised cells. This feature is required for the diagnosis under WHO 5th edition criteria. MCN occurs almost exclusively in women and almost always in the pancreatic body or tail, but these are demographic features rather than defining histological criteria. IPMN, by contrast, arises within the pancreatic duct system without ovarian-type stroma, and may occur in either sex. The distinction matters because management differs — MCN is generally resected even in low-grade cases given the malignant potential, while branch-duct IPMN management depends on size, symptoms, and high-risk features per Fukuoka guidelines.

Option A is a demographic feature that supports MCN but does not define it. Option B (dysplasia grade) does not discriminate between MCN and IPMN. Option C (female sex) is supportive but not defining. Option E (mucinous epithelium) is common to both MCN and IPMN.

Q14.2. Solid pseudopapillary neoplasm (SPN) of the pancreas has characteristic morphological and molecular features that distinguish it from other pancreatic neoplasms. A 25-year-old woman has a 6 cm pancreatic body mass resected. Histology shows discohesive cells around fibrovascular cores forming pseudopapillae, with uniform monomorphic cells, abundant pale cytoplasm, and intracellular hyaline globules. Which single immunohistochemistry pattern is most specific for this diagnosis?

A. Diffuse nuclear beta-catenin, abnormal E-cadherin (loss of membrane staining with nuclear or cytoplasmic relocalisation), CD10 positive, cyclin D1 positive.

B. Synaptophysin and chromogranin positive with INSM1 nuclear positivity.

C. Trypsin and chymotrypsin positive with BCL10 positive.

D. CK7 positive, MUC1 positive, CDX2 negative.

E. Calretinin, WT1, and D2-40 positive.

Answer: A

Solid pseudopapillary neoplasm has a characteristic immunohistochemistry signature reflecting its underlying CTNNB1 mutation with WNT pathway activation. Nuclear beta-catenin accumulation is the diagnostic IHC — present in over 90 per cent of SPN. E-cadherin shows characteristic abnormal pattern with loss of membrane staining and nuclear or cytoplasmic relocalisation. CD10 is positive in the majority of SPN. Cyclin D1 is positive reflecting the WNT pathway activation. Other supportive markers include vimentin, NSE, and alpha-1 antitrypsin (resistant to diastase, often producing characteristic intracellular hyaline globules). The combination of morphology and IHC supports the definitive diagnosis.

Option B describes the IHC pattern of pancreatic neuroendocrine tumour. Option C describes acinar cell carcinoma. Option D describes pancreaticobiliary-type ampullary carcinoma. Option E describes mesothelial cell IHC pattern.

Q14.3. Autoimmune pancreatitis is sub-classified into type 1 (IgG4-related) and type 2 (idiopathic duct-centric) with distinct clinical and pathological features. A 55-year-old man with no IBD history has a focal pancreatic mass resected on suspicion of carcinoma. Histology shows lymphoplasmacytic sclerosing pancreatitis with storiform fibrosis, obliterative phlebitis, and IgG4-positive plasma cells in excess of 20 per high-power field. The patient's serum IgG4 is elevated. Which single statement best describes the diagnosis and the implication?

A. Pancreatic ductal adenocarcinoma — complete resection sufficient.

B. Type 1 autoimmune pancreatitis (IgG4-related disease); systemic involvement should be assessed; corticosteroids are first-line therapy.

C. Type 2 autoimmune pancreatitis — IBD screening recommended.

D. Chronic pancreatitis from alcohol — abstinence advised.

E. Lymphoma of the pancreas — chemotherapy required.

Answer: B

Type 1 autoimmune pancreatitis is part of IgG4-related disease, a systemic fibroinflammatory condition affecting multiple organ systems. The diagnostic histology shows lymphoplasmacytic sclerosing pancreatitis with abundant IgG4-positive plasma cells (over 10 per high-power field in pancreatic tissue), storiform fibrosis, and obliterative phlebitis — the three features supporting the diagnosis. Serum IgG4 is typically elevated. Recognition is important because the disease responds dramatically to corticosteroid therapy, in contrast to malignancy. The clinical management includes systemic assessment for IgG4-related involvement of other organs (sclerosing cholangitis, retroperitoneal fibrosis, salivary gland disease, lacrimal gland disease, lymphadenopathy, aortitis) and corticosteroid initiation. Surgical resection performed for suspected malignancy is the unfortunately common scenario.

Option A is incorrect — PDAC would show infiltrative adenocarcinoma with desmoplastic stroma and the specific features described are diagnostic of IgG4-AIP rather than PDAC. Option C describes type 2 with granulocytic epithelial lesions and IBD association, not matching the features described. Option D would show different features (fibrosis with calcification, ductal dilatation, lobular atrophy with preserved islets). Option E is inconsistent with the lymphoplasmacytic sclerosing morphology.

14.10 Chapter EMQ

EMQ 14.1. Pancreatic pathology. For each scenario, select the single most appropriate diagnosis from the option list. Each option may be used once, more than once, or not at all.

A. Acute pancreatitis

B. Chronic pancreatitis

C. Type 1 autoimmune pancreatitis

D. Serous cystadenoma

E. Mucinous cystic neoplasm (MCN)

F. Intraductal papillary mucinous neoplasm (IPMN)

G. Solid pseudopapillary neoplasm

H. Pancreatic ductal adenocarcinoma

I. Pancreatic neuroendocrine tumour (NET)

J. Acinar cell carcinoma

(1) A 28-year-old woman has a 5 cm pancreatic tail mass with mixed solid and pseudopapillary architecture, discohesive cells around fibrovascular cores, uniform monomorphic cells, and intracellular hyaline globules. Nuclear beta-catenin is positive. **Answer: G**

(2) A 65-year-old man has a 3 cm pancreatic head mass. Histology shows infiltrative ductal carcinoma with dense desmoplastic stroma, perineural invasion, and characteristic glandular architecture. KRAS G12D is detected. **Answer: H**

(3) A 55-year-old patient has a multicystic lesion in the pancreatic body with characteristic central stellate scar on imaging. Histology shows multiple small cysts lined by cuboidal epithelium with clear cytoplasm, PAS-positive and diastase-sensitive. **Answer: D**

(4) A 45-year-old woman has a 4 cm cystic lesion in the pancreatic tail. Histology shows tall columnar mucinous epithelium with low-grade dysplasia, and the underlying stroma comprises spindle cells with elongated nuclei, ER and PR positive on IHC. **Answer: E**

(5) A 60-year-old man has hypoglycaemia and a 1 cm pancreatic body mass. Histology shows uniform cells in nested architecture, synaptophysin and chromogranin positive, with insulin immunohistochemistry positive, Ki-67 of 1 per cent. **Answer: I**

Chapter 15 — Lung

Lung pathology occupies a large proportion of histopathology workload, dominated by lung cancer in resection and biopsy material — by interstitial lung disease in transbronchial and surgical biopsy specimens, and and by infectious and inflammatory entities throughout. The FRCPath Part 1 candidate is expected to interpret the patterns of lung injury, recognise the principal entities, apply the WHO 5th edition classification of lung tumours, apply the dominant predictive biomarker pathways for lung adenocarcinoma, and use the AJCC 8 TNM framework. This chapter sets out the discipline against current international standards.

15.1 Normal lung histology

Lung histology comprises the airway-conducting and gas-exchanging compartments. The trachea and major bronchi are lined by ciliated pseudostratified columnar epithelium with goblet cells, supported by hyaline cartilage rings and mucous submucosal glands. Bronchi progressively lose cartilage support as they branch into bronchioles distally — terminal bronchioles are lined by simple cuboidal to columnar ciliated epithelium without cartilage or submucosal glands. Respiratory bronchioles transition to alveolar ducts and ultimately to alveoli — the gas-exchanging units lined by type I pneumocytes (thin, flat cells covering most of the surface area) and type II pneumocytes — cuboidal, surfactant-producing, the progenitor cells for type I regeneration. The pulmonary capillary network in the alveolar walls supports gas exchange. The visceral pleura covers the lung surface; the parietal pleura lines the chest wall.

15.2 Patterns of lung injury

Lung pathology often presents as a pattern of injury rather than a specific entity — and the candidate is expected to recognise the dominant patterns and their differential. Acute interstitial pneumonia (AIP — the histological pattern of acute respiratory distress syndrome) shows diffuse alveolar damage (DAD) with hyaline membranes lining alveolar surfaces, intra-alveolar oedema, type II pneumocyte hyperplasia, and progression through proliferative and fibrotic phases. The aetiology may be idiopathic or secondary to viral pneumonia, sepsis, aspiration, drug toxicity, or radiation. Organising pneumonia (formerly bronchiolitis obliterans organising pneumonia, BOOP) shows characteristic plugs of organising granulation tissue — Masson bodies — within bronchioles and alveolar ducts, with preserved alveolar architecture and mild chronic inflammation. The pattern is steroid-responsive and may be cryptogenic or secondary to infection, drug, autoimmune disease, or radiation.

Usual interstitial pneumonia (UIP) is the histological pattern of idiopathic pulmonary fibrosis (IPF) — and is also seen in connective tissue disease, asbestosis, and chronic hypersensitivity pneumonitis. The defining features are patchy fibrosis with temporal and spatial heterogeneity — fibrotic and normal areas adjacent, older dense fibrosis adjacent to younger fibroblastic foci — peripheral and subpleural distribution, honeycomb change with cystically dilated airspaces lined by bronchiolar epithelium within dense fibrosis, and architectural distortion. The 2018 ATS/ERS/JRS/ALAT IPF guidelines define UIP, probable UIP, indeterminate, and alternative diagnosis categories on the histological pattern, in conjunction with HRCT findings.

Other interstitial patterns include non-specific interstitial pneumonia (NSIP — temporally uniform interstitial inflammation and fibrosis, more cellular pattern in cellular NSIP and more fibrotic in fibrotic NSIP), desquamative interstitial pneumonia (DIP — intra-alveolar macrophage accumulation, smoking-related), respiratory bronchiolitis-interstitial lung disease (RB-ILD — similar to DIP but more bronchiolar centric, smoking-related), lymphocytic interstitial pneumonia (LIP — lymphoid infiltrate; associated with Sjogren's, HIV in some), and pulmonary Langerhans cell histiocytosis — smoking-related, with characteristic CD1a-positive Langerhans cells in stellate fibrotic scars.

Interstitial lung disease patterns at a glance

UIP: patchy fibrosis with temporal/spatial heterogeneity, fibroblastic foci, honeycomb. IPF and CTD-ILD.

NSIP: temporally uniform interstitial inflammation/fibrosis; cellular vs fibrotic. Often CTD-associated.

OP: Masson bodies in bronchioles and alveolar ducts, preserved architecture. Steroid-responsive.

DAD: hyaline membranes, type II hyperplasia. ARDS / AIP pattern.

DIP/RB-ILD: intra-alveolar pigmented macrophages, smoking-related.

Hypersensitivity pneumonitis: bronchiolocentric chronic inflammation with poorly-formed granulomas.

PLCH: stellate scars with CD1a+ Langerhans cells, smoking-related.

15.3 Granulomatous disease

Pulmonary tuberculosis remains a global health priority and a recurring item in lung biopsy practice. The histological hallmark is caseating granulomas with central necrosis, epithelioid macrophages, Langhans giant cells, and surrounding lymphocytic infiltrate — distributed throughout the parenchyma. Acid-fast bacilli are demonstrated on Ziehl-Neelsen staining, with molecular detection (PCR for Mycobacterium tuberculosis complex) increasingly used as confirmatory tool. Sarcoidosis shows non-caseating granulomas with characteristic Schaumann bodies (laminated calcium-containing inclusions) and asteroid bodies (star-shaped cytoplasmic inclusions) — distributed along lymphatic routes (bronchovascular, septal, pleural). The differential between TB and sarcoidosis is supported by clinical context, geographical risk, and microbiological investigation.

Granulomatosis with polyangiitis (GPA, formerly Wegener's) is a small-vessel vasculitis — with characteristic pulmonary involvement. Histology shows necrotising granulomas with geographic necrosis, mixed inflammatory infiltrate including neutrophils, multinucleated giant cells, and necrotising vasculitis affecting small to medium vessels. Serological correlation with c-ANCA (anti-PR3) is the typical pattern. Other granulomatous diseases include hypersensitivity pneumonitis (small poorly-formed granulomas in a bronchiolocentric distribution with chronic inflammation), fungal infections (Aspergillus, Cryptococcus, Histoplasma — with characteristic morphology supported by Grocott methenamine silver staining), and rare entities such as berylliosis and chronic granulomatous disease.

15.4 Lung cancer — adenocarcinoma

Adenocarcinoma is the dominant lung malignancy in most Western populations, with rising incidence in never-smokers — particularly women in East Asian populations. The WHO 5th edition classifies lung adenocarcinoma into preinvasive (atypical adenomatous hyperplasia, adenocarcinoma in situ), minimally invasive (under 5 mm invasive focus), and invasive categories, with invasive disease sub-classified by predominant architectural pattern (lepidic, acinar, papillary, micropapillary, solid, with rare patterns including mucinous, colloid, fetal, enteric). The predominant pattern is determined by which is most extensive on histological assessment — and the percentage of each pattern is reported. Lepidic-predominant tumours have the best prognosis; micropapillary and solid patterns have the worst.

Lung adenocarcinoma is the most molecularly-stratified solid tumour in routine practice — with reflex testing for actionable variants now standard at diagnosis. EGFR mutation — exon 19 deletion, L858R, and others, with T790M as the dominant resistance mutation — drives first, second, and third-generation TKI selection. ALK rearrangement — companion diagnostic IHC plus FISH or NGS confirmation — drives alectinib, brigatinib, and lorlatinib selection. ROS1 rearrangement drives crizotinib and entrectinib. BRAF V600E drives dabrafenib plus trametinib. MET exon 14 skipping and high-level MET amplification drive capmatinib and tepotinib. RET fusion drives selpercatinib and pralsetinib. NTRK fusion drives larotrectinib and entrectinib. KRAS G12C drives sotorasib and adagrasib. HER2 mutation drives trastuzumab deruxtecan. Each variant has defined IHC and molecular pathways for detection; many laboratories deploy NGS panels to test the full set in a single assay, supporting broad reflex testing.

PD-L1 testing using tumour proportion score (TPS — percentage of viable tumour cells with membrane staining) informs immune checkpoint inhibitor selection. TPS thresholds include 1 per cent for some indications, 50 per cent for first-line pembrolizumab monotherapy in metastatic disease. The 22C3 PharmDx assay is the dominant companion diagnostic — inter-laboratory variation has been documented and supports regular EQA participation. The IASLC PD-L1 atlas provides reference images for scoring.

Lung adenocarcinoma — actionable molecular targets

EGFR: exon 19 del, L858R most common. Osimertinib first-line; T790M resistance.

ALK: fusion. IHC screen, FISH/NGS confirm. Alectinib first-line.

ROS1: fusion. Crizotinib, entrectinib.

BRAF V600E: Dabrafenib + trametinib.

MET ex14 skip / amplification: Capmatinib, tepotinib.

RET fusion: Selpercatinib, pralsetinib.

NTRK fusion: Larotrectinib, entrectinib.

KRAS G12C: Sotorasib, adagrasib.

HER2 mutation: Trastuzumab deruxtecan.

PD-L1 TPS: ≥1% (some indications); ≥50% for first-line pembrolizumab monotherapy.

15.5 Squamous cell carcinoma and other histologies

Lung squamous cell carcinoma typically arises in central airways from squamous metaplasia and dysplasia in chronic smokers, although peripheral cases are increasingly recognised. The histology shows squamous differentiation with keratinisation, intercellular bridges, and keratin pearls in well-differentiated cases; poorly-differentiated tumours lose these features and require IHC (p40, p63, CK5/6 positive; TTF-1 and napsin A negative) for confirmation. Squamous dysplasia is the preinvasive lesion, graded into mild, moderate, severe, and carcinoma in situ. Molecular profile features FGFR1 amplification and PIK3CA mutations more often than adenocarcinoma; EGFR and ALK alterations are rare. Lung squamous carcinoma is typically not reflex-tested for the full lung adenocarcinoma panel, except in selected centres.

Other histological types include adenosquamous carcinoma — with both adenocarcinoma and squamous components, each comprising at least 10 per cent of the tumour — large cell carcinoma (a diagnosis of exclusion when no specific differentiation is demonstrable), sarcomatoid carcinoma (with malignant spindle cell or giant cell components), and pulmonary salivary gland-type tumours (mucoepidermoid carcinoma, adenoid cystic carcinoma — rare but with characteristic morphology and molecular drivers including MAML2 fusion for mucoepidermoid).

15.6 Neuroendocrine tumours of the lung

Lung neuroendocrine neoplasms form a four-tier spectrum — from indolent typical carcinoid to aggressive small cell carcinoma. Typical carcinoid (TC) shows uniform monomorphic cells in organoid nests, no necrosis, fewer than 2 mitoses per 2 mm squared, and Ki-67 typically under 5 per cent. Atypical carcinoid (AC) shows 2 to 10 mitoses per 2 mm squared or focal necrosis (less than 10 per cent of the tumour) — with intermediate prognosis. Large cell neuroendocrine carcinoma (LCNEC) shows larger cells with abundant cytoplasm, prominent nucleoli, over 10 mitoses per 2 mm squared, prominent necrosis, and aggressive behaviour. Small cell carcinoma (SCLC) shows small cells with scant cytoplasm, fine granular chromatin, nuclear moulding, and very high mitotic and necrosis rates — molecular drivers include TP53 and RB1 inactivation in over 90 per cent of cases.

Neuroendocrine markers (synaptophysin, chromogranin, INSM1, CD56) confirm the lineage, with TTF-1 nuclear positivity supporting pulmonary origin. The WHO 5th edition recognises a category of high-grade carcinoma with neuroendocrine differentiation but without classical small cell or large cell features — sometimes called combined small cell carcinoma when admixed with non-small-cell components.

15.7 TNM staging and reporting

AJCC 8 staging for lung cancer records T based on tumour size and local extension — T1a under 1 cm, T1b 1-2 cm, T1c 2-3 cm, T2a 3-4 cm, T2b 4-5 cm, T3 5-7 cm or invasion of pleura, parietal pericardium, or chest wall, T4 over 7 cm or invasion of mediastinum, diaphragm, heart, great vessels, vertebra. N category records regional lymph node involvement at hilar (N1), ipsilateral mediastinal (N2), and contralateral mediastinal or supraclavicular (N3) stations. M category distinguishes M1a (within thorax including separate nodule in contralateral lobe and pleural disease), M1b (single extrathoracic metastasis), and M1c (multiple extrathoracic metastases).

Reporting follows the RCPath dataset. Core items include specimen type, tumour location, histological type and subtype with quantification of each pattern in adenocarcinoma, tumour size, depth and extent of invasion, pleural invasion (PL0 none; PL1 visceral pleura without serosa breach; PL2 visceral pleura with serosa breach; PL3 parietal pleura), margins, lymphovascular invasion, perineural invasion, lymph node count and status by station, treatment effect where applicable, and biomarker results (PD-L1, EGFR, ALK, ROS1, BRAF, MET, RET, NTRK, KRAS, HER2 in adenocarcinoma). The synoptic block supports MDT presentation.

15.8 Key points

Chapter 15 — key points

Adenocarcinoma patterns: Lepidic, acinar, papillary, micropapillary, solid; predominant pattern reported. Lepidic (formerly BAC) has best prognosis; micropapillary and solid the worst.

Squamous carcinoma: p40/p63 + CK5/6 + TTF-1 negative. Keratinising, non-keratinising, basaloid.

IASLC 2020 grading: Adenocarcinoma grade 1 (lepidic predominant, no high-grade), grade 2 (acinar/papillary predominant, no high-grade), grade 3 (any solid, micropapillary, complex glandular ≥20%).

Molecular alterations: EGFR (Asian, never-smoker, female), ALK fusion, ROS1 fusion, KRAS G12C, BRAF V600E, MET exon 14, RET fusion, NTRK fusion, HER2.

PD-L1: Tumour proportion score (TPS) for lung. 22C3 pharmDx for pembrolizumab; cut-offs 1% and 50%.

ILD patterns: UIP (patchy subpleural fibrosis, fibroblastic foci, honeycomb), NSIP (uniform fibrosis), OP (intra-luminal Masson bodies), DIP/RBILD (smoker macrophages), DAD (acute, hyaline membranes).

Neuroendocrine: Typical carcinoid (<2 mitoses/2 mm^2), atypical carcinoid (2–10 + necrosis), small cell, LCNEC; CK ± synaptophysin ± chromogranin ± INSM1.

15.9 Chapter SBAs

Q15.1. Routine molecular profiling of lung adenocarcinoma identifies actionable variants that drive first-line treatment selection. A 65-year-old never-smoker woman has metastatic lung adenocarcinoma. Reflex testing identifies an EGFR exon 19 deletion. Which single statement best describes the first-line therapeutic implication?

A. Cytotoxic chemotherapy with platinum doublet is first-line.

B. Osimertinib (third-generation EGFR-TKI) is first-line.

C. Immunotherapy with pembrolizumab monotherapy regardless of PD-L1.

D. First-line ALK inhibitor.

E. Trastuzumab deruxtecan first-line.

Answer: B

EGFR exon 19 deletion is one of the two commonest activating EGFR mutations (alongside L858R) in lung adenocarcinoma and confers sensitivity to EGFR-TKI therapy. Osimertinib (the third-generation EGFR-TKI) is the standard first-line agent in the UK following the FLAURA trial demonstrating superior progression-free and overall survival compared to first-generation TKIs. Osimertinib also covers the T790M resistance mutation that emerges in the majority of patients progressing on first/second-generation TKIs. The clinical pathway is reflex molecular testing at diagnosis followed by first-line osimertinib for EGFR-mutant disease.

Option A (chemotherapy) is reserved for patients without actionable mutations or after TKI exhaustion. Option C (immunotherapy monotherapy) is the standard for PD-L1 high disease without driver mutations; in EGFR-mutant disease, immunotherapy single agent shows poor response. Option D applies to ALK rearrangement, not EGFR mutation. Option E applies to HER2-mutant disease.

Q15.2. Histological pattern recognition guides interpretation of interstitial lung disease biopsies in the context of clinical and HRCT findings. A 60-year-old man has a surgical lung biopsy showing patchy fibrosis with adjacent normal lung parenchyma, peripheral and subpleural distribution, fibroblastic foci at the interface between fibrotic and normal lung, and honeycomb change. Which single statement best describes the diagnosis?

A. Usual interstitial pneumonia (UIP) — consistent with idiopathic pulmonary fibrosis.

B. Cellular non-specific interstitial pneumonia.

C. Organising pneumonia.

D. Hypersensitivity pneumonitis.

E. Diffuse alveolar damage.

Answer: A

The combination of patchy fibrosis with temporal and spatial heterogeneity (fibrotic and normal areas adjacent), peripheral and subpleural distribution, fibroblastic foci (small clusters of myofibroblasts at the interface between fibrotic and normal lung — the marker of active fibrosis), and honeycomb change (cystically dilated airspaces lined by bronchiolar epithelium within dense fibrosis) defines the usual interstitial pneumonia (UIP) pattern. UIP is the histological substrate of idiopathic pulmonary fibrosis (IPF) when no other cause is identifiable, but the same pattern occurs in connective tissue disease-associated ILD, asbestosis, and chronic hypersensitivity pneumonitis. The 2018 ATS/ERS/JRS/ALAT IPF guidelines define UIP, probable UIP, indeterminate, and alternative diagnosis categories based on histology in conjunction with HRCT.

Option B (cellular NSIP) shows temporally uniform pattern without fibroblastic foci. Option C (OP) shows Masson bodies in bronchioles. Option D (hypersensitivity pneumonitis) shows bronchiolocentric inflammation with poorly-formed granulomas. Option E (DAD) shows hyaline membranes and type II hyperplasia.

Q15.3. Classification of lung neuroendocrine tumours is based on a combination of mitotic count, necrosis, and morphology under the WHO 5th edition framework. A 55-year-old man has a 3 cm lung mass. Histology shows uniform monomorphic cells in organoid nests with characteristic chromatin pattern, 3 mitoses per 2 mm squared (averaged across multiple high-power fields), and a focus of necrosis comprising less than 5 per cent of the tumour. Which single diagnosis is most appropriate?

A. Typical carcinoid.

B. Atypical carcinoid.

C. Large cell neuroendocrine carcinoma.

D. Small cell carcinoma.

E. Adenocarcinoma with neuroendocrine differentiation.

Answer: B

Atypical carcinoid (AC) is defined by 2 to 10 mitoses per 2 mm squared and/or focal necrosis (less than 10 per cent of the tumour), in a tumour with carcinoid morphology (uniform monomorphic cells in organoid architecture). The described tumour has 3 mitoses per 2 mm squared (within the AC range) and focal necrosis under 5 per cent (also within the AC range). Typical carcinoid (TC) by contrast requires fewer than 2 mitoses per 2 mm squared and no necrosis. Large cell neuroendocrine carcinoma requires over 10 mitoses per 2 mm squared, larger cell size, prominent nucleoli, and extensive necrosis. The atypical carcinoid carries intermediate prognosis, with five-year survival around 60-70 per cent.

Option A (TC) is excluded by the mitotic count exceeding 2 per 2 mm squared and the presence of necrosis. Option C (LCNEC) requires over 10 mitoses per 2 mm squared. Option D (SCLC) shows small cells with scant cytoplasm and very high mitotic rate. Option E (adenocarcinoma with neuroendocrine differentiation) requires glandular component with focal neuroendocrine differentiation.

15.10 Chapter EMQ

EMQ 15.1. Lung pathology — diagnosis. For each scenario, select the single most appropriate diagnosis from the option list. Each option may be used once, more than once, or not at all.

A. Usual interstitial pneumonia (UIP)

B. Non-specific interstitial pneumonia (NSIP)

C. Organising pneumonia

D. Diffuse alveolar damage

E. Sarcoidosis

F. Granulomatosis with polyangiitis (GPA)

G. Lung adenocarcinoma (lepidic-predominant)

H. Lung squamous cell carcinoma

I. Small cell lung carcinoma

J. Typical carcinoid

(1) A 28-year-old non-smoker has bilateral upper-lobe nodules and mediastinal lymphadenopathy. Surgical biopsy of a mediastinal node shows non-caseating granulomas with Schaumann and asteroid bodies, distributed along lymphatic routes. **Answer: E**

(2) A 65-year-old man with arthralgia and haematuria presents with cavitating lung nodules. Lung biopsy shows necrotising granulomas with geographic necrosis, mixed inflammatory infiltrate including neutrophils, and necrotising vasculitis affecting small to medium vessels. c-ANCA is positive. **Answer: F**

(3) A 50-year-old woman with rapid-onset respiratory failure has a lung biopsy showing hyaline membranes lining alveolar surfaces with type II pneumocyte hyperplasia and intra-alveolar oedema. **Answer: D**

(4) A 45-year-old never-smoker has a 1.5 cm subpleural pulmonary nodule. The histology shows tumour cells growing along intact alveolar septa (lepidic pattern) without invasion, comprising over 90 per cent of the tumour with focal acinar pattern. **Answer: G**

(5) A 40-year-old non-smoker has a 2 cm central bronchial lesion. Histology shows uniform monomorphic cells in organoid nests with characteristic stippled chromatin, no necrosis, and 1 mitosis per 2 mm squared. Synaptophysin and chromogranin are positive. **Answer: J**

Chapter 16 — Pleura

Pleural pathology occupies a focused but high-stakes section of the syllabus, dominated by the diagnosis of malignant mesothelioma and its differential against reactive mesothelial hyperplasia and metastatic adenocarcinoma. The clinical consequences are real — mesothelioma diagnosis triggers medicolegal proceedings linked to occupational asbestos exposure, drives prognostic discussion, and informs systemic therapy decisions. The discipline of pleural diagnosis combines careful morphology, a targeted immunohistochemistry panel, and molecular ancillaries (CDKN2A/MTAP loss, BAP1 loss) that have transformed the diagnostic certainty in difficult cases. This chapter sets out the syllabus against the WHO 5th edition classification of pleural tumours and current UK reporting standards.

16.1 Normal pleural anatomy

The pleura comprises two serosal membranes — visceral pleura covering the lung surface and parietal pleura lining the chest wall, mediastinum, and diaphragm — separated by a potential space containing a thin film of serous fluid. Both surfaces are lined by a single layer of mesothelial cells overlying a thin subserosal connective tissue layer with vessels, lymphatics, and scattered fibroblasts. The visceral pleura is intimately attached to the lung parenchyma without an intervening adipose layer; the parietal pleura sits on a layer of subpleural adipose tissue and is innervated (giving rise to pleuritic pain).

16.2 Reactive pleural changes

Reactive mesothelial hyperplasia follows pleural irritation from any cause — pneumothorax, infection, surgery, trauma, malignant effusion. The histology shows proliferation of mesothelial cells in papillary or solid sheet pattern, with mild nuclear atypia, occasional mitotic figures, and an inflammatory background. The distinction from mesothelioma is the central diagnostic challenge in pleural pathology and is supported by morphology (reactive changes lack stromal invasion, retain orderly architecture), immunohistochemistry (BAP1 retained, MTAP retained in reactive disease; lost in most mesothelioma), and clinical and radiological context. The molecular ancillaries (BAP1 IHC, MTAP IHC for CDKN2A surrogate, and FISH for CDKN2A) have made the distinction markedly more reliable than in earlier decades.

Pleural plaques are the characteristic asbestos-related pleural lesion — discrete circumscribed thickenings of the parietal pleura, often calcified, with a 'basket-weave' pattern of hyalinised collagen on histology and minimal cellularity. They are typically symptomatic but indicate documented asbestos exposure and elevated mesothelioma risk over decades. Diffuse pleural thickening is a distinct entity, more often symptomatic, involving the visceral pleura more extensively, and arising on a background of asbestos exposure or post-inflammatory aetiology.

16.3 Malignant mesothelioma

Epidemiology and aetiology

Malignant mesothelioma is the principal pleural malignancy, with a long latency (often 20-50 years) following asbestos exposure. Occupational exposure (shipbuilding, construction, asbestos manufacture, lagging, electrical work) accounts for the majority of cases; environmental and household exposures are recognised. Crocidolite (blue asbestos) is the most strongly mesothelioma-genic, with chrysotile less so. The disease is more common in men (reflecting occupational exposure patterns) and incidence varies by region depending on historical asbestos use. SV40 virus has been investigated as a potential co-factor but the evidence is not conclusive.

Histological subtypes — WHO 5

The WHO 5th edition recognises three principal histological subtypes of diffuse malignant pleural mesothelioma. Epithelioid mesothelioma (around 60-70 per cent) shows polygonal cells with eosinophilic cytoplasm in tubulopapillary, solid, or microcystic patterns. Sarcomatoid mesothelioma (around 10-20 per cent) shows spindle cell morphology resembling sarcoma with high pleomorphism and pleural-based growth. Biphasic mesothelioma (around 20-30 per cent) shows both epithelioid and sarcomatoid components, each comprising at least 10 per cent of the tumour. Desmoplastic mesothelioma is a sarcomatoid variant with dense collagenised stroma resembling fibrous pleurisy — a particularly difficult diagnostic challenge requiring careful sampling and ancillary studies. Other rare variants include lymphohistiocytoid mesothelioma. The WHO 5th edition introduced grading for epithelioid mesothelioma based on nuclear grade and necrosis, with grade predicting prognosis.

Immunohistochemistry panel

Confirming mesothelioma versus the principal differentials (adenocarcinoma metastasis, reactive mesothelial hyperplasia) uses a structured IHC panel of two or more mesothelial markers and two or more carcinoma markers. Mesothelial markers include calretinin (nuclear and cytoplasmic, the most sensitive), WT1 (nuclear), D2-40/podoplanin (membranous), and CK5/6 (cytoplasmic). Adenocarcinoma markers depend on the suspected primary — TTF-1 and napsin A for lung adenocarcinoma, MOC31 and BerEp4 as broad-spectrum carcinoma markers, claudin 4 (specific for carcinoma), GATA3 (for urothelial and breast), CDX2 (for GI primary), PAX8 (for renal/Mullerian/thyroid). The pattern of differential positivity supports the diagnosis. Pankeratin AE1/AE3 is positive in both mesothelioma and carcinoma and supports excluding sarcoma or melanoma.

The distinction between mesothelioma and reactive mesothelial hyperplasia relies on BAP1 IHC (BAP1 loss is highly specific for mesothelioma, demonstrating bi-allelic BAP1 inactivation, present in around 60 per cent of epithelioid mesothelioma), MTAP IHC (MTAP loss is a surrogate for CDKN2A homozygous deletion, present in around 70 per cent of epithelioid mesothelioma and over 90 per cent of sarcomatoid mesothelioma), and supportive markers (mesothelioma shows EZH2 over-expression in many cases; merlin/NF2 loss in some). FISH for CDKN2A homozygous deletion is the molecular gold standard for the MTAP-LOH-equivalent test. These ancillaries have transformed the diagnostic certainty — most cases that previously triggered 'atypical mesothelial proliferation, distinction from mesothelioma cannot be made' can now be classified definitively.

Mesothelioma diagnosis essentials

Mesothelial IHC: calretinin, WT1, D2-40, CK5/6 — at least two positive.

Adenocarcinoma IHC: TTF-1, napsin A, MOC31, BerEp4, claudin 4, GATA3, CDX2, PAX8 by suspected primary.

BAP1 loss: specific for mesothelioma vs reactive; present in ~60% of epithelioid.

MTAP loss: surrogate for CDKN2A homozygous deletion; ~70% epithelioid, >90% sarcomatoid.

FISH CDKN2A: molecular gold standard; homozygous deletion confirms mesothelioma.

Subtypes: epithelioid (60-70%), sarcomatoid (10-20%), biphasic (20-30%); desmoplastic variant of sarcomatoid.

Grading (WHO 5): nuclear grade + necrosis for epithelioid mesothelioma — prognostic.

16.4 Mesothelioma in situ and well-differentiated papillary mesothelial tumour

Mesothelioma in situ is a recently recognised category — bona fide neoplastic mesothelial proliferation without stromal invasion, defined by BAP1 loss and/or CDKN2A deletion in the absence of invasive component. The entity is uncommon but increasingly identified on aggressive biopsy sampling of recurrent effusions or mass-forming pleural disease. Well-differentiated papillary mesothelial tumour (WDPMT, formerly well-differentiated papillary mesothelioma) is a separate entity with characteristic morphology (papillary architecture with bland mesothelial cells, no invasion, no significant atypia) and indolent behaviour. The 2021 WHO 5 update renamed the entity to remove 'mesothelioma' from the name in recognition of its borderline behaviour.

16.5 Solitary fibrous tumour

Solitary fibrous tumour (SFT, formerly called localised fibrous tumour of pleura or benign fibrous mesothelioma) is a distinct mesenchymal tumour arising from submesothelial fibroblasts rather than mesothelial cells. The histology shows a 'patternless' arrangement of bland spindle cells with intervening collagen, varying cellularity, and characteristic 'staghorn' branching vessels. The defining molecular feature is NAB2-STAT6 fusion, with nuclear STAT6 IHC positivity as the diagnostic surrogate. The tumour is also CD34, CD99, BCL2 positive and pankeratin negative — supporting the distinction from epithelioid mesothelioma which is pankeratin positive. The Demicco risk model (age, size, mitotic count, necrosis) predicts malignant behaviour, with high-risk tumours warranting closer surveillance.

16.6 Pleural metastases and other entities

Metastatic disease to the pleura accounts for the majority of pleural malignancies in clinical practice — far exceeding mesothelioma in absolute numbers. Lung adenocarcinoma and breast cancer are the commonest sources, with ovarian, gastric, renal, and other primaries also recognised. The IHC panel is directed by the suspected primary as outlined above, and the IHC profile supports identification of the source. Other pleural entities include pleural-based lymphoma (rare; primary effusion lymphoma associated with HHV-8 in immunocompromised patients), pleural fibrosis from prior infection or inflammation, and rare pleural tumours including epithelioid haemangioendothelioma and angiosarcoma.

16.7 Reporting and staging

Mesothelioma staging follows the AJCC 8 system with separate stage groupings for pleural mesothelioma. T category records local extension — T1 (parietal pleura only), T2 (involving visceral pleura, lung parenchyma, or diaphragm), T3 (locally advanced but resectable; involving endothoracic fascia, mediastinal fat, single chest wall focus, non-transmural pericardial involvement), T4 (locally advanced unresectable; transmural pericardial, contralateral pleural, peritoneal, spine, brachial plexus, vertebral body, mediastinal organ involvement). N category records lymph node involvement (N0, N1 — ipsilateral mediastinal/internal mammary; N2 — contralateral or supraclavicular). M0/M1 records distant metastasis.

Reporting follows the RCPath dataset for pleural mesothelioma. Core items include specimen type, tumour location and extent, histological subtype with quantification in biphasic disease, grade (for epithelioid), BAP1 and MTAP IHC status, CDKN2A FISH result where performed, presence of necrosis, lymphovascular invasion, lymph node involvement, and tumour at margins. The medicolegal context drives the importance of clear documentation of asbestos-related changes (pleural plaques, asbestos bodies in parenchymal lung tissue where available) for compensation claims.

16.8 Key points

Chapter 16 — key points

Mesothelioma subtypes: Epithelioid (best prognosis), sarcomatoid (worst), biphasic. Desmoplastic and lymphohistiocytoid are rare epithelioid variants.

Diagnostic panel: Mesothelial: calretinin, CK5/6, WT1, D2-40, EMA membranous. Adenocarcinoma exclusion: MOC-31, BerEP4, CEA, BG8, TTF-1, claudin-4.

BAP1 and MTAP: BAP1 loss (nuclear) and MTAP loss (cytoplasmic) support mesothelioma over benign reactive proliferation. CDKN2A deletion by FISH is the most specific molecular marker.

Reporting: Subtype, invasion (chest wall, diaphragm, lung, pericardium), pT stage (TNM 8), grade for epithelioid (nuclear features, mitotic count, necrosis).

Benign mimics: Reactive mesothelial hyperplasia, fibrous pleurisy, well-differentiated papillary mesothelial tumour. Lack of invasion and intact BAP1/MTAP favour benign.

Solitary fibrous tumour: STAT6 nuclear positive; NAB2::STAT6 fusion. Risk stratification by modified four-variable Demicco model.

16.9 Chapter SBAs

Q16.1. Distinction between malignant mesothelioma and reactive mesothelial hyperplasia is the central diagnostic challenge in pleural pathology. A 70-year-old man with prior occupational asbestos exposure has a thoracoscopic pleural biopsy showing atypical mesothelial proliferation with mild nuclear pleomorphism. The morphology alone is equivocal between reactive and neoplastic processes. Which single ancillary test result would most strongly support a diagnosis of mesothelioma?

A. Calretinin positivity in tumour cells.

B. Pankeratin AE1/AE3 positivity.

C. BAP1 loss demonstrated by IHC.

D. Increased Ki-67 proliferation index.

E. Positive WT1 nuclear staining.

Answer: C

BAP1 immunohistochemistry has transformed the diagnostic certainty in pleural pathology. BAP1 (BRCA1-Associated Protein 1) is a tumour suppressor gene on chromosome 3p21; bi-allelic BAP1 inactivation occurs in around 60 per cent of epithelioid mesothelioma and is essentially never seen in reactive mesothelial proliferations. BAP1 loss on IHC — defined as complete loss of nuclear staining in tumour cells with retained internal control staining in lymphocytes or stromal cells — is therefore a highly specific marker for mesothelioma versus reactive disease. The negative interpretation requires careful technical assessment because patchy or weak loss can be artefact. When combined with MTAP loss (surrogate for CDKN2A homozygous deletion, present in around 70 per cent of epithelioid mesothelioma) and FISH for CDKN2A, the molecular ancillaries support definitive classification in most previously equivocal cases.

Option A (calretinin) confirms mesothelial origin but does not distinguish reactive from neoplastic mesothelial proliferation. Option B (pankeratin) confirms epithelial differentiation in both reactive and neoplastic mesothelium. Option D (Ki-67) is non-specific and overlaps between reactive and neoplastic. Option E (WT1) similarly confirms mesothelial lineage but does not discriminate.

Q16.2. Distinction between solitary fibrous tumour and mesothelioma drives different management and prognosis. A 50-year-old patient has a 6 cm well-circumscribed pleural-based mass resected. Histology shows bland spindle cells in a 'patternless' arrangement with intervening collagen and characteristic 'staghorn' branching vessels. Which single immunohistochemistry pattern is most consistent with the diagnosis?

A. Calretinin, WT1, and pankeratin positive — consistent with sarcomatoid mesothelioma.

B. Nuclear STAT6, CD34, and BCL2 positive; pankeratin negative — consistent with solitary fibrous tumour.

C. S100 and SOX10 positive — consistent with schwannoma.

D. Desmin and myogenin positive — consistent with rhabdomyosarcoma.

E. CD117/KIT and DOG1 positive — consistent with GIST.

Answer: B

The defining morphological features described — bland spindle cells in a 'patternless' arrangement with intervening collagen and 'staghorn' branching vessels — are classical for solitary fibrous tumour (SFT). The molecular driver is NAB2-STAT6 fusion arising from an intrachromosomal inversion on chromosome 12q. Nuclear STAT6 immunohistochemistry is the diagnostic surrogate for the underlying fusion and is positive in over 95 per cent of SFT. CD34 is positive in around 95 per cent; CD99 and BCL2 are typically positive. Pankeratin AE1/AE3 is negative — distinguishing SFT from sarcomatoid mesothelioma which is pankeratin positive. The Demicco risk stratification model (combining age, tumour size, mitotic count, and necrosis) predicts malignant behaviour.

Option A is incorrect — sarcomatoid mesothelioma would be pankeratin positive. Option C describes schwannoma morphology different from the described features. Option D describes rhabdomyosarcoma which has skeletal muscle differentiation markers. Option E describes GIST which has different morphology and is rare in the pleura.

Q16.3. WHO 5th edition grading of epithelioid mesothelioma drives prognostic discussion. A 65-year-old man with prior asbestos exposure has a pleural decortication specimen showing epithelioid mesothelioma. Histology shows polygonal cells with moderate nuclear pleomorphism, prominent nucleoli, 8 mitoses per 2 mm squared, and necrosis affecting 20 per cent of the tumour. Which single statement best describes the WHO 5 grade?

A. Grade 1 epithelioid mesothelioma — favourable prognosis.

B. Grade 2 epithelioid mesothelioma — intermediate prognosis.

C. Grade 3 epithelioid mesothelioma — adverse prognosis.

D. Sarcomatoid mesothelioma — grading not applied.

E. Grading is no longer recommended for epithelioid mesothelioma.

Answer: C

The WHO 5th edition introduced grading of epithelioid mesothelioma based on nuclear grade (combining nuclear pleomorphism with mitotic count) and necrosis. Nuclear grade is scored 1 (mild atypia, fewer than 1 mitosis per 2 mm squared), 2 (moderate atypia, 1 to 4 mitoses per 2 mm squared), or 3 (severe atypia, more than 5 mitoses per 2 mm squared). Necrosis is scored absent or present. The combined WHO grade integrates these: grade 1 (nuclear grade 1 or 2 without necrosis), grade 2 (nuclear grade 2 with necrosis or grade 3 without necrosis), grade 3 (nuclear grade 3 with necrosis). The described tumour with 8 mitoses per 2 mm squared (nuclear grade 3) and necrosis is therefore grade 3 epithelioid mesothelioma, carrying adverse prognosis. Grade strongly predicts survival.

Options A and B understate the grade given the high mitotic count and necrosis. Option D is incorrect — the morphology is epithelioid, not sarcomatoid. Option E is factually incorrect; WHO 5 introduced grading for epithelioid mesothelioma.

16.10 Chapter EMQ

EMQ 16.1. Pleural pathology — diagnosis. For each scenario, select the single most appropriate diagnosis from the option list. Each option may be used once, more than once, or not at all.

A. Reactive mesothelial hyperplasia

B. Pleural plaque (asbestos-related)

C. Epithelioid mesothelioma

D. Sarcomatoid mesothelioma

E. Biphasic mesothelioma

F. Desmoplastic mesothelioma

G. Well-differentiated papillary mesothelial tumour

H. Solitary fibrous tumour

I. Pleural metastasis from lung adenocarcinoma

J. Pleural metastasis from breast carcinoma

(1) A 75-year-old shipyard worker has bilateral parietal pleural thickening. Biopsy shows discrete acellular plaques of hyalinised collagen with basket-weave pattern and focal calcification. **Answer: B**

(2) A 70-year-old man with asbestos exposure history has a pleural biopsy showing polygonal mesothelial cells in tubulopapillary architecture with eosinophilic cytoplasm. IHC: calretinin, WT1, D2-40 positive; BAP1 lost in tumour cells; MTAP lost; pankeratin positive. **Answer: C**

(3) A 55-year-old woman has a 5 cm circumscribed pleural-based mass. Histology shows bland spindle cells in patternless arrangement with collagen and staghorn vessels. STAT6 nuclear, CD34, and BCL2 positive; pankeratin negative. **Answer: H**

(4) A 75-year-old man has pleural biopsy showing diffuse spindle cell proliferation with high nuclear pleomorphism and pleural-based growth. Calretinin and pankeratin are positive; D2-40 is positive in some cells. MTAP is lost. No epithelioid component is identified on multiple blocks. **Answer: D**

(5) A 60-year-old woman has a pleural effusion with metastatic disease. Biopsy shows glandular architecture with mucin production. IHC: GATA3 positive, mammaglobin positive, oestrogen receptor positive; TTF-1 negative, calretinin negative. **Answer: J**

Chapter 17 — Cardiac pathology

Cardiac histopathology is concentrated in three principal areas of practice: native cardiac valve surgical specimens, endomyocardial biopsy (predominantly for transplant rejection monitoring and selected cardiomyopathy or infiltrative disease investigation), and autopsy assessment of the heart in sudden cardiac death and other contexts. The discipline is supported by a focused histological technique — a small but well-defined IHC and special stain panel — and the Banff and ISHLT classifications for transplant rejection. The FRCPath Part 1 candidate is expected to know the principal entities encountered in routine practice — ischaemic heart disease and its complications, the valvular disease spectrum, the cardiomyopathies, the inflammatory and infiltrative disorders of the myocardium, and the framework for transplant biopsy assessment.

17.1 Normal cardiac histology

The cardiac wall comprises three layers — endocardium, myocardium, and epicardium. The endocardium is a thin layer of endothelium overlying a subendothelial connective tissue layer and the subendocardial loose tissue. The myocardium is the dominant component, composed of branching striated muscle fibres with central nuclei, intercalated discs (visible on high-power examination as transverse dark lines representing specialised intercellular junctions), and supporting capillary network. Cardiomyocytes are larger than skeletal muscle fibres, have central rather than peripheral nuclei, branch and anastomose with each other, and contain a single nucleus per cell (rarely two). The epicardium (visceral pericardium) is a layer of mesothelium overlying subepicardial fat with vessels and nerves. The heart valves comprise a fibrous core with characteristic three-layered structure — fibrosa, spongiosa, ventricularis or atrialis — covered by endothelium.

17.2 Ischaemic heart disease

Myocardial infarction (MI) shows a defined sequence of histological changes over time, useful at autopsy for age determination. Within the first 4-6 hours, the gross and microscopic appearance is unchanged. From 6 to 12 hours, wavy fibres and early coagulative necrosis develop. From 12 to 24 hours, coagulative necrosis advances with hypereosinophilic fibres, pyknotic nuclei, and the onset of neutrophilic infiltration. From 24 to 72 hours, the neutrophilic infiltration is maximal with prominent necrosis. From 3 to 7 days, macrophages replace neutrophils and remove necrotic debris. From 7 to 14 days, granulation tissue with neovascularisation appears at the margins. From 2 to 4 weeks, fibrous tissue replaces granulation. From 6 weeks onward, dense collagenous scar is the dominant histology. The sequence is approximate and is modulated by reperfusion, patient factors, and infarct size; contraction band necrosis, in particular, is the classical histological signature of reperfusion injury (whether spontaneous, thrombolytic, or interventional) rather than of any specific time point in untreated infarction, and its presence in a regional infarct supports recent reperfusion.

Complications of MI include arrhythmia — a common cause of early mortality — pump failure with cardiogenic shock, mural thrombus formation, free wall rupture (typically days 3-7), septal rupture (similar timeframe), papillary muscle rupture (causing acute mitral regurgitation), Dressler syndrome (post-MI autoimmune pericarditis weeks later), ventricular aneurysm (months-years later), and the late ventricular remodelling that drives chronic heart failure. The autopsy reporting of MI documents the age of the lesion, the extent and distribution, the responsible coronary lesion (if identifiable), and any complications.

Myocardial infarction — histological time course

0-6 hours: no light microscopy changes; electron microscopy may show early features.

6-12 hours: wavy fibres, coagulative necrosis early.

12-24 hours: hypereosinophilic fibres, pyknotic nuclei, early neutrophilic infiltration. Contraction band necrosis is a reperfusion signature, not a fixed time point.

24-72 hours: maximal neutrophilic infiltration, prominent necrosis.

3-7 days: macrophage infiltration replacing neutrophils, removal of necrotic debris.

7-14 days: granulation tissue at margins with neovascularisation.

2-4 weeks: fibrous tissue replacing granulation.

6+ weeks: dense collagenous scar.

17.3 Valvular heart disease

Surgical valve specimens come most commonly from aortic stenosis, mitral regurgitation, and combined disease, with mitral stenosis (predominantly post-rheumatic in current practice) less common in Western populations. Degenerative aortic stenosis shows progressive calcification of valve cusps with thickening, distortion, and reduced mobility — the histology shows dystrophic calcification with chronic inflammation, neoangiogenesis, and lipid accumulation in the cusps in a pattern resembling atherosclerosis. Bicuspid aortic valve (a congenital variant in 1-2 per cent of the population) accelerates the calcification process and presents at younger age than the tricuspid form.

Mitral valve disease has a diverse aetiological spectrum. Rheumatic valvular disease (now rare in the UK but common globally) shows characteristic features — fibrous thickening with fusion of commissures, calcification, contracted chordae tendineae, and Aschoff bodies in active rheumatic carditis (granulomatous lesions with central fibrinoid material, surrounding macrophages, and the characteristic 'Anitschkow cells' with caterpillar-like nuclei). Mitral valve prolapse (myxomatous degeneration) shows expansion of the spongiosa layer with mucinous matrix accumulation, thinning of the fibrosa, redundant leaflet tissue, and chordal elongation. Infective endocarditis shows vegetations composed of fibrin, platelets, neutrophils, and microorganisms (with characteristic Gram-positive cocci, Gram-negative organisms, or fungi depending on aetiology).

17.4 Cardiomyopathy

The cardiomyopathies are primary diseases of the myocardium, classified by the European Society of Cardiology into five categories — hypertrophic, dilated, restrictive, arrhythmogenic right ventricular cardiomyopathy, and unclassified — with each having genetic, idiopathic, and acquired forms.

Hypertrophic cardiomyopathy (HCM) shows hypertrophied cardiomyocytes with bizarre nuclear morphology, myocyte disarray — where fibres lose parallel orientation and appear scattered at angles — interstitial fibrosis, and mural thickening. The disease is most commonly autosomal dominant from sarcomeric protein mutations (MYH7, MYBPC3, TNNT2, TNNI3, MYL2, MYL3, ACTC1).

Dilated cardiomyopathy (DCM) shows ventricular dilatation with attenuated myocardial wall, attenuation of cardiomyocytes with elongated nuclei, interstitial fibrosis, and sometimes endocardial fibrosis. The disease is genetic in around a third of cases — TTN truncating variants are the commonest single cause — and acquired causes include alcohol, anthracycline chemotherapy, peripartum disease, viral myocarditis (often parvovirus or HHV-6 in children, more variable in adults), and idiopathic. Arrhythmogenic right ventricular cardiomyopathy (ARVC) shows characteristic fibrofatty replacement of the right ventricular myocardium, particularly in the 'triangle of dysplasia' (RV inflow, outflow, and apex). The genetic basis is dominated by desmosomal protein mutations (PKP2, DSG2, DSP, DSC2, JUP).

Restrictive cardiomyopathies show reduced ventricular compliance with normal or near-normal wall thickness and ventricular dimensions. Causes include cardiac amyloidosis (light chain AL or transthyretin ATTR — distinguished by IHC and mass spectrometry subtyping; Congo red apple-green birefringence under polarised light) — idiopathic restrictive cardiomyopathy, endomyocardial fibrosis, hypereosinophilic syndrome with Loffler endocarditis, sarcoidosis, and storage diseases (haemochromatosis, Fabry disease, mucopolysaccharidoses). The diagnostic workup combines endomyocardial biopsy with specific stains, IHC, and increasingly molecular tissue subtyping for amyloid.

17.5 Myocarditis

Myocarditis is inflammation of the myocardium, classified by the predominant inflammatory cell population. Lymphocytic myocarditis (the commonest form, typically viral — parvovirus B19, HHV-6, enterovirus, adenovirus, and SARS-CoV-2 implicated) shows mononuclear cell infiltration with associated cardiomyocyte injury and necrosis — the Dallas Criteria for diagnosis require both. Eosinophilic myocarditis is associated with hypersensitivity reactions, drugs, parasitic infection, and hypereosinophilic syndrome. Giant cell myocarditis (rare, aggressive) shows multinucleated giant cells with diffuse myocardial necrosis and severe heart failure; the prognosis is poor without transplantation. Sarcoid involvement of the heart shows characteristic non-caseating granulomas and may be the dominant presentation of systemic sarcoidosis or an isolated cardiac entity.

17.6 Cardiac transplantation pathology

Endomyocardial biopsies in heart transplant recipients monitor for acute cellular rejection, antibody-mediated rejection, and recurrent or de novo cardiac pathology. The ISHLT 2004 working formulation grades acute cellular rejection on a four-grade scale: Grade 0R (no rejection), Grade 1R (mild — interstitial and/or perivascular lymphocytic infiltrate without myocyte necrosis), Grade 2R (moderate — multiple foci of lymphocytic infiltrate with associated myocyte necrosis), Grade 3R (severe — diffuse lymphocytic infiltrate with multifocal myocyte necrosis with or without oedema, haemorrhage, or vasculitis). Quilty effect — dense endocardial lymphocytic aggregates without underlying myocyte necrosis — is a non-rejection finding that should not be misinterpreted as rejection.

Antibody-mediated rejection (AMR) is identified by immunohistochemistry for CD68 (capillary intravascular macrophage accumulation), C4d (capillary endothelial deposition), and CD31 (vessel marker). AMR grading uses the ISHLT 2013 AMR grading system: pAMR 0 (negative), pAMR 1(H+) (histological only, capillary macrophage accumulation without C4d), pAMR 1(I+) (immunological only, C4d positive without histological changes), pAMR 2 (both histological and immunological), pAMR 3 (severe with associated tissue injury). Donor-specific antibody (DSA) testing in serum complements the tissue findings. Chronic rejection presents as cardiac allograft vasculopathy with concentric intimal thickening of coronary arteries.

17.7 Sudden cardiac death and other autopsy considerations

Sudden cardiac death (SCD) in adults is dominated by ischaemic heart disease (atherosclerotic coronary disease with acute coronary thrombosis or remote infarction) and hypertensive heart disease, with smaller contributions from cardiomyopathies, valvular disease, and arrhythmogenic conditions. In young SCD (under 35 years), the principal entities are HCM, ARVC, dilated cardiomyopathy, ion channelopathies (long QT syndrome, Brugada, CPVT — diagnosed by molecular testing on tissue stored from autopsy in 'molecular autopsy' workflows), myocarditis, anomalous coronary arteries, and aortic dissection. The autopsy heart is dissected systematically — short-axis slicing through the ventricles from apex to base — to allow assessment of infarct distribution and intramural lesions. Cardiac amyloidosis is increasingly recognised at autopsy as a contributor to heart failure and SCD in elderly patients (predominantly ATTR amyloidosis).

17.8 Cardiac tumours

Primary cardiac tumours are rare. Cardiac myxoma is the commonest primary cardiac tumour in adults, typically affecting the left atrium and presenting with embolic complications, obstruction, or constitutional symptoms. Histology shows polygonal myxoma cells (lepidic-like cells) within a myxoid stroma, with characteristic perivascular cuffing. Carney complex (germline PRKAR1A mutation) is the autosomal dominant syndrome that produces multiple recurrent myxomas with other features (skin and mucosal pigmentation, endocrine tumours). Cardiac fibroma occurs predominantly in children. Rhabdomyoma is associated with tuberous sclerosis. Metastatic disease to the heart is more common than primary tumour, with melanoma, lung cancer, breast cancer, and renal cell carcinoma frequent sources. Pericardial mesothelioma is rare but recognised in asbestos-exposed patients.

17.9 Reporting and key points

Chapter 17 — key points

Endomyocardial biopsy: Acute cellular rejection graded by ISHLT 2004: 0R, 1R, 2R, 3R. Quilty effect (endocardial lymphocytic infiltrate) mimics rejection.

Antibody-mediated rejection: C4d immunostaining of capillaries, intravascular macrophages (CD68), donor-specific antibody. ISHLT pAMR0–3.

Myocarditis: Lymphocytic (viral, hypersensitivity); giant cell (fulminant, life-threatening); eosinophilic (hypersensitivity, parasites); granulomatous (sarcoid).

Cardiac amyloidosis: Congo red apple-green birefringence; subtype: AL (immunoglobulin light chain), ATTR-wild type (senile), ATTR-variant (TTR mutation). Mass spec typing is gold standard.

Hypertrophic cardiomyopathy: Asymmetric septal hypertrophy with myocyte disarray, interstitial fibrosis, dysplastic intramural arteries. Sarcomere gene mutations (MYH7, MYBPC3).

Valvular pathology: Calcific aortic stenosis (age-related); rheumatic mitral disease (commissural fusion, Aschoff bodies in active phase); infective endocarditis (vegetations with organisms).

Sudden cardiac death: Conduction system review; retain tissue for genetic testing where appropriate.

17.10 Chapter SBAs

Q17.1. Histological dating of myocardial infarction is a recurring autopsy task. A 65-year-old man dies suddenly at home. Autopsy of the heart shows an area of left ventricular wall thinning with granulation tissue at the margins, neovascularisation, and early fibrous tissue extending from the periphery. Macrophages dominate the inflammatory infiltrate; neutrophils are scant. Which single estimate of infarct age is most consistent?

A. Less than 6 hours.

B. 12-24 hours.

C. 24-72 hours.

D. 7-14 days.

E. Greater than 6 weeks (old scar).

Answer: D

The appearance of granulation tissue at the margins of an infarct with neovascularisation, macrophages dominating the inflammatory infiltrate, and early fibrous tissue dates the lesion to approximately 7-14 days post-infarction. The histological time course follows a defined sequence: 0-6 hours shows no light microscopic changes; 12-24 hours shows hypereosinophilic fibres with pyknotic nuclei and early neutrophilic infiltration; 24-72 hours shows maximal neutrophilic infiltration with prominent coagulative necrosis; 3-7 days shows macrophage infiltration replacing neutrophils; 7-14 days shows granulation tissue with neovascularisation at the margins; 2-4 weeks shows fibrous tissue replacing granulation; 6 weeks onward shows dense collagenous scar. Contraction band necrosis is a reperfusion-injury feature and is not tied to a specific stage of untreated infarction. The described features fit the 7-14 day window most closely.

Option A would show no detectable changes by light microscopy. Option B would show hypereosinophilic fibres with pyknotic nuclei and early neutrophilic infiltration. Option C would show maximal neutrophilic infiltration. Option E would show dense collagenous scar without granulation tissue or active inflammation.

Q17.2. ISHLT grading of acute cellular rejection in cardiac transplant biopsies drives immunosuppression decisions. A heart transplant recipient at 3 months post-transplant has a routine endomyocardial biopsy showing multiple foci of perivascular lymphocytic infiltrate with associated myocyte necrosis identified in two of the four biopsy fragments. Which single ISHLT 2004 grade is most appropriate?

A. Grade 0R (no rejection).

B. Grade 1R (mild rejection).

C. Grade 2R (moderate rejection).

D. Grade 3R (severe rejection).

E. Quilty effect — benign finding, not rejection.

Answer: C

The ISHLT 2004 working formulation grades acute cellular rejection in heart transplant biopsies on a four-grade scale. Grade 0R indicates no rejection. Grade 1R (mild) shows interstitial and/or perivascular lymphocytic infiltrate without myocyte necrosis. Grade 2R (moderate) shows multiple foci of lymphocytic infiltrate with associated myocyte necrosis — the diagnostic feature distinguishing 2R from 1R is myocyte necrosis. Grade 3R (severe) shows diffuse lymphocytic infiltrate with multifocal myocyte necrosis, often with oedema, haemorrhage, or vasculitis. The described biopsy with multiple foci of lymphocytic infiltrate and associated myocyte necrosis fits Grade 2R.

Option A (0R) is excluded by the presence of inflammation. Option B (1R) is excluded by the myocyte necrosis. Option D (3R) requires diffuse rather than multifocal involvement with more extensive necrosis. Option E (Quilty effect) describes a different entity — dense endocardial lymphocytic aggregates without underlying myocyte necrosis — and is not the appropriate diagnosis here.

Q17.3. Cardiac amyloidosis is increasingly recognised as a cause of heart failure and sudden cardiac death, and subtyping is essential because management differs markedly. An 80-year-old man has restrictive cardiomyopathy and an endomyocardial biopsy showing extensive eosinophilic amorphous deposits in the interstitium with apple-green birefringence on Congo red staining under polarised light. Mass spectrometry on the tissue identifies transthyretin as the principal amyloid protein. Which single statement best describes the diagnosis and the implication?

A. AL (light chain) amyloidosis — chemotherapy and stem cell transplantation considered.

B. ATTR (transthyretin) amyloidosis — tafamidis approved as disease-modifying therapy.

C. AA (serum amyloid A) amyloidosis — treat underlying inflammation.

D. Beta-2 microglobulin amyloidosis — review dialysis-related causes.

E. Amyloid subtype cannot be determined.

Answer: B

Cardiac amyloidosis is dominated in current practice by two principal subtypes — light chain (AL) amyloidosis from plasma cell dyscrasia, and transthyretin (ATTR) amyloidosis from misfolded transthyretin protein. ATTR is further subdivided into wild-type (formerly senile systemic amyloidosis, predominantly affecting elderly men) and hereditary (autosomal dominant TTR mutation). Mass spectrometry on tissue is the gold standard for amyloid subtyping, with the identification of transthyretin defining the case as ATTR. The clinical implication is real because tafamidis (a transthyretin stabiliser) is approved disease-modifying therapy for ATTR cardiomyopathy with demonstrated mortality benefit (the ATTR-ACT trial). Patisiran and other RNA-targeting therapies are emerging additional options for hereditary ATTR amyloidosis.

Option A describes AL amyloidosis with different management. Option C describes AA amyloidosis associated with chronic inflammatory disease, not the typical cardiac amyloid pattern described. Option D describes beta-2 microglobulin amyloidosis associated with long-term dialysis. Option E is incorrect because mass spectrometry has already identified the subtype.

17.11 Chapter EMQ

EMQ 17.1. Cardiac pathology. For each scenario, select the single most appropriate diagnosis from the option list. Each option may be used once, more than once, or not at all.

A. Hypertrophic cardiomyopathy

B. Dilated cardiomyopathy

C. Arrhythmogenic right ventricular cardiomyopathy

D. Cardiac AL amyloidosis

E. Cardiac ATTR amyloidosis

F. Lymphocytic myocarditis (viral)

G. Giant cell myocarditis

H. Sarcoid heart disease

I. ISHLT 2R acute cellular rejection

J. Cardiac myxoma

(1) A 25-year-old man dies suddenly during sport. Autopsy shows ventricular wall thickening up to 25 mm in the septum. Histology shows hypertrophied cardiomyocytes with bizarre nuclei, myocyte disarray, and interstitial fibrosis. Genetic testing identifies an MYBPC3 truncating variant. **Answer: A**

(2) An 80-year-old man with progressive heart failure has an endomyocardial biopsy showing extensive eosinophilic amorphous deposits in the interstitium. Congo red staining shows apple-green birefringence. Mass spectrometry identifies transthyretin as the principal amyloid protein. **Answer: E**

(3) A 30-year-old woman with rapidly progressive heart failure has an endomyocardial biopsy showing multinucleated giant cells with diffuse myocardial necrosis and severe inflammation. **Answer: G**

(4) A 35-year-old man dies suddenly. Autopsy shows fibrofatty replacement of the right ventricular myocardium predominantly in the inflow, outflow, and apical regions. Genetic testing identifies a PKP2 truncating variant. **Answer: C**

(5) A 55-year-old heart transplant recipient at 4 months post-transplant has a surveillance endomyocardial biopsy. Multiple foci of perivascular lymphocytic infiltrate with associated cardiomyocyte necrosis are identified in three of four fragments. **Answer: I**

Chapter 18 — Vascular pathology

Vascular pathology covers a defined syllabus dominated by atherosclerosis and its complications, the vasculitides classified by vessel size, aneurysmal disease, venous pathology, and the surgical specimens (predominantly temporal artery biopsies for suspected giant cell arteritis) that come through routine histopathology practice. The FRCPath Part 1 candidate is expected to recognise the principal entities, apply the Chapel Hill Consensus Conference classification of vasculitis, and interpret temporal artery biopsy with the appropriate structured assessment. This chapter sets out the discipline against current consensus frameworks and UK reporting standards.

18.1 Normal vascular histology

Arteries are classified by size and structure into three categories. Large elastic arteries (aorta, pulmonary, brachiocephalic) have a thick media composed predominantly of elastic lamellae alternating with smooth muscle — supporting the windkessel function during cardiac systole. Medium muscular arteries — renal, coronary, mesenteric, femoral — have a thick media of smooth muscle with internal and external elastic laminae as distinct elastic structures separating intima from media and media from adventitia. Small arteries and arterioles have progressively thinner walls with reducing elastic content; arterioles have one or two smooth muscle layers and serve as the principal resistance vessels for blood pressure regulation. Capillaries have an endothelial layer with pericyte support; post-capillary venules show the first lymphocyte transmigration features and are the principal site of leukocyte adhesion molecule expression. Veins have a thinner wall than the corresponding artery with less elastic and smooth muscle content, frequently with valves in the limbs.

18.2 Atherosclerosis

Atherosclerosis is the systemic disease of large and medium arteries — characterised by progressive intimal accumulation of lipid, inflammatory cells, smooth muscle cells, and extracellular matrix. The lesion progression follows the AHA classification: type I (initial lesion — isolated foam cells in the intima), type II (fatty streak — multiple foam cells with lipid droplets), type III (intermediate — extracellular lipid pools), type IV (atheroma — confluent lipid core, fibrous cap not yet developed), type V (fibroatheroma — lipid core covered by fibrous cap, the classical mature plaque), type VI (complicated plaque with surface defect, haematoma, haemorrhage, or thrombosis), type VII (calcified plaque), type VIII (fibrous plaque without lipid core, the burnt-out lesion).

Plaque complications drive clinical events. Plaque rupture or fissure exposes the highly thrombogenic lipid core and tissue factor to circulating blood — triggering platelet activation and thrombus formation — the principal mechanism of acute coronary syndromes and most ischaemic strokes. Plaque erosion (intact fibrous cap with surface endothelial denudation and overlying thrombus) is a smaller fraction. Stable plaques produce flow-limiting stenosis and exertional symptoms (angina, claudication). Atherosclerotic aneurysm formation — particularly in the infrarenal abdominal aorta — follows from medial weakening with adventitial inflammation and matrix degradation.

18.3 Aneurysmal disease

True aneurysms involve all three layers of the vessel wall and are classified by aetiology and morphology. Atherosclerotic aneurysms (the dominant form, particularly in the infrarenal abdominal aorta) show medial atrophy with disruption of elastic lamellae, adventitial fibrosis, and chronic inflammatory infiltrate; the classical appearance includes a mural thrombus filling the lumen with central blood flow channel. Mycotic (infected) aneurysms show acute and chronic inflammation with organism identification on special stains and microbiological culture. Inflammatory aortic aneurysm shows prominent periaortic inflammation and fibrosis. Connective tissue disease — Marfan syndrome, Ehlers-Danlos vascular type, Loeys-Dietz syndrome — drives aneurysm formation in younger patients, often affecting the ascending aorta.

Aortic dissection follows entry of blood into the medial layer through an intimal tear, with propagation of the dissection plane along the media for variable distance. The Stanford classification distinguishes type A (involving the ascending aorta — surgical emergency) and type B (limited to the descending aorta — medical management is often initial). The histology of the resected dissection shows the intimal tear, the dissection plane in the media, and often pre-existing medial degeneration (cystic medial degeneration with mucoid pools and loss of elastic lamellae, especially in connective tissue disease).

18.4 Vasculitis

The Chapel Hill Consensus Conference (CHCC) classification of vasculitis (2012, with subsequent revisions) groups vasculitides primarily by vessel size, with additional categories for variable-vessel and single-organ vasculitis. The size-based classification informs the histological pattern, serological associations, and clinical features. Large vessel vasculitis (giant cell arteritis, Takayasu arteritis) affects the aorta and its major branches. Medium vessel vasculitis (polyarteritis nodosa, Kawasaki disease) affects medium muscular arteries. Small vessel vasculitis (ANCA-associated and immune complex) affects arterioles, capillaries, and venules.

Chapel Hill Consensus — vasculitis classification

Large vessel: giant cell arteritis (GCA), Takayasu arteritis.

Medium vessel: polyarteritis nodosa (PAN), Kawasaki disease.

Small vessel ANCA-associated: granulomatosis with polyangiitis (GPA), microscopic polyangiitis (MPA), eosinophilic granulomatosis with polyangiitis (EGPA).

Small vessel immune complex: IgA vasculitis (Henoch-Schonlein), cryoglobulinaemic, anti-GBM (Goodpasture).

Variable vessel: Behcet syndrome, Cogan syndrome.

Single-organ: primary CNS vasculitis, cutaneous vasculitis, others.

Vasculitis with systemic disease: rheumatoid, lupus, sarcoid.

Giant cell arteritis and temporal artery biopsy

Giant cell arteritis (GCA) is the principal large vessel vasculitis in older adults (typically over 50 years), with predilection for branches of the external carotid artery — the temporal artery being the standard biopsy site. The classical histology shows transmural inflammation with prominent lymphocytic, plasma cell, and macrophage infiltrate, fragmentation of the internal elastic lamina, and characteristic multinucleated giant cells. Giant cells are present in around 75 per cent of biopsy-positive cases and are not required for the diagnosis when the other features are present. Skip lesions occur — meaning that a negative biopsy does not exclude GCA — and the recommendation is for an adequate length of artery — at least 1 cm formalin-fixed — with serial sectioning through multiple levels of each block to maximise detection. Elastic stains (Van Gieson, EVG) demonstrate the fragmentation of the internal elastic lamina even when inflammation is subtle.

Healed arteritis (post-treatment or healed primary disease) shows fibrous intimal thickening, fibrosis in the media, sometimes residual focal fragmentation of the internal elastic lamina, and the absence of active inflammation. The temporal artery biopsy report should comment on the length of the specimen, the number of levels examined, the presence or absence of active vasculitis (with the type of inflammatory infiltrate), giant cells, internal elastic lamina fragmentation, and any features supporting healed arteritis. The 2022 ACR/EULAR criteria for GCA classification integrate biopsy with clinical findings.

ANCA-associated vasculitis

ANCA-associated vasculitis (AAV) comprises three principal entities. Granulomatosis with polyangiitis (GPA, formerly Wegener's) shows necrotising granulomas, mixed inflammatory infiltrate including neutrophils, and necrotising vasculitis affecting small and medium vessels; c-ANCA (anti-PR3) is the typical pattern. Upper respiratory, lower respiratory, and renal involvement are characteristic. Microscopic polyangiitis (MPA) shows necrotising small vessel vasculitis without granulomas — p-ANCA (anti-MPO) is the typical pattern. Renal involvement with pauci-immune crescentic glomerulonephritis is dominant; lung involvement is common. Eosinophilic granulomatosis with polyangiitis (EGPA, formerly Churg-Strauss) shows eosinophilic infiltrate, necrotising small vessel vasculitis, and granulomas with eosinophils; asthma and eosinophilia are clinical hallmarks; ANCA is positive in around 40 per cent (usually p-ANCA/anti-MPO).

18.5 Venous pathology

Varicose veins are the dominant venous surgical specimen — with histology showing intimal thickening, smooth muscle hyperplasia and disarray, fibrosis with replacement of normal venous wall structure, calcification in chronic lesions, and chronic inflammation. Deep vein thrombosis (DVT) is a common autopsy finding and an occasional histological identification when associated with surgical complications. Acute thrombus shows the characteristic 'Zahn lines' of alternating platelet/fibrin and red cell layers in propagating thrombi, with organisation through endothelial overgrowth and recanalisation over weeks. Pulmonary embolism complications include the saddle embolus at the pulmonary artery bifurcation in fatal cases, with smaller distal emboli causing infarcts. Phlebitis and thrombophlebitis are inflammatory and infectious conditions of the venous system.

18.6 Other vascular conditions

Fibromuscular dysplasia affects medium and small arteries — renal, carotid, vertebral being most common — with characteristic 'string of beads' appearance on angiography and histology showing layered fibrosis or smooth muscle proliferation in the media. The disease is most common in young to middle-aged women and may present with hypertension, stroke, or dissection. Thromboangiitis obliterans (Buerger disease) is a segmental occlusive disease of small and medium arteries in young smokers — with histology showing inflammatory thrombus with surrounding panvasculitis but preserved internal elastic lamina (unlike atherosclerosis). Vascular tumours — angiosarcoma (the principal malignant vascular tumour), epithelioid haemangioendothelioma (intermediate-grade malignancy with characteristic WWTR1-CAMTA1 fusion), Kaposi sarcoma (HHV-8 driven), capillary haemangioma, cavernous haemangioma, and pyogenic granuloma — span a wide histological spectrum.

18.7 Reporting and key points

Chapter 18 — key points

Vasculitis classification: Chapel Hill 2012 by vessel size: large (GCA, Takayasu); medium (PAN, Kawasaki); small ANCA-associated (GPA, MPA, EGPA); small immune-complex (IgA vasculitis, anti-GBM, cryoglobulinaemic).

Giant cell arteritis: Temporal artery biopsy ≥2 cm; serial sections; granulomatous transmural inflammation with multinucleated giant cells; internal elastic lamina fragmentation.

ANCA-associated vasculitis: GPA (necrotising granulomas, upper airway, kidney, c-ANCA/PR3); MPA (no granulomas, p-ANCA/MPO); EGPA (asthma, eosinophilia, p-ANCA in 40%).

Atherosclerosis: Foam cells, cholesterol clefts, fibrous cap, calcification. Complications: rupture, thrombosis, embolism, aneurysm.

Aortic disease: Cystic medial degeneration (Marfan, vEDS); aortitis (GCA, Takayasu, syphilis, IgG4); dissection (intimal tear, false lumen).

Peripheral nerve biopsy: Vasculitic neuropathy (mononeuritis multiplex); amyloid (Congo red); CIDP (onion-bulb formation); sural nerve standard biopsy site.

IgG4-related disease: Storiform fibrosis, obliterative phlebitis, IgG4+/IgG+ >40% with >10 IgG4+ cells/HPF.

18.8 Chapter SBAs

Q18.1. Temporal artery biopsy interpretation in suspected giant cell arteritis requires structured assessment of multiple features. A 75-year-old woman with new-onset headache, jaw claudication, and elevated ESR has a temporal artery biopsy. The 1.2 cm specimen shows segmental transmural lymphocytic and macrophage infiltration with focal multinucleated giant cells, fragmentation of the internal elastic lamina demonstrated on elastic stain, and intimal thickening. Which single statement best describes the diagnosis?

A. Giant cell arteritis — confirmed.

B. Polyarteritis nodosa — typical features.

C. Healed arteritis — no active disease.

D. Atherosclerosis with chronic inflammation.

E. Fibromuscular dysplasia.

Answer: A

Giant cell arteritis (GCA) is confirmed by the constellation of transmural lymphocytic and macrophage infiltration, fragmentation of the internal elastic lamina (best demonstrated on elastic stain), multinucleated giant cells, and intimal thickening — all of which are present in the described biopsy. Giant cells are present in around 75 per cent of biopsy-positive cases; their presence is supportive but not required when the other features are present. The clinical context (older patient, headache, jaw claudication, elevated inflammatory markers) further supports the diagnosis. The adequate biopsy length (over 1 cm) and the absence of skip-lesion concern in this case make the diagnosis straightforward. Management with high-dose corticosteroids should be initiated promptly given the risk of visual loss.

Option B (PAN) is medium-vessel vasculitis affecting different vessels — temporal artery involvement is not characteristic. Option C (healed arteritis) would lack active inflammation. Option D (atherosclerosis) lacks the transmural inflammation and giant cells. Option E (FMD) shows layered fibrosis or smooth muscle proliferation without transmural inflammation.

Q18.2. Aortic dissection assessment integrates anatomical classification with histological evidence of predisposing factors. A 45-year-old man with Marfan syndrome dies suddenly from rupture of a type A aortic dissection. The resected ascending aorta shows the entry tear and dissection plane in the media. Histology of the adjacent aortic wall shows accumulation of mucoid material in pools within the media, loss of elastic lamellae, and apoptotic smooth muscle cells. Which single statement best describes the predisposing histological abnormality?

A. Atherosclerotic plaque rupture.

B. Cystic medial degeneration (medial mucoid degeneration).

C. Necrotising vasculitis.

D. Healed previous dissection.

E. Inflammatory aortitis.

Answer: B

Cystic medial degeneration (also called medial mucoid degeneration, Erdheim-Gsell degeneration, or by the descriptive term medial cystic necrosis though no true necrosis is present) is the principal histological substrate of aortic dissection in connective tissue disease. The features include accumulation of mucopolysaccharide-rich material in pools within the aortic media, loss of elastic lamellae, and apoptotic smooth muscle cells. The pattern is highly characteristic of Marfan syndrome (FBN1 mutation) and other connective tissue diseases (Loeys-Dietz syndrome with TGFBR1/2 mutations, Ehlers-Danlos vascular type with COL3A1 mutations). The histological abnormality weakens the medial wall and predisposes to dissection.

Option A (atherosclerotic plaque rupture) involves intimal disease rather than the medial degeneration described. Option C (necrotising vasculitis) involves inflammatory infiltrate that is not described. Option D would show fibrotic and inflammatory features of healed disease. Option E (inflammatory aortitis) would show prominent inflammatory cell infiltrate which is absent in cystic medial degeneration.

Q18.3. ANCA-associated vasculitis (AAV) sub-classification informs the differential and the management. A 50-year-old woman with sinusitis, haemoptysis, and renal failure has a renal biopsy showing pauci-immune crescentic glomerulonephritis. A lung biopsy shows necrotising granulomas with mixed inflammatory infiltrate and necrotising vasculitis. ANCA serology is positive with a cytoplasmic staining pattern (c-ANCA) and positive for anti-PR3. Which single diagnosis is most consistent?

A. Microscopic polyangiitis (MPA).

B. Granulomatosis with polyangiitis (GPA).

C. Eosinophilic granulomatosis with polyangiitis (EGPA).

D. Polyarteritis nodosa (PAN).

E. Goodpasture syndrome (anti-GBM disease).

Answer: B

The combination of upper respiratory disease (sinusitis), lower respiratory disease (haemoptysis), renal involvement (pauci-immune crescentic glomerulonephritis), necrotising granulomas on lung biopsy, necrotising vasculitis, and positive c-ANCA with anti-PR3 specificity is characteristic of granulomatosis with polyangiitis (GPA, formerly Wegener's). The triad of upper respiratory, lower respiratory, and renal involvement is the classical clinical presentation. The histological features of necrotising granulomas combined with necrotising small vessel vasculitis distinguish GPA from MPA, which shows the same vasculitic features without granulomas. EGPA additionally requires asthma and eosinophilia. The serological pattern (c-ANCA/anti-PR3) is most strongly associated with GPA, although a sizeable minority of GPA cases show p-ANCA/anti-MPO.

Option A (MPA) lacks the granulomas. Option C (EGPA) requires asthma and eosinophilia which are not described. Option D (PAN) affects medium vessels with different features. Option E (Goodpasture) shows linear IgG deposition on direct immunofluorescence rather than pauci-immune pattern.

18.9 Chapter EMQ

EMQ 18.1. Vascular pathology. For each scenario, select the single most appropriate diagnosis from the option list. Each option may be used once, more than once, or not at all.

A. Giant cell arteritis (active)

B. Giant cell arteritis (healed)

C. Takayasu arteritis

D. Polyarteritis nodosa

E. Granulomatosis with polyangiitis

F. Microscopic polyangiitis

G. Eosinophilic granulomatosis with polyangiitis

H. Atherosclerotic abdominal aortic aneurysm

I. Aortic dissection with cystic medial degeneration

J. Buerger disease

(1) A 30-year-old male smoker has occlusive ischaemic disease of the digital arteries of the hands. Biopsy shows inflammatory thrombus with surrounding panvasculitis but preserved internal elastic lamina. **Answer: J**

(2) A 60-year-old man with poorly-controlled asthma, eosinophilia, and mononeuritis multiplex has a sural nerve biopsy showing necrotising small vessel vasculitis with prominent eosinophilic infiltrate and granulomas with eosinophils. p-ANCA is positive. **Answer: G**

(3) A 28-year-old woman has bilateral upper limb claudication and an absent right radial pulse. Imaging shows segmental narrowing of the subclavian arteries. A surgical specimen of the affected segment shows mononuclear inflammation in the media and adventitia of a large elastic artery, with intimal fibrosis. **Answer: C**

(4) A 75-year-old woman has 2 weeks of headache and jaw claudication. Temporal artery biopsy of 1.5 cm specimen shows segmental transmural lymphocytic and macrophage infiltration, internal elastic lamina fragmentation, focal multinucleated giant cells, and intimal thickening. **Answer: A**

(5) A 65-year-old man with diabetes and hypertension dies suddenly from rupture of a 7 cm infrarenal aortic aneurysm. The aorta wall shows extensive atherosclerotic plaque with adventitial fibrosis and chronic inflammation. Histology of the wall shows medial atrophy with disruption of elastic lamellae but no cystic medial degeneration. **Answer: H**

Chapter 19 — Thyroid and parathyroid

Thyroid pathology occupies a large fraction of endocrine pathology workload, dominated by the surgical specimen for nodular disease — by the increasing volume of thyroidectomies for differentiated carcinoma, and by FNA cytology assessment under the Bethesda framework. Parathyroid pathology is concentrated on the surgical specimen for primary or secondary hyperparathyroidism — with intraoperative parathyroid identification frozen sections as a recurring practical task. The FRCPath Part 1 candidate is expected to know the WHO 5th edition classification of thyroid tumours, the Bethesda system for FNA cytology, the molecular framework for thyroid carcinoma, and the distinguishing features of parathyroid adenoma, hyperplasia, and carcinoma.

19.1 Normal thyroid histology

The thyroid gland comprises lobules of follicles — closed spherical structures lined by a single layer of cuboidal follicular epithelium, with the lumen containing colloid (PAS-positive proteinaceous material, predominantly thyroglobulin). Follicle size varies — smaller follicles in active glands, larger and colloid-distended follicles in suppressed or atrophic glands. Subtle regional differences are recognised. Scattered parafollicular cells (C cells, calcitonin-producing) are derived embryologically from the ultimobranchial body and are concentrated at the junction of the upper third and lower two-thirds of each lateral lobe; they may be difficult to identify on routine H&E and are demonstrated by calcitonin immunohistochemistry. The thyroid receives extensive vascularity and lymphatic drainage — the latter important in carcinoma spread. The capsule is a thin fibrous layer separating the gland from surrounding structures.

19.2 Thyroiditis

Hashimoto thyroiditis (chronic lymphocytic thyroiditis) is the commonest autoimmune thyroid disease — predominantly affecting women — and shows characteristic histology — diffuse lymphocytic infiltration with germinal centres, follicular atrophy with reduced colloid, Hurthle cell change (oncocytic metaplasia of follicular epithelium with abundant pink granular cytoplasm), and progressive fibrosis. Anti-thyroid peroxidase (anti-TPO) and anti-thyroglobulin antibodies support the diagnosis serologically. The fibrotic variant shows extensive fibrous replacement; the differential includes Riedel thyroiditis (a distinct entity with dense fibrosis extending beyond the gland into surrounding tissues, part of the IgG4-related disease spectrum in many cases).

Subacute (de Quervain) thyroiditis is a self-limited post-viral inflammatory thyroiditis — with characteristic granulomatous foreign-body-type reaction to extravasated colloid, multinucleated giant cells, and follicular destruction. Painless (silent) thyroiditis and postpartum thyroiditis share features with Hashimoto thyroiditis — but with a more transient course. Graves disease is the autoimmune cause of hyperthyroidism mediated by TSH receptor-stimulating antibodies; the thyroid shows diffuse hyperplasia with tall papillary infoldings of follicular epithelium, depleted colloid (with characteristic scalloping at the colloid-cell interface), and patchy lymphoid infiltrate. Treatment with anti-thyroid drugs and radioiodine modifies the histology toward more inactive appearance.

19.3 Nodular goitre

Multinodular goitre is the commonest surgical thyroid specimen in many endocrine pathology services, and a frequent source of incidental findings. The gland shows multiple nodules of varying size with intervening relatively normal parenchyma, often with cystic change and haemorrhage. Histology of individual nodules ranges from cellular nodules with crowded follicles to colloid-distended nodules with atrophic epithelium, with frequent calcification, fibrosis, and haemosiderin-laden macrophages. Differentiating a dominant nodule in a multinodular goitre from a follicular adenoma can be challenging — the adenoma has a complete fibrous capsule and uniform architecture, while a hyperplastic nodule typically lacks a complete capsule and shows variable architecture compared with adjacent nodules. The distinction matters more for follicular carcinoma assessment. The distinction has limited clinical impact when both are benign, but the discipline of capsule and architectural assessment is also the basis for distinguishing adenoma from follicular carcinoma — the principal diagnostic challenge.

19.4 Thyroid carcinoma — WHO 5

Thyroid carcinoma classification was reorganised in the WHO 5th edition (2022) — introducing the umbrella categories of differentiated thyroid carcinoma (DTC) of follicular cell origin (further subdivided), poorly differentiated thyroid carcinoma, high-grade differentiated thyroid carcinoma (a new category), and anaplastic thyroid carcinoma. Medullary thyroid carcinoma derives from parafollicular C cells and is classified separately.

Papillary thyroid carcinoma

Papillary thyroid carcinoma (PTC) is the commonest thyroid malignancy, accounting for around 80% of cases in most series. The diagnostic features are nuclear — the classical Orphan Annie nuclei (large, oval, with cleared or 'powdery' chromatin), nuclear grooves (longitudinal indentations of nuclear membrane), nuclear pseudoinclusions (cytoplasmic invaginations into nuclei appearing as round inclusions), nuclear overlap, and crowding. These features can occur in classical, follicular, tall cell, columnar cell, hobnail, diffuse sclerosing, and other architectural variants. Psammoma bodies (laminated calcifications) are characteristic. The follicular variant of PTC — composed entirely of follicles with PTC nuclear features — is a recognised diagnostic challenge and led to the introduction of non-invasive follicular thyroid neoplasm with papillary-like nuclear features (NIFTP) for tumours previously categorised as encapsulated non-invasive follicular variant PTC with no capsular or vascular invasion. Aggressive variants — tall cell, columnar cell, hobnail, diffuse sclerosing, solid trabecular — carry worse prognosis. Molecular drivers include BRAF V600E (around 60 per cent of classical PTC) — and RAS family mutations.

Follicular thyroid carcinoma

Follicular thyroid carcinoma (FTC) shows follicular architecture without PTC nuclear features and is distinguished from follicular adenoma by the demonstration of capsular invasion (the tumour breaches the full thickness of its fibrous capsule) or vascular invasion (tumour cells within vessels of the capsule or beyond). Without invasion, the lesion is a follicular adenoma. Under WHO 5th edition

(2022), FTC is sub-classified by the type and extent of invasion into three categories. Minimally invasive FTC is defined by capsular invasion only, with no vascular invasion of any kind. Encapsulated angio-invasive FTC is defined by the presence of vascular invasion within or beyond the capsule, and is further subdivided into focal (fewer than 4 involved vessels) and extensive (4 or more involved vessels). Widely invasive FTC shows broad infiltration of adjacent thyroid parenchyma with extensive capsular and parenchymal breach. The molecular drivers are RAS mutations — NRAS, HRAS, KRAS — and PAX8::PPARG fusion. Hurthle cell (oncocytic) thyroid carcinoma — now reclassified by WHO 5 as a separate entity 'oncocytic carcinoma of thyroid' — shares many features with FTC but has a distinct molecular profile and somewhat different behaviour. The distinct designation reflects accumulated evidence.

Medullary thyroid carcinoma

Medullary thyroid carcinoma (MTC) derives from parafollicular C cells. The histology shows nests and trabeculae of polygonal or spindle cells in a vascular stroma with amyloid deposition (demonstrable on Congo red — amyloid derived from calcitonin). Calcitonin immunohistochemistry is the diagnostic IHC, with chromogranin, synaptophysin, INSM1, and TTF-1 also positive (CEA is positive and serves as a serum marker in addition to calcitonin). MTC is sporadic in around 70 per cent — and germline RET mutation in around 30 per cent (MEN2A, MEN2B, and familial MTC syndromes). Bilateral and multifocal MTC suggests germline disease. C-cell hyperplasia is the precursor lesion of MEN2-associated MTC.

Anaplastic thyroid carcinoma

Anaplastic thyroid carcinoma (ATC) is the highly aggressive undifferentiated thyroid malignancy of older patients, with median survival of months from diagnosis. Histology shows pleomorphic spindle, giant, or epithelioid cells with high mitotic activity, extensive necrosis, and invasion of surrounding structures. The differential includes high-grade sarcoma, metastatic carcinoma, and lymphoma, and the IHC panel includes thyroid markers (TTF-1, PAX8, thyroglobulin — typically negative in ATC despite the follicular cell derivation), epithelial markers (pankeratin variably positive), and exclusion markers. BRAF V600E mutation is present in around 40 per cent, and is the principal current targeted therapy opportunity (dabrafenib plus trametinib have approved indications). Routine BRAF and other molecular testing is now standard for ATC.

19.5 NIFTP and indeterminate lesions

Non-invasive follicular thyroid neoplasm with papillary-like nuclear features (NIFTP) is the WHO entity introduced in 2017 for tumours previously called non-invasive encapsulated follicular variant papillary thyroid carcinoma. The diagnostic criteria require encapsulation or clear demarcation from surrounding thyroid, follicular architecture without papillae, nuclear features of PTC (Orphan Annie nuclei, grooves, occasional pseudoinclusions), absence of capsular invasion, absence of vascular invasion, and no necrosis or high mitotic activity. The entity is treated as a low-risk lesion (effectively a borderline/indolent tumour rather than carcinoma) and managed by lobectomy alone in most cases. Recognition is important because mis-classification as PTC drives over-treatment with total thyroidectomy and adjuvant radioactive iodine.

19.6 Bethesda system for FNA cytology

The Bethesda System for Reporting Thyroid Cytopathology classifies FNA results into six categories with defined cytological features and recommended management. Category I (non-diagnostic or unsatisfactory) requires repeat FNA. Category II (benign) shows colloid nodule, lymphocytic thyroiditis, or other benign findings — surveillance without surgery. Category III (atypia of undetermined significance / follicular lesion of undetermined significance, AUS/FLUS) is the indeterminate category for ambiguous cytology, with repeat FNA or molecular testing recommended. Category IV (follicular neoplasm / suspicious for follicular neoplasm) shows a microfollicular architecture with crowded follicles and scant colloid, raising the question of follicular neoplasm; molecular testing or lobectomy is recommended. Category V (suspicious for malignancy) shows features suggesting but not diagnostic of malignancy. Category VI (malignant) confirms malignancy (typically papillary, medullary, anaplastic, or metastatic).

19.7 Parathyroid pathology

Normal parathyroid glands comprise chief cells (small polygonal cells with central round nuclei and pale or finely granular cytoplasm, the dominant cell type), oxyphil cells (larger cells with abundant eosinophilic granular cytoplasm rich in mitochondria, increasing with age), and stromal adipose tissue (typically 30-50 per cent of the gland by weight in adults). The four parathyroid glands lie behind the thyroid lobes (typically), with occasional ectopic locations (mediastinum, thymus, within the thyroid, retro-oesophageal). Parathyroid adenoma is the commonest cause of primary hyperparathyroidism (around 85 per cent of cases) and is typically a single gland enlargement with absence of stromal fat, increased chief cell density, and a rim of compressed normal parathyroid at the periphery. Parathyroid hyperplasia (around 10 per cent of primary hyperparathyroidism) involves multiple glands with similar histology — a distinction from adenoma is sometimes difficult on a single specimen and may require intraoperative assessment of all four glands. Parathyroid carcinoma (around 1 per cent) shows characteristic features — fibrous bands traversing the tumour, vascular or capsular invasion, mitotic activity over 5 per 10 HPF, marked nuclear pleomorphism — and may require parafibromin (CDC73) IHC loss for confirmation in difficult cases. The diagnostic threshold is high.

19.8 Reporting and key points

Chapter 19 — key points

Thyroid carcinoma — WHO 5: Papillary (PTC) and variants, NIFTP, follicular thyroid carcinoma (FTC), oncocytic (Hürthle) carcinoma, poorly differentiated, anaplastic, medullary.

PTC molecular: BRAF V600E (classical PTC, aggressive); RAS (follicular variant, NIFTP); RET fusions (paediatric, radiation-associated).

NIFTP: Non-invasive follicular thyroid neoplasm with papillary-like nuclear features. Strict criteria: encapsulated, no invasion, follicular architecture, PTC-type nuclei, no necrosis, low mitoses.

Follicular carcinoma: Diagnosis requires capsular or vascular invasion on the resected lesion — cytology cannot make the distinction. Minimally invasive vs widely invasive.

Medullary thyroid carcinoma: Calcitonin and CEA positive; amyloid stroma. Sporadic or MEN 2A/2B (RET germline). Pre-operative serum calcitonin diagnostic.

Anaplastic: Undifferentiated, often pan-keratin focal; BRAF and TP53 mutations common; rapidly fatal.

Bethesda TBSRTC: I non-diagnostic, II benign, III AUS, IV follicular neoplasm, V suspicious, VI malignant. Risk of malignancy and management mapped to each category.

Parathyroid: Adenoma (single gland, suppression of others), hyperplasia (multi-gland), carcinoma (capsular/vascular invasion, fibrous bands, mitoses).

19.9 Chapter SBAs

Q19.1. Distinction between follicular adenoma and follicular carcinoma is based on demonstration of invasion. A 50-year-old woman has a 3 cm thyroid nodule lobectomy. The lesion is encapsulated with follicular architecture without papillary thyroid carcinoma nuclear features. Histology shows tumour cells within a vessel located beyond the fibrous capsule. Which single statement best describes the diagnosis?

A. Follicular adenoma — benign behaviour.

B. Encapsulated angio-invasive follicular carcinoma (focal vascular invasion).

C. Widely invasive follicular carcinoma.

D. Follicular variant papillary carcinoma.

E. NIFTP.

Answer: B

The presence of unequivocal vascular invasion (tumour cells within a vessel of the capsule or beyond) defines follicular carcinoma rather than follicular adenoma. Under WHO 5th edition (2022), any vascular invasion shifts the diagnosis to encapsulated angio-invasive FTC; minimally invasive FTC is reserved for capsular invasion only, with no vascular invasion of any kind. Encapsulated angio-invasive FTC is further subdivided into focal (fewer than 4 involved vessels) and extensive (4 or more). The single focus of vascular invasion described here therefore places the lesion in the encapsulated angio-invasive (focal) category. The distinction matters prognostically: focal angio-invasive FTC has better outcomes than extensive angio-invasive disease, and both differ from widely invasive FTC, which warrants more aggressive completion thyroidectomy and adjuvant radioactive iodine.

Option A (follicular adenoma) is excluded by the presence of vascular invasion. Option C (widely invasive) requires extensive parenchymal invasion not described. Option D (follicular variant PTC) requires PTC nuclear features (Orphan Annie nuclei, grooves, pseudoinclusions) which are absent. Option E (NIFTP) requires PTC nuclear features and explicitly excludes any invasion.

Q19.2. Medullary thyroid carcinoma identification triggers specific clinical and family workup. A 40-year-old man has a 2 cm thyroid mass biopsy showing nests and trabeculae of polygonal cells with eosinophilic cytoplasm in a vascular stroma. Congo red staining demonstrates amyloid deposition with apple-green birefringence under polarised light. Calcitonin immunohistochemistry is strongly positive. Which single statement best describes the most important next clinical action?

A. Total thyroidectomy alone — no further workup needed.

B. Test for germline RET mutation to identify MEN2 / familial MTC; assess for phaeochromocytoma; assess for primary hyperparathyroidism.

C. BRAF V600E testing.

D. Radioactive iodine ablation.

E. Lobectomy alone is sufficient.

Answer: B

Medullary thyroid carcinoma (MTC) requires germline RET testing to identify MEN2 (MEN2A, MEN2B, or familial MTC) which accounts for around 30 per cent of MTC cases. The implications are real: MEN2A is associated with phaeochromocytoma (typically bilateral, in adrenal medulla, with up to 50 per cent lifetime risk) and primary hyperparathyroidism; MEN2B is associated with phaeochromocytoma, mucosal neuromas, marfanoid habitus, and characteristically younger-onset more aggressive MTC. Prior to thyroidectomy, plasma metanephrines and 24-hour urinary catecholamines should be measured to exclude phaeochromocytoma — operating on a patient with an unrecognised phaeochromocytoma carries serious anaesthetic risk. Calcium and PTH should be measured to assess for primary hyperparathyroidism. Family screening follows confirmation of germline mutation.

Option A is incomplete because the germline assessment changes prognosis and family screening implications. Option C (BRAF V600E) is not relevant to MTC (it is relevant to PTC and ATC). Option D (radioactive iodine) is not effective in MTC because C cells do not concentrate iodine. Option E (lobectomy) is inadequate — total thyroidectomy with central neck dissection is standard for MTC.

Q19.3. Bethesda system categorisation drives the management of indeterminate thyroid FNA results. A 45-year-old woman has a thyroid FNA showing a microfollicular architecture with crowded follicles and scant colloid, in the absence of papillary thyroid carcinoma nuclear features. Which single Bethesda category is most appropriate?

A. Bethesda I (non-diagnostic).

B. Bethesda II (benign).

C. Bethesda III (AUS/FLUS).

D. Bethesda IV (follicular neoplasm / suspicious for follicular neoplasm).

E. Bethesda VI (malignant).

Answer: D

Bethesda Category IV (follicular neoplasm or suspicious for follicular neoplasm) is the appropriate category for cytology showing a microfollicular architecture with crowded follicles and scant colloid, in the absence of definitive PTC nuclear features. The cytology cannot distinguish between follicular adenoma and follicular carcinoma because the diagnosis of carcinoma requires demonstration of capsular or vascular invasion on histology — which is not assessable on FNA. The recommended management is either molecular testing (with commercial assays including Afirma, ThyroSeq, or others to refine the malignancy risk) or diagnostic surgical lobectomy. The risk of malignancy in Bethesda IV is around 25-40 per cent.

Option A (non-diagnostic) would have insufficient cells for assessment. Option B (benign) would show abundant colloid with macrofollicles. Option C (AUS/FLUS) is a heterogeneous category for ambiguous cytology that does not meet the criteria for follicular neoplasm. Option E (malignant) requires definitive features of carcinoma which are absent.

19.10 Chapter EMQ

EMQ 19.1. Thyroid and parathyroid pathology. For each scenario, select the single most appropriate diagnosis from the option list. Each option may be used once, more than once, or not at all.

A. Hashimoto thyroiditis

B. Graves disease

C. Subacute (de Quervain) thyroiditis

D. Multinodular goitre

E. Follicular adenoma

F. Papillary thyroid carcinoma (classical)

G. Follicular thyroid carcinoma (minimally invasive)

H. Medullary thyroid carcinoma

I. Anaplastic thyroid carcinoma

J. Parathyroid adenoma

(1) A 40-year-old woman with progressive hypothyroidism has a total thyroidectomy. Histology shows diffuse lymphocytic infiltrate with germinal centres, follicular atrophy with reduced colloid, Hurthle cell change, and progressive fibrosis. **Answer: A**

(2) A 75-year-old man presents with rapidly enlarging neck mass and stridor. Biopsy shows highly pleomorphic spindle and giant cells with high mitotic activity and extensive necrosis. Thyroglobulin and TTF-1 are negative; pankeratin is variably positive. BRAF V600E is detected. **Answer: I**

(3) A 35-year-old woman has a 1.5 cm thyroid mass. Histology shows papillary architecture with cells having clear oval nuclei with longitudinal grooves and intranuclear pseudoinclusions. Psammoma bodies are present. BRAF V600E is detected. **Answer: F**

(4) A 50-year-old man has a 2.5 cm thyroid mass biopsy showing nests of polygonal cells with eosinophilic cytoplasm in a vascular stroma. Amyloid deposition is identified. Calcitonin is strongly positive. **Answer: H**

(5) A 60-year-old woman with primary hyperparathyroidism has a parathyroidectomy. Histology shows a 1.5 cm well-circumscribed nodule comprising chief cells with absent stromal fat, surrounded by a rim of compressed normal parathyroid tissue at the periphery. **Answer: J**

Chapter 20 — Adrenal, pituitary, paraganglioma

The remaining endocrine pathology syllabus covers the pituitary gland (neuroendocrine adenomas now reclassified as pituitary neuroendocrine tumours under WHO 5), the adrenal cortex and medulla (cortical adenomas, cortical carcinoma, phaeochromocytoma), and the paragangliomas (sympathetic and parasympathetic) with their important genetic associations. The discipline is supported by a focused IHC panel — hormone immunohistochemistry, transcription factor immunohistochemistry for pituitary lineage determination, and SDHB IHC for SDH-deficient paragangliomas — and a structured set of grading and risk stratification tools (Weiss criteria for adrenal cortical neoplasms, PASS and GAPP scores for phaeochromocytoma/paraganglioma). The FRCPath Part 1 candidate is expected to know the principal entities, the molecular and genetic framework, and the recurrent diagnostic challenges in each compartment.

20.1 Pituitary

Normal histology

The anterior pituitary (adenohypophysis) comprises endocrine cells arranged in nests and cords supported by a delicate reticulin framework. The cells are conventionally classified by H&E staining into acidophil (eosinophilic granular cytoplasm — predominantly somatotrophs and lactotrophs), basophil (basophilic cytoplasm — corticotrophs, thyrotrophs, gonadotrophs), and chromophobe (sparse cytoplasm) groups. Modern classification follows transcription factor immunohistochemistry — PIT1 drives somatotroph, lactotroph, and thyrotroph lineages; TPIT drives corticotroph lineage; SF1 drives gonadotroph lineage. The posterior pituitary (neurohypophysis) is composed of axonal terminals from hypothalamic magnocellular neurones, supporting glial cells (pituicytes), and Herring bodies (axonal swellings containing neurosecretory granules). Reticulin staining is essential for assessing adenohypophysial architecture — the normal reticulin pattern shows individual nest contours, while pituitary adenomas typically show effacement of the reticulin framework.

Pituitary neuroendocrine tumours (PitNETs)

The WHO 5th edition (2022) reclassified pituitary adenomas as pituitary neuroendocrine tumours (PitNETs), aligning the terminology with neuroendocrine tumours elsewhere. The tumours are classified by cell of origin using a structured IHC panel: hormone IHC (growth hormone, prolactin, ACTH, FSH, LH, TSH, alpha-subunit) and transcription factor IHC (PIT1, TPIT, SF1). The combined panel assigns the lineage even when hormone production is limited or absent. Functional PitNETs produce clinical syndromes — prolactinoma (the commonest functional tumour, presenting with galactorrhoea, amenorrhoea, or hypogonadism), somatotroph adenoma (acromegaly or gigantism), corticotroph adenoma (Cushing disease), thyrotroph adenoma (TSH-secreting, with thyrotoxicosis), gonadotroph adenoma (often clinically silent despite hormone production).

Non-functional PitNETs present with mass effect (visual field defect from optic chiasm compression, headache, pituitary insufficiency) without hormone-related symptoms despite gonadotroph or null cell differentiation in many cases. Aggressive variants include sparsely granulated somatotroph adenoma, lactotroph carcinoma, Crooke cell adenoma (with characteristic hyaline change), silent corticotroph adenoma, and the genetically defined plurihormonal PIT1-positive tumour (formerly silent subtype III). The 2022 WHO emphasised lineage-based classification with high-risk subtypes flagged for closer surveillance. Pituitary carcinoma is defined by the demonstration of metastasis (craniospinal or systemic) and is rare; aggressive PitNETs without metastasis are not classified as carcinoma despite their behaviour.

20.2 Adrenal cortex

Normal histology

The adrenal cortex comprises three concentric zones with distinct histology and hormonal output. Zona glomerulosa (outermost, narrow band of small cells in nests) produces aldosterone under renin-angiotensin control. Zona fasciculata (middle, broad zone of large clear cells in radial cords — 'lipid-laden' cells with prominent lipid vacuolation) produces cortisol under ACTH control. Zona reticularis (innermost, compact eosinophilic cells in irregular cord arrangement with lipofuscin pigment) produces adrenal androgens.

Cortical hyperplasia and adenoma

Diffuse and nodular cortical hyperplasia is common in patients with hypercortisolism or hypertension and may be incidentally identified at adrenalectomy or autopsy. Cushing disease (ACTH-dependent hypercortisolism from a corticotroph PitNET) drives bilateral diffuse cortical hyperplasia with cortical thickening and proliferation. Ectopic ACTH syndrome (often from small cell lung carcinoma) produces similar findings. Conn syndrome (primary hyperaldosteronism) often shows a small (under 2 cm) zona glomerulosa-derived adenoma with characteristic spironolactone bodies (eosinophilic intracytoplasmic inclusions) in treated patients, or bilateral adrenal hyperplasia with multiple aldosterone-producing micronodules.

Adrenal cortical adenoma is the principal cortical neoplasm and is typically discovered incidentally on imaging or following clinical hypercortisolism (cortisol-producing), hyperaldosteronism (aldosterone-producing), or virilisation (androgen-producing); non-functional adenomas are also common. The histology shows a circumscribed nodule of cortical cells (resembling zona fasciculata most often, with lipid-laden cytoplasm) without significant pleomorphism, necrosis, or atypical mitoses. Size is the principal feature that drives the differential between adenoma and carcinoma — most cortical lesions under 5 cm with no concerning histological features are adenomas; lesions over 5 cm or with atypical features warrant detailed assessment for carcinoma.

Adrenal cortical carcinoma — Weiss criteria

Adrenal cortical carcinoma (ACC) is uncommon and aggressive, with overall five-year survival under 50 per cent. The Weiss histological scoring system (modified Weiss) provides the diagnostic framework, with nine criteria: nuclear grade 3 or 4 (Fuhrman-like nuclear scoring), mitotic rate over 5 per 50 HPF, atypical mitoses, eosinophilic cytoplasm in over 75 per cent of cells, diffuse architecture in over 33 per cent, necrosis, venous invasion, sinusoidal invasion, and capsular invasion. A score of 3 or more supports the diagnosis of carcinoma; 0-2 supports adenoma. The reticulin pattern assessment supplements Weiss — reticulin loss/disruption supports carcinoma. The molecular landscape includes TP53 mutations (around 25 per cent), CTNNB1 mutations with WNT pathway activation (around 15 per cent), and IGF2 over-expression (frequent). Inheritance includes Li-Fraumeni syndrome (germline TP53), Beckwith-Wiedemann syndrome (chromosome 11p15), MEN1, and others. Staging follows AJCC 8 with size and extent criteria.

20.3 Adrenal medulla — phaeochromocytoma

Phaeochromocytoma is the catecholamine-producing tumour of adrenal medullary chromaffin cells. The histology shows nests and cords of polygonal cells in characteristic 'zellballen' architecture with surrounding sustentacular cells highlighted by S100 immunohistochemistry. Diagnostic IHC includes chromogranin, synaptophysin, GATA3, and tyrosine hydroxylase — the latter supporting catecholamine-producing tumour. Clinical features include hypertension (paroxysmal or sustained), tachycardia, headache, sweating, and the characteristic 'spells' from catecholamine surges.

The 2022 WHO 5 endorses the principle that 'all phaeochromocytomas have malignant potential' and abandons the prior dichotomy of benign versus malignant phaeochromocytoma in favour of risk-stratification scoring. The PASS score (Pheochromocytoma of the Adrenal gland Scaled Score) and GAPP score (Grading of Adrenal Pheochromocytoma and Paraganglioma) combine histological features (large nest size, central tumour necrosis, high cellularity, cellular monotony, tumour cell spindling, mitoses, atypical mitoses, vascular invasion, capsular invasion, profound nuclear pleomorphism, nuclear hyperchromasia) into a composite score that predicts metastatic risk. The principal risk feature in clinical practice is the presence of metastasis at distant sites without normal chromaffin tissue (lymph nodes, bone, liver, lung) — the only proof of malignant behaviour.

Hereditary phaeochromocytoma is recognised in around 30-40 per cent of cases — markedly higher than previous estimates. The key inherited syndromes include MEN2 (germline RET mutation, often bilateral adrenal phaeochromocytoma), von Hippel-Lindau syndrome (germline VHL mutation), neurofibromatosis type 1 (NF1 mutation), and the SDH-related syndromes (SDHA, SDHB, SDHC, SDHD, SDHAF2 mutations, with SDHB carrying the highest metastatic risk). SDHB IHC loss in tumour cells is the surrogate for SDH gene mutation and triggers genetic counselling and family screening. Composite phaeochromocytoma (with ganglioneuroma or ganglioneuroblastoma component) is recognised but uncommon.

20.4 Paragangliomas

Paragangliomas are tumours of paraganglia — extra-adrenal chromaffin tissue (sympathetic, predominantly thoracic and abdominal) and parasympathetic ganglia (predominantly head and neck — carotid body, jugulotympanic, vagal). Sympathetic paragangliomas are typically catecholamine-producing and present with hypertension; parasympathetic head and neck paragangliomas are typically non-functional and present with mass effect. The histology is identical to phaeochromocytoma with zellballen architecture, chromogranin and synaptophysin positivity, and S100-positive sustentacular cells.

SDH-deficient paragangliomas form a clinically distinct group — typically extra-adrenal, often multifocal, with elevated metastatic risk (SDHB mutations particularly), and identifiable by loss of SDHB immunohistochemistry. Other inherited syndromes parallel those of phaeochromocytoma. The 2022 WHO emphasises the inseparable consideration of phaeochromocytoma and paraganglioma in a single conceptual framework — sometimes denoted 'PPGL' — given their shared origin, molecular and inherited substrate, and clinical and pathological assessment.

Phaeochromocytoma and paraganglioma essentials

Architecture: zellballen — nests of polygonal cells with surrounding sustentacular cells.

IHC: chromogranin, synaptophysin, GATA3, tyrosine hydroxylase positive; S100 in sustentacular cells.

Risk scoring: PASS and GAPP integrate histological features; only metastasis proves malignant behaviour.

Hereditary: up to 30-40% — MEN2 (RET), VHL, NF1, SDHA-D, SDHAF2.

SDHB IHC loss: surrogate for SDH gene mutation; triggers genetic counselling.

SDHB mutation: highest metastatic risk among SDH genes.

WHO 5 framework: all PPGL have malignant potential; metastasis is the only proof.

20.5 Neuroblastic tumours (paediatric)

Neuroblastic tumours of the paediatric adrenal medulla and sympathetic chain form a developmental spectrum from neuroblastoma (the most undifferentiated, composed of small round blue cells with Homer Wright rosettes) through ganglioneuroblastoma (mixed component with maturing ganglion-like cells) to ganglioneuroma (fully mature, indolent). The international neuroblastoma pathology classification (INPC, also called Shimada classification) integrates histological grade with patient age to risk-stratify. MYCN amplification (assessed by FISH) is the principal adverse prognostic molecular feature and drives high-risk treatment intensification. Other adverse features include 1p deletion and 11q deletion. Neuroblastoma is the commonest extracranial solid tumour of childhood and the commonest cancer in infants.

20.6 Reporting and key points

Chapter 20 — key points

Pituitary adenomas (PitNETs): Lineage by transcription factor (PIT1, TPIT, SF1) plus hormone immunoprofile. Granularity (sparsely vs densely granulated) and aggressive markers reported.

Adrenal cortex: Adrenocortical adenoma vs carcinoma. Weiss criteria (≥3 of 9): high grade, mitoses >5/50 HPF, atypical mitoses, clear cells <25%, diffuse architecture, necrosis, venous invasion, sinusoidal invasion, capsular invasion.

Phaeochromocytoma: PASS and GAPP scores assess malignant potential but no histology reliably predicts behaviour — all are now PHEO 'with metastatic potential'. SDHB IHC screens for hereditary disease.

Hereditary syndromes: VHL, MEN 2 (RET), NF1, SDH-deficient, HIF2A. Refer all phaeochromocytoma and paraganglioma for genetic testing.

Paragangliomas: Head and neck (parasympathetic, often SDHD); thoracic and abdominal (sympathetic). Synaptophysin and chromogranin positive; S100 highlights sustentacular cells.

Neuroblastoma: INPC/Shimada favourable vs unfavourable by age, MKI, differentiation, schwannian stroma. MYCN amplification predicts poor prognosis.

INRG staging: L1 (localised, no risk factors), L2 (localised, with risk factors), M (metastatic), MS (special metastatic pattern <18 months).

20.7 Chapter SBAs

Q20.1. Adrenal cortical neoplasm differential between adenoma and carcinoma uses defined histological criteria. A 45-year-old man has a 7 cm adrenal mass resected for clinical hypercortisolism. Histology shows a partially encapsulated cortical neoplasm with nuclear grade 3, 8 mitoses per 50 HPF, atypical mitoses identified, eosinophilic cytoplasm in over 90 per cent of cells, diffuse architecture in over 50 per cent of the tumour, focal necrosis, and capsular invasion. Which single statement best describes the diagnosis under the modified Weiss criteria?

A. Adrenal cortical adenoma — Weiss score below threshold.

B. Adrenal cortical carcinoma — Weiss score 6, exceeds threshold of 3.

C. Pheochromocytoma.

D. Phaeochromocytoma with metastatic potential.

E. Adrenal myelolipoma.

Answer: B

The modified Weiss criteria assess nine histological features for adrenal cortical neoplasm classification: nuclear grade 3 or 4, mitotic rate over 5 per 50 HPF, atypical mitoses, eosinophilic cytoplasm in over 75 per cent of cells, diffuse architecture in over 33 per cent, necrosis, venous invasion, sinusoidal invasion, and capsular invasion. A score of 3 or more supports the diagnosis of carcinoma. The described tumour meets at least six criteria (nuclear grade 3, mitoses over 5/50 HPF, atypical mitoses, eosinophilic cytoplasm over 75%, diffuse architecture over 33%, necrosis, capsular invasion) — markedly exceeding the threshold and confirming adrenal cortical carcinoma. The clinical context (large size, hypercortisolism) supports the diagnosis. Reticulin loss/disruption assessment supplements the Weiss score in difficult cases.

Option A is incorrect because the Weiss score exceeds the threshold. Option C describes a different tumour type from the adrenal medulla with chromaffin cell origin. Option D similarly describes a different entity. Option E (myelolipoma) shows mature adipose tissue with haematopoietic elements.

Q20.2. SDH-deficient paragangliomas have distinct clinical and management implications. A 28-year-old woman has a 4 cm paraganglioma of the carotid body resected, with histology showing characteristic zellballen architecture, chromogranin and synaptophysin positivity, and S100 in sustentacular cells. SDHB immunohistochemistry shows complete loss of staining in the tumour cells with retained internal control. Which single statement best describes the implication?

A. No additional workup needed; tumour is sporadic.

B. Refer for germline SDHx testing and family screening; elevated risk of multifocal disease and metastasis (particularly with SDHB mutation).

C. Adjuvant chemotherapy is mandatory.

D. Radioactive iodine ablation.

E. Continue surveillance with annual catecholamines only.

Answer: B

Loss of SDHB immunohistochemistry in a paraganglioma is the surrogate marker for an underlying SDH-related germline mutation (SDHA, SDHB, SDHC, SDHD, or SDHAF2). The finding triggers clinical genetics referral, germline mutation testing, family screening, and long-term surveillance for synchronous and metachronous tumours — these mutations carry elevated risk of multifocal paraganglioma, phaeochromocytoma, and other tumours (renal cell carcinoma, GIST in SDH syndrome). SDHB mutations specifically carry the highest metastatic risk among the SDH genes (around 30-40 per cent metastatic rate), driving the importance of identifying these patients for closer surveillance. The 2022 WHO 5 emphasises that the SDH-deficient paragangliomas form a distinct clinical and pathological group.

Option A understates the implications. Option C is premature without metastasis assessment. Option D is not applicable to paraganglioma (radioactive iodine works for differentiated thyroid carcinoma). Option E understates the surveillance required.

Q20.3. Pituitary neuroendocrine tumour (PitNET) classification under WHO 5 uses lineage-based criteria. A 35-year-old man with bitemporal hemianopia and elevated growth hormone has a transsphenoidal resection of a 1.2 cm pituitary tumour. Histology shows monomorphic cells arranged in nests and cords, with marked GH positivity and PIT1 transcription factor positivity. Which single PitNET classification is most appropriate?

A. Corticotroph adenoma (PitNET).

B. Somatotroph adenoma (PitNET) — densely or sparsely granulated subtype based on cytokeratin pattern.

C. Lactotroph adenoma (PitNET).

D. Gonadotroph adenoma (PitNET).

E. Null cell adenoma (PitNET).

Answer: B

Growth hormone positivity with PIT1 transcription factor positivity classifies the tumour as a somatotroph adenoma (somatotroph PitNET). PIT1 drives the somatotroph, lactotroph, and thyrotroph lineages — discrimination among these is by hormone profile, with somatotroph adenomas characterised by GH dominance. The clinical context (acromegaly with elevated GH) confirms the functional designation. Somatotroph adenomas are further classified into densely granulated (CAM5.2 keratin positivity throughout the cytoplasm, more indolent course) and sparsely granulated (CAM5.2 fibrous body positivity, more aggressive behaviour and lower response to somatostatin analogue therapy) subtypes. The 2022 WHO 5 emphasises this lineage-and-subtype classification as informing management decisions.

Option A (corticotroph) would show TPIT positivity and ACTH production. Option C (lactotroph) would show predominant prolactin positivity with PIT1. Option D (gonadotroph) would show SF1 positivity with FSH/LH or alpha-subunit production. Option E (null cell) shows absence of all lineage transcription factors.

20.8 Chapter EMQ

EMQ 20.1. Adrenal, pituitary, and paraganglioma pathology. For each scenario, select the single most appropriate diagnosis from the option list. Each option may be used once, more than once, or not at all.

A. Somatotroph PitNET

B. Corticotroph PitNET

C. Lactotroph PitNET

D. Adrenal cortical adenoma

E. Adrenal cortical carcinoma

F. Phaeochromocytoma (sporadic)

G. Phaeochromocytoma (MEN2-associated, RET germline)

H. SDH-deficient paraganglioma (SDHB mutation)

I. Neuroblastoma

J. Ganglioneuroma

(1) A 35-year-old woman with bilateral phaeochromocytoma has germline RET M918T mutation identified on clinical genetics testing. She also has features of mucosal neuromas and marfanoid habitus. **Answer: G**

(2) A 2-year-old child has a 6 cm retroperitoneal mass. Histology shows small round blue cells with Homer Wright rosettes and high mitotic rate. MYCN FISH shows amplification with >10 copies per cell. **Answer: I**

(3) A 50-year-old man has a 4 cm adrenal mass resected. Modified Weiss assessment: nuclear grade 3, 12 mitoses per 50 HPF, atypical mitoses present, eosinophilic cytoplasm in 80% of cells, focal necrosis, capsular invasion. Score is 6. **Answer: E**

(4) A 30-year-old man with bitemporal hemianopia and acromegaly has a transsphenoidal resection. Histology shows monomorphic cells with growth hormone positivity and PIT1 positivity. CAM5.2 shows fibrous body pattern. **Answer: A**

(5) A 30-year-old woman has a 4 cm carotid body paraganglioma resected. Zellballen architecture with chromogranin and synaptophysin positivity. SDHB IHC shows complete loss of staining in tumour cells with retained internal control in stromal cells. **Answer: H**

Chapter 21 — Medical renal disease

Medical renal pathology is one of the most technique-dependent subspecialties of histopathology — combining light microscopy, immunofluorescence, and electron microscopy. The native kidney biopsy is processed with light microscopy with multiple stains (H&E, PAS, silver methenamine, trichrome), immunofluorescence covering IgA, IgG, IgM, C3, C4, kappa, lambda, fibrinogen, C1q — and electron microscopy as standard. The transplant biopsy adds C4d immunoperoxidase, BK virus assessment, and Banff classification. The FRCPath Part 1 candidate is expected to recognise the principal patterns of glomerular and tubulointerstitial disease, interpret the immunofluorescence and electron microscopy findings, and apply the Banff schema for transplant rejection. This chapter focuses on the core entities encountered in routine practice.

21.1 Normal renal histology

The renal cortex contains glomeruli and adjacent tubules with a typical glomerular density. Each glomerulus is a tuft of capillaries supported by mesangial matrix and cells — surrounded by Bowman's capsule with its parietal epithelial cells. The capillary tuft is lined by fenestrated endothelium and visceral epithelial cells (podocytes) with characteristic foot processes interdigitating across a glomerular basement membrane (GBM). The mesangium provides structural support and contains contractile mesangial cells and matrix. The peritubular interstitium contains capillaries, fibroblasts, and dendritic cells. Tubular segments include proximal tubule (brush border, abundant eosinophilic cytoplasm), thin loops of Henle, distal tubule (cuboidal), connecting tubule, and collecting duct (principal cells and intercalated cells). The renal medulla is dominated by tubular segments with vasa recta supplying the countercurrent multiplier system.

21.2 Glomerular diseases — nephrotic syndromes

Nephrotic syndrome — proteinuria over 3.5 g/24h, hypoalbuminaemia, oedema, hyperlipidaemia — reflects podocyte injury with disruption of the glomerular filtration barrier. The principal entities are minimal change disease, focal segmental glomerulosclerosis (FSGS), membranous nephropathy, and diabetic nephropathy.

Minimal change disease

Minimal change disease (MCD) is the commonest cause of nephrotic syndrome in children — and a large fraction in adults. Light microscopy shows normal glomeruli; immunofluorescence is negative or shows trace mesangial IgM; electron microscopy shows the defining finding — diffuse effacement of podocyte foot processes without electron-dense deposits. The disease is highly steroid-responsive and may remit and relapse over years. Secondary MCD is associated with NSAIDs, lithium, and lymphoma, particularly Hodgkin lymphoma.

Focal segmental glomerulosclerosis

FSGS shows focal (some glomeruli) and segmental (part of each affected glomerulus) sclerosis with hyalinosis, podocyte foot process effacement on electron microscopy, and variable immunofluorescence (often IgM and C3 in sclerotic segments). The Columbia classification identifies five histological variants — collapsing (worst prognosis, associated with HIV and APOL1 risk alleles in patients of African ancestry), tip lesion (best prognosis, more steroid-responsive), perihilar, cellular, and not otherwise specified. Primary FSGS is driven by a circulating permeability factor — suPAR among the candidates — while secondary FSGS arises from glomerular hyperfiltration in the context of obesity, reflux nephropathy, oligonephronia, or sickle cell disease. Genetic FSGS — NPHS1, NPHS2/podocin, ACTN4, TRPC6, INF2, others — is recognised particularly in steroid-resistant disease.

Membranous nephropathy

Membranous nephropathy shows characteristic GBM thickening with subepithelial 'spikes' on silver staining (the spikes represent GBM extensions between subepithelial immune complex deposits). Electron microscopy shows subepithelial electron-dense deposits with overlying foot process effacement, evolving through four Ehrenreich-Churg stages. Immunofluorescence shows granular IgG (predominantly IgG4 in primary disease) and C3 along the GBM. Primary (idiopathic) membranous nephropathy is driven by autoantibodies to phospholipase A2 receptor — anti-PLA2R, around 70 per cent of primary cases — or thrombospondin type-1 domain-containing 7A (THSD7A, around 5-10 per cent). PLA2R staining on tissue (and serum autoantibody) is the principal diagnostic marker. Secondary membranous nephropathy is associated with hepatitis B and C, lupus, drugs (gold, penicillamine, NSAIDs), and malignancy (often gastrointestinal or pulmonary in adults).

21.3 Glomerular diseases — nephritic syndromes

Nephritic syndrome — haematuria with red cell casts, variable proteinuria, hypertension, sometimes acute kidney injury — reflects glomerular inflammation. The principal entities are IgA nephropathy, post-infectious glomerulonephritis, membranoproliferative glomerulonephritis, anti-GBM disease, and ANCA-associated pauci-immune crescentic glomerulonephritis.

IgA nephropathy

IgA nephropathy is the commonest primary glomerulonephritis worldwide, particularly in East Asia. Light microscopy shows mesangial hypercellularity with variable segmental sclerosis, crescents, and tubulointerstitial changes. Immunofluorescence is the defining feature — dominant or co-dominant mesangial IgA deposition, with C3 and often IgG and IgM also present. Electron microscopy shows mesangial electron-dense deposits. The Oxford MEST-C classification grades mesangial hypercellularity (M0/M1), endocapillary hypercellularity (E0/E1), segmental sclerosis (S0/S1), tubular atrophy/interstitial fibrosis (T0/T1/T2), and crescents (C0/C1/C2), with each component contributing to prognostic stratification. IgA vasculitis (formerly Henoch-Schonlein purpura) is the systemic form with cutaneous purpura, arthralgia, and gastrointestinal symptoms; the renal histology is indistinguishable from primary IgA nephropathy.

Membranoproliferative glomerulonephritis

Membranoproliferative glomerulonephritis (MPGN) shows characteristic GBM 'double contour' or 'tram-track' appearance from mesangial cell interposition along the GBM — with mesangial proliferation, lobular accentuation of the glomerular tuft, and variable crescents. Modern classification distinguishes immune complex MPGN (driven by chronic antigenic stimulation — hepatitis C, monoclonal gammopathy, lupus, chronic infections) from C3 glomerulopathy — driven by alternative complement pathway dysregulation, autoantibodies to C3 convertase or genetic complement gene variants. Immunofluorescence is the principal discriminator — immune complex MPGN shows immunoglobulin (IgG, IgM) and complement deposition, while C3 glomerulopathy shows dominant C3 with minimal immunoglobulin.

Lupus nephritis

Lupus nephritis is classified by ISN/RPS into six classes that drive treatment decisions. Class I (minimal mesangial — normal LM, mesangial deposits on IF/EM only) and Class II (mesangial proliferative) are mild forms. Class III (focal proliferative — affecting under 50 per cent of glomeruli) and Class IV (diffuse proliferative — over 50 per cent of glomeruli) are the immunologically active proliferative classes, with active and chronic indices reported. Class V (membranous lupus nephritis — subepithelial deposits resembling primary membranous) may coexist with III or IV (denoted III+V or IV+V). Class VI is advanced sclerosing (over 90 per cent global glomerulosclerosis). Immunofluorescence shows the characteristic 'full-house' pattern (IgG, IgM, IgA, C3, C1q deposits) reflecting immune complex disease. Electron microscopy may show tubuloreticular inclusions in endothelial cells (interferon-induced structures).

ANCA-associated and anti-GBM disease

ANCA-associated vasculitis (granulomatosis with polyangiitis, microscopic polyangiitis, eosinophilic granulomatosis with polyangiitis) produces pauci-immune crescentic glomerulonephritis with necrotising features and segmental fibrinoid necrosis. Immunofluorescence shows little or no immune deposition (the 'pauci-immune' descriptor). Anti-GBM disease — Goodpasture syndrome when there is pulmonary involvement — shows linear IgG along the GBM on immunofluorescence with extensive crescent formation. Both entities are medical emergencies requiring immunosuppression and often plasma exchange.

Glomerular IF patterns at a glance

Linear IgG: anti-GBM disease (Goodpasture).

Pauci-immune: ANCA-associated vasculitis (GPA, MPA, EGPA).

Dominant mesangial IgA: IgA nephropathy or IgA vasculitis.

Granular IgG + C3 along GBM: membranous nephropathy (PLA2R+ in primary).

'Full house' (IgG, IgM, IgA, C3, C1q): lupus nephritis.

Dominant C3 alone: C3 glomerulopathy (dense deposit disease, C3GN).

Negative or trace IgM: minimal change disease.

21.4 Tubulointerstitial disease and other entities

Acute tubular necrosis (ATN) shows tubular epithelial cell flattening, loss of brush border in proximal tubule, sloughing of cells into the lumen, mitotic figures (regeneration), and intratubular casts. Ischaemic and toxic ATN are the principal forms, with renal failure recovery over days to weeks in most cases. Acute interstitial nephritis shows interstitial oedema with mononuclear (often with eosinophils) inflammatory infiltrate and tubulitis (lymphocytes within tubular epithelium); drug hypersensitivity (especially antibiotics, NSAIDs, proton pump inhibitors) is the common cause. Diabetic nephropathy shows characteristic mesangial expansion with nodular sclerosis (Kimmelstiel-Wilson nodules), GBM thickening, hyaline arteriolosclerosis (afferent and efferent), and progressive glomerulosclerosis. Hypertensive nephrosclerosis shows ischaemic glomerular changes with wrinkled GBM, tubular atrophy, interstitial fibrosis, and hyaline arteriolosclerosis with intimal fibroplasia.

21.5 Renal transplant pathology — Banff

Renal transplant biopsies follow the Banff classification, with sequential updates (Banff 2017, 2019, 2022) refining the categories. Acute T-cell-mediated rejection (TCMR) is graded based on tubulitis (lymphocytes within tubular epithelium — Banff t scores t1-t3 by severity), interstitial inflammation (i scores i1-i3 by extent), and intimal arteritis (v scores v1-v3). Banff IA (tubulitis with significant interstitial inflammation), Banff IB (severe tubulitis), Banff IIA (mild to moderate intimal arteritis), Banff IIB (severe intimal arteritis), and Banff III (transmural arteritis with fibrinoid necrosis) form the classical TCMR grades.

Antibody-mediated rejection (AMR) requires three criteria — histological features (microvascular inflammation with glomerulitis g score, peritubular capillaritis ptc score, transplant glomerulopathy chronic feature), evidence of antibody interaction (C4d deposition in peritubular capillaries, or microvascular inflammation g+ptc score 2 or greater, or specific gene expression), and donor-specific antibody. C4d immunohistochemistry on peritubular capillaries is the classical marker of complement-mediated antibody-mediated injury; C4d-negative AMR is now recognised with high microvascular inflammation scores. Chronic active TCMR and chronic active AMR are the chronic categories with active inflammation superimposed on chronic damage (transplant glomerulopathy, peritubular capillary basement membrane multilayering on EM, interstitial fibrosis and tubular atrophy).

BK virus nephropathy is identified by characteristic tubular epithelial nuclear viral inclusions ('owl-eye' appearance) with positive SV40 large T antigen immunohistochemistry. The diagnosis triggers reduction of immunosuppression. Calcineurin inhibitor toxicity shows striped interstitial fibrosis, isometric tubular vacuolisation, and arteriolar hyalinosis. Recurrent or de novo primary renal disease (FSGS, IgA nephropathy, MPGN, membranous nephropathy, lupus nephritis, anti-GBM disease) is recognised in transplants and identified by the histological features of the underlying disease alongside transplant-specific changes.

21.6 Reporting and key points

Chapter 21 — key points

Native renal biopsy: Adequate sample: ≥10 glomeruli on light microscopy. Light, immunofluorescence (IgG, IgA, IgM, C3, C1q, kappa, lambda), and electron microscopy on every case.

Nephrotic syndromes: Minimal change (EM foot process effacement, no immune deposits); FSGS (segmental sclerosis, podocyte stress markers); membranous (subepithelial deposits, PLA2R IHC); diabetic (mesangial expansion, Kimmelstiel-Wilson nodules).

Nephritic syndromes: Post-infectious (subepithelial humps); IgA nephropathy (mesangial IgA); lupus nephritis (ISN/RPS class I–VI, full-house IF); ANCA-pauci-immune crescentic; anti-GBM (linear IgG).

Thrombotic microangiopathy: Endothelial swelling, fragmented red cells, glomerular and arteriolar fibrin; aetiologies: TTP, HUS (Shiga toxin), atypical HUS (complement), drugs, malignant hypertension.

Tubulointerstitial: Acute tubular injury, acute interstitial nephritis (eosinophils, drug-related), pyelonephritis, granulomatous (sarcoid, TB, drug).

Banff transplant: T-cell-mediated rejection (tubulitis, interstitial inflammation, arteritis); antibody-mediated rejection (peritubular capillaritis, glomerulitis, C4d, DSA); recurrent disease; BK virus nephropathy.

Special techniques: EM essential for podocytopathies, Alport, MIDD; IF subtype distinguishes lupus, IgA, membranous.

21.7 Chapter SBAs

Q21.1. Immunofluorescence pattern interpretation in glomerular disease is one of the most discriminating tools in renal pathology. A 45-year-old man with nephrotic syndrome has a native kidney biopsy. Light microscopy shows uniform GBM thickening with subepithelial spikes on silver stain. Immunofluorescence shows granular IgG and C3 along the glomerular basement membrane. PLA2R immunoperoxidase on tissue is strongly positive. Which single diagnosis is most likely?

A. Minimal change disease.

B. Focal segmental glomerulosclerosis (FSGS).

C. Primary (PLA2R-associated) membranous nephropathy.

D. Secondary membranous nephropathy from hepatitis B.

E. IgA nephropathy.

Answer: C

The combination of GBM thickening with subepithelial spikes on silver stain, granular IgG and C3 along the GBM on immunofluorescence, and PLA2R tissue positivity is diagnostic of primary membranous nephropathy associated with phospholipase A2 receptor autoantibodies. Anti-PLA2R is present in around 70 per cent of primary membranous nephropathy and is a highly specific marker —

tissue PLA2R staining and serum anti-PLA2R autoantibody both support the diagnosis. The presence of PLA2R positivity distinguishes primary from secondary membranous nephropathy (the latter associated with hepatitis B and C, lupus, drugs, malignancy — all typically PLA2R-negative). The clinical implication is that anti-PLA2R-positive primary membranous nephropathy carries elevated immunosuppression and rituximab responsiveness.

Option A would show normal light microscopy and foot process effacement on EM. Option B would show focal/segmental sclerosis without the membranous features. Option D shows a different IF pattern with often full-house deposits including IgA and C1q. Option E shows dominant mesangial IgA deposition with mesangial hypercellularity.

Q21.2. Lupus nephritis ISN/RPS classification drives treatment decisions and prognosis. A 30-year-old woman with systemic lupus erythematosus has a native kidney biopsy. Light microscopy shows endocapillary proliferation and crescents affecting 60 per cent of glomeruli, with mesangial expansion and segmental necrosis. Immunofluorescence shows granular IgG, IgM, IgA, C3, and C1q (full-house pattern) in mesangial and subendothelial locations. Electron microscopy shows tubuloreticular inclusions in endothelial cells. Which single ISN/RPS class is most appropriate?

A. Class I (minimal mesangial).

B. Class II (mesangial proliferative).

C. Class III (focal proliferative).

D. Class IV (diffuse proliferative).

E. Class V (membranous).

Answer: D

Class IV lupus nephritis is defined by diffuse proliferative glomerulonephritis affecting 50 per cent or more of glomeruli. The described biopsy with proliferative changes and crescents affecting 60 per cent of glomeruli fits Class IV. Active and chronic indices are reported separately to inform treatment (active features include endocapillary hypercellularity, fibrinoid necrosis, cellular crescents; chronic features include glomerulosclerosis, fibrous crescents, interstitial fibrosis). The 'full-house' IF pattern (IgG, IgM, IgA, C3, C1q) and tubuloreticular inclusions on EM are characteristic of lupus nephritis. Class IV typically requires intensive immunosuppression with combination therapy (corticosteroids plus mycophenolate or cyclophosphamide induction, followed by mycophenolate or azathioprine maintenance).

Option A shows mesangial deposits only without proliferation. Option B shows mesangial proliferation without endocapillary proliferation. Option C requires under 50 per cent of glomeruli to be affected. Option E shows membranous features only (subepithelial deposits) without proliferative changes.

Q21.3. Banff classification of renal transplant rejection drives management decisions. A renal transplant recipient at 6 months has a biopsy for rising creatinine. The biopsy shows tubulitis with 5 or more lymphocytes within multiple tubular cross-sections (Banff t2-t3), interstitial inflammation involving 30 per cent of unscarred cortex (Banff i2), and intimal arteritis with mononuclear cells beneath the endothelium of one arteriole (Banff v1). C4d staining of peritubular capillaries is negative. Donor-specific antibody testing is negative. Which single Banff category is most appropriate?

A. Banff IA (tubulitis-only).

B. Banff IIA (mild to moderate intimal arteritis with TCMR features).

C. Antibody-mediated rejection.

D. BK virus nephropathy.

E. Calcineurin inhibitor toxicity.

Answer: B

Banff classification of acute T-cell-mediated rejection (TCMR) integrates tubulitis (t score), interstitial inflammation (i score), and intimal arteritis (v score). The presence of intimal arteritis (lymphocytes beneath the endothelium of arteries) defines vascular rejection and shifts the classification to Banff IIA (mild to moderate intimal arteritis) or Banff IIB (severe intimal arteritis or transmural disease). The described biopsy with significant tubulitis (t2-t3), interstitial inflammation (i2), and mild intimal arteritis (v1) meets the criteria for Banff IIA TCMR. The vascular features predict poorer response to standard treatment than purely interstitial TCMR (Banff IA or IB) and influence treatment intensification decisions. The absence of C4d staining and donor-specific antibody excludes antibody-mediated rejection.

Option A (IA) lacks the intimal arteritis. Option C requires C4d positivity or high microvascular inflammation plus donor-specific antibody. Option D would show characteristic intra-tubular epithelial nuclear viral inclusions with SV40 IHC positivity. Option E shows striped interstitial fibrosis and isometric vacuolisation rather than tubulitis with intimal arteritis.

21.8 Chapter EMQ

EMQ 21.1. Medical renal pathology. For each scenario, select the single most appropriate diagnosis from the option list. Each option may be used once, more than once, or not at all.

A. Minimal change disease

B. Focal segmental glomerulosclerosis (FSGS)

C. Primary membranous nephropathy (PLA2R+)

D. IgA nephropathy

E. Membranoproliferative GN (immune complex)

F. C3 glomerulopathy

G. Lupus nephritis class IV

H. ANCA-associated pauci-immune crescentic GN

I. Anti-GBM disease (Goodpasture)

J. Banff IIA T-cell-mediated rejection

(1) A 35-year-old man with haemoptysis and rapidly progressive renal failure has a biopsy showing crescents in 80 per cent of glomeruli. Immunofluorescence shows linear IgG along the glomerular basement membrane. **Answer: I**

(2) A 25-year-old man has microscopic haematuria with red cell casts after an upper respiratory infection. Biopsy shows mesangial hypercellularity. Immunofluorescence shows dominant mesangial IgA deposition with co-deposition of C3. **Answer: D**

(3) A 4-year-old boy with nephrotic syndrome has a biopsy showing normal light microscopy. Immunofluorescence is negative. Electron microscopy shows diffuse podocyte foot process effacement. The disease remits with corticosteroid therapy. **Answer: A**

(4) A 60-year-old man on transplant immunosuppression has rising creatinine at 6 months. Biopsy shows significant tubulitis, interstitial inflammation in 30 per cent of cortex, and intimal arteritis with mononuclear cells. C4d is negative; DSA is negative. **Answer: J**

(5) A 65-year-old woman with sinusitis, haemoptysis, and renal failure has a biopsy showing necrotising glomerulonephritis with crescents. Immunofluorescence shows scant immune deposition. Serum c-ANCA is positive. **Answer: H**

Chapter 22 — Renal tumours

Renal tumour pathology has undergone extensive revision in the WHO 5th edition (2022) — with introduction of new molecularly defined entities, abandonment of the previous papillary RCC type 1/type 2 subtyping, and emphasis on a molecularly informed framework for the inherited renal cancer syndromes. The FRCPath Part 1 candidate is expected to know the principal entities, apply the integrated histological and molecular classification, apply the WHO/ISUP grading and AJCC 8 staging, and recognise the inherited cancer syndromes that drive germline testing referrals. This chapter sets out the discipline against the current consensus framework.

22.1 Normal renal tumour-relevant anatomy

The renal cortex and medulla form the parenchyma, with the renal sinus containing the collecting system (calyces and renal pelvis), vessels, and surrounding fat. Renal tumours arise from each compartment — with predominantly cortical origin in the conventional renal cell carcinomas, medullary origin in collecting duct and renal medullary carcinoma, and renal pelvis origin in urothelial carcinoma. The capsule of the kidney is a thin fibrous layer — perinephric fat surrounds the capsule and is the next anatomical level for staging. Gerota fascia surrounds the perinephric fat with the pararenal fat lying outside. These layers underpin the AJCC 8 T-staging conventions.

22.2 Clear cell RCC

Clear cell renal cell carcinoma (ccRCC) is the dominant adult renal malignancy — around 70 per cent of RCC. The histology shows nests of polygonal cells with abundant clear or eosinophilic cytoplasm rich in lipid and glycogen — separated by a delicate vascular network ('chicken-wire' vascular pattern). The clear cytoplasm is due to lipid and glycogen extraction during processing — the cells appear clear on H&E with thin cytoplasmic outlines. Some cases show predominantly eosinophilic cytoplasm (the 'high-grade' eosinophilic variant). The molecular driver is loss of function of the VHL gene on chromosome 3p25 — germline VHL mutation produces von Hippel-Lindau syndrome with bilateral and multifocal ccRCC; sporadic cases show somatic VHL mutation or hypermethylation in over 80 per cent. VHL inactivation drives HIF stabilisation — angiogenesis, and the characteristic vascular pattern. Additional 3p21 alterations affect PBRM1, BAP1, and SETD2 in subsets of ccRCC — with BAP1 loss carrying worse prognosis.

Immunohistochemistry supports the diagnosis. Pan-RCC markers include PAX8 (nuclear, positive in most renal epithelial tumours), CA9 (membranous, dominant in ccRCC), CD10 (membranous, positive), vimentin (cytoplasmic). Differential negative markers include CK7 (typically negative in ccRCC, positive in chromophobe and papillary), CD117/KIT (negative). Sarcomatoid and rhabdoid differentiation may occur in any RCC subtype — and indicates aggressive behaviour. PD-L1 testing increasingly informs immunotherapy decisions in advanced ccRCC.

22.3 Papillary RCC and other epithelial RCCs

Papillary RCC accounts for around 10-15 per cent of adult RCC — the second commonest RCC subtype. The WHO 5th edition no longer subtypes papillary RCC into type 1 versus type 2 (recognising that the type 2 category encompassed multiple molecularly distinct entities — including FH-deficient RCC, MiT family translocation RCC, and high-grade papillary RCC NOS — that are now classified separately). The remaining entity 'papillary RCC' is characterised by papillary architecture with fibrovascular cores covered by single or multiple layers of cuboidal to columnar cells, often with foamy macrophages in the cores, psammoma bodies, and haemosiderin pigment. The molecular landscape includes MET pathway alterations (germline MET mutation in hereditary papillary RCC syndrome).

Chromophobe RCC shows characteristic large polygonal cells with pale eosinophilic granular cytoplasm and prominent cell membranes ('plant cell' appearance) — perinuclear halos, raisinoid nuclei, and binucleation. Hale colloidal iron staining shows diffuse cytoplasmic positivity — a useful marker but technically demanding. CK7 is diffusely positive — in contrast to ccRCC. The molecular landscape includes loss of multiple chromosomes (Y, 1, 2, 6, 10, 13, 17, 21) with TP53 and PTEN mutations. Birt-Hogg-Dube syndrome (germline FLCN mutation) is the inherited syndrome predisposing to chromophobe RCC — oncocytic-chromophobe hybrid tumours, and other renal tumours; cutaneous fibrofolliculomas and pulmonary cysts complete the syndrome.

Oncocytoma is the principal benign renal tumour — comprising nests of cells with abundant eosinophilic granular cytoplasm (mitochondria-rich), uniform round nuclei, and small nucleoli. Hybrid oncocytic-chromophobe tumours occur, particularly in Birt-Hogg-Dube syndrome. Renal medullary carcinoma is a rare highly aggressive tumour of young patients with sickle cell trait — characterised by SMARCB1 (INI1) loss on immunohistochemistry and very poor prognosis. Collecting duct carcinoma is a rare aggressive medullary tumour with tubulopapillary architecture and desmoplastic stroma.

22.4 Molecularly defined RCC entities

The WHO 5th edition formalised several molecularly defined RCC entities previously called variants. MiT family translocation RCC (TFE3-rearranged and TFEB-altered) is driven by gene fusions of the TFE3 or TFEB transcription factors with various partners. The TFE3-rearranged variant occurs predominantly in young patients and shows papillary architecture with abundant clear cytoplasm — TFE3 nuclear IHC positivity is the diagnostic marker. TFEB-altered RCC (with TFEB amplification or alternative rearrangement) is also recognised. SDH-deficient RCC (germline SDHA, SDHB, SDHC, or SDHD mutation — paralleling the SDH-deficient paraganglioma syndromes) shows distinctive cytoplasmic vacuoles or 'bubbles' with characteristic eosinophilic-cell morphology; SDHB IHC loss is the diagnostic marker.

FH-deficient RCC is driven by germline FH (fumarate hydratase) mutation in hereditary leiomyomatosis and renal cell carcinoma (HLRCC) syndrome — autosomal dominant. The tumour shows aggressive behaviour with papillary or sometimes tubular architecture, large cells with abundant eosinophilic cytoplasm, and characteristic large nucleoli with perinuclear halos (sometimes called 'inclusion-like' nucleoli — viral-like in appearance). FH IHC loss and 2-succinyl-cysteine (2SC) IHC positivity (the latter a metabolic surrogate for FH deficiency) support the diagnosis. The syndromic context (cutaneous leiomyomas, uterine fibroids at younger age in women) and family history support germline testing. ELOC-mutant RCC, ALK-rearranged RCC, and TFEB-amplified RCC are other recognised molecular entities. Tubulocystic RCC and acquired cystic disease-associated RCC are histologically defined entities.

WHO/ISUP grading of renal cell carcinoma

Grade 1: nucleoli absent or inconspicuous at high magnification.

Grade 2: nucleoli visible at high magnification (>40x).

Grade 3: nucleoli prominent at low magnification (>10x).

Grade 4: marked nuclear pleomorphism, multinucleate cells, rhabdoid or sarcomatoid differentiation.

Applies to: clear cell RCC and papillary RCC; routine grading not currently recommended for chromophobe RCC.

22.5 TNM staging and reporting

AJCC 8 staging for renal cell carcinoma records T based on size and extension — T1a (4 cm or less, confined to kidney), T1b (4-7 cm, confined), T2a (7-10 cm, confined), T2b (over 10 cm, confined), T3a (extending into perinephric or renal sinus fat, or into the renal vein, or into segmental or pelvicalyceal system), T3b (extending into vena cava below the diaphragm), T3c (extending into vena cava above the diaphragm or invading caval wall), T4 (invading beyond Gerota fascia or into ipsilateral adrenal). N category records regional lymph node involvement. M0/M1 records distant metastasis.

Reporting follows the RCPath dataset. Core items include specimen type, tumour size, histological subtype (per WHO 5), WHO/ISUP grade for clear cell and papillary RCC (with separate grading for chromophobe), sarcomatoid or rhabdoid components, presence of necrosis, lymphovascular invasion, renal sinus invasion, perinephric fat invasion, renal vein involvement, margin status, lymph node count and status, and biomarker results (SDHB IHC if SDH-deficient suspected, FH IHC and 2SC for HLRCC suspected, TFE3 IHC for translocation RCC suspected). The synoptic block supports MDT presentation and clinical genetics referral when hereditary disease is identified.

22.6 Wilms tumour

Wilms tumour (nephroblastoma) is the commonest paediatric renal tumour — predominantly affecting children under 5 years. The histology shows three components — blastema (densely packed small round blue cells), epithelial component (tubular structures, sometimes with primitive glomerular-like structures), and stroma (mesenchymal — fibroblastic, myxoid, or with smooth muscle or skeletal muscle differentiation). The proportion of each component varies; favourable histology Wilms tumour comprises around 90 per cent of cases and has excellent prognosis. Anaplastic Wilms tumour (around 5 per cent) shows nuclear enlargement (over 3x normal), hyperchromasia, and atypical mitotic figures, indicating poor prognosis. Inherited Wilms tumour syndromes include WAGR (germline WT1 deletion with aniridia, genitourinary abnormalities, intellectual disability), Denys-Drash (WT1 point mutation with renal disease and gonadal dysgenesis), Beckwith-Wiedemann (11p15 abnormalities, overgrowth syndrome), and BRCA2-associated familial Wilms.

22.7 Angiomyolipoma and other entities

Angiomyolipoma (AML) is a benign mesenchymal tumour of the kidney — composed of variable proportions of abnormal vessels, smooth muscle, and adipose tissue. The entity is part of the PEComa family (perivascular epithelioid cell neoplasms) and shows distinctive melanocytic and smooth muscle differentiation (HMB45, melan-A, SMA positivity). The smooth muscle and adipose components may predominate in different cases ('predominantly muscular' or 'predominantly fatty' variants). Epithelioid angiomyolipoma is a recognised variant with malignant potential. Tuberous sclerosis complex (germline TSC1 or TSC2 mutation) is the inherited syndrome predisposing to angiomyolipoma — typically bilateral and multifocal — with other features including cortical tubers, subependymal nodules, cardiac rhabdomyoma, and skin findings (facial angiofibromas, shagreen patches).

Urothelial carcinoma of the renal pelvis is the principal malignancy of the collecting system and is classified by the urothelial WHO framework (parallel to bladder urothelial carcinoma — covered in Vol 2). Renal pelvis urothelial tumours present with haematuria and may be associated with concurrent bladder urothelial carcinoma. Other renal entities include metanephric adenoma (a benign tubular neoplasm) and metanephric stromal tumour. Renal lymphoma is rare as primary disease but more common as part of disseminated lymphoma. Metastatic disease to the kidney is recognised (lung, breast, melanoma, and other primaries).

22.8 Reporting and key points

Chapter 22 — key points

Clear cell RCC: Commonest. VHL inactivation; 3p loss. WHO/ISUP grade 1–4 by nucleolar prominence; sarcomatoid and rhabdoid components recorded separately.

Papillary RCC: Type 1 (MET-associated, basophilic, hereditary papillary syndrome) vs type 2 (heterogeneous; HLRCC FH-deficient subgroup). Removed as distinct entities in WHO 2022 — now graded and described.

Chromophobe RCC: Plant-cell-like membranes, raisinoid nuclei, perinuclear halo; Hale colloidal iron positive; CK7+/CAIX– distinguishes from clear cell.

Molecularly defined entities: TFE3-rearranged (Xp11), TFEB-rearranged (t(6;11)), SDH-deficient, FH-deficient (HLRCC), ELOC-mutated, SMARCB1-deficient renal medullary carcinoma.

AJCC TNM 8: pT1 ≤7 cm (a/b at 4 cm), pT2 >7 cm (a/b at 10 cm), pT3a (sinus fat, renal vein), pT3b (IVC below diaphragm), pT3c (IVC above diaphragm or wall), pT4 (beyond Gerota's, adrenal direct).

Wilms tumour: Triphasic blastemal, epithelial, stromal. Anaplasia (focal/diffuse) is the principal prognostic histology; nephrogenic rests recorded.

AML and oncocytoma: AML: HMB-45, melan-A, smooth muscle actin positive. Oncocytoma: CD117+/CK7− (focal only); distinct from chromophobe RCC which is CD117+/CK7+ (diffuse).

22.9 Chapter SBAs

Q22.1. Inherited renal cancer syndromes drive distinct treatment and surveillance pathways. A 40-year-old woman with cutaneous leiomyomas and a history of uterine fibroid at age 28 has a 4 cm renal mass resected. Histology shows papillary architecture with large cells, abundant eosinophilic cytoplasm, and characteristic large nucleoli with perinuclear halos ('viral-like' inclusion-like nucleoli). FH immunohistochemistry shows loss of staining in tumour cells; 2-succinyl-cysteine (2SC) IHC is strongly positive. Which single statement best describes the implication?

A. Sporadic papillary renal cell carcinoma — no further workup.

B. FH-deficient renal cell carcinoma; refer for germline FH testing for HLRCC syndrome; family screening required.

C. Clear cell RCC — VHL-pathway driven.

D. MiT family translocation RCC — TFE3 IHC needed.

E. SDH-deficient RCC — SDHx germline testing.

Answer: B

The clinical and histological features are diagnostic of FH-deficient renal cell carcinoma in the context of hereditary leiomyomatosis and renal cell carcinoma (HLRCC) syndrome. The syndrome is driven by germline FH (fumarate hydratase) mutation with autosomal dominant inheritance, characterised by cutaneous and uterine leiomyomas (often at younger age than sporadic disease) and an aggressive type 2 papillary-like RCC with characteristic inclusion-like nucleoli. FH IHC loss and 2-succinyl-cysteine (2SC) IHC positivity (the latter a metabolic surrogate reflecting fumarate accumulation) support the diagnosis. Clinical genetics referral and germline FH testing are indicated. The implications include intensive renal surveillance, consideration of prophylactic nephron-sparing surgery, and family screening for at-risk relatives. The FH-deficient RCC is biologically aggressive and metastasises early.

Option A misses the inherited syndrome. Option C is incorrect — VHL pathway drives ccRCC, not this entity. Option D would show TFE3 nuclear positivity and is unrelated to the FH pathway. Option E describes a different inherited syndrome with different histology and SDHx mutations.

Q22.2. Histological recognition of renal medullary carcinoma is important because the entity is highly aggressive and associated with a specific clinical setting. A 25-year-old man with sickle cell trait has a 5 cm renal mass with poor prognosis on imaging. Histology shows tubulopapillary architecture with high-grade nuclei, prominent nucleoli, mitoses, and tumour necrosis. SMARCB1 (INI1) immunohistochemistry shows complete loss of staining in tumour cells with retained internal control. Which single diagnosis is most appropriate?

A. Clear cell renal cell carcinoma.

B. Papillary renal cell carcinoma.

C. Renal medullary carcinoma.

D. Collecting duct carcinoma.

E. MiT family translocation RCC.

Answer: C

Renal medullary carcinoma is a rare highly aggressive renal tumour characterised by SMARCB1 (INI1) loss on immunohistochemistry and strong association with sickle cell trait or, less commonly, sickle cell disease. The tumour typically affects young patients (median age 28 years) with male predominance and presents with advanced disease. The histology shows tubulopapillary architecture with high-grade cytology, mitoses, necrosis, and desmoplastic stroma. SMARCB1 loss (with retained staining in internal control cells confirming the tissue was preserved) is the defining feature. The prognosis is very poor — median survival under 1 year despite aggressive treatment. The 2022 WHO 5 emphasises the recognition of this entity for the implications of further workup (sickling screen if not known, family education about sickle cell trait).

Option A typically shows clear cytoplasm and a different molecular profile. Option B lacks the specific features and SMARCB1 loss. Option D is medullary but lacks the specific SMARCB1 loss and sickle cell trait association. Option E shows TFE3 or TFEB rearrangement with different morphology.

Q22.3. Differential diagnosis between angiomyolipoma and renal cell carcinoma is occasionally challenging when the AML is predominantly muscular. A 30-year-old woman with tuberous sclerosis complex has bilateral renal masses. A representative 4 cm lesion is resected. Histology shows abnormal thick-walled vessels, smooth muscle with epithelioid morphology, and small foci of adipose tissue. Immunohistochemistry shows positive HMB45, melan-A, and smooth muscle actin, with negative pankeratin, PAX8, and CA9. Which single statement best describes the diagnosis?

A. Renal cell carcinoma with sarcomatoid differentiation.

B. Angiomyolipoma — benign PEComa-family lesion; tuberous sclerosis is the inherited driver (TSC1/TSC2 germline).

C. Leiomyosarcoma.

D. Renal medullary carcinoma.

E. Solitary fibrous tumour.

Answer: B

The combination of abnormal thick-walled vessels, smooth muscle (sometimes predominantly epithelioid), variable adipose tissue, and positivity for HMB45, melan-A, and smooth muscle actin with negativity for pankeratin, PAX8, and CA9 is diagnostic of angiomyolipoma — a benign mesenchymal tumour of the PEComa (perivascular epithelioid cell tumour) family. Tuberous sclerosis complex (germline TSC1 or TSC2 mutation, autosomal dominant) is the inherited syndrome predisposing to bilateral and multifocal angiomyolipoma, with other features including cortical tubers, subependymal nodules, cardiac rhabdomyoma, and characteristic skin findings (facial angiofibromas, shagreen patches, hypomelanotic macules). Epithelioid angiomyolipoma is a recognised variant with malignant potential and is closely related to PEComa elsewhere; classical angiomyolipoma has benign behaviour.

Option A would show carcinomatous components positive for PAX8 and pankeratin. Option C would show high-grade smooth muscle malignant features and would not express melanocytic markers. Option D shows SMARCB1 loss with sickle trait association. Option E shows STAT6 nuclear positivity from NAB2-STAT6 fusion with different morphology.

22.10 Chapter EMQ

EMQ 22.1. Renal tumour pathology. For each scenario, select the single most appropriate diagnosis from the option list. Each option may be used once, more than once, or not at all.

A. Clear cell renal cell carcinoma

B. Papillary renal cell carcinoma

C. Chromophobe renal cell carcinoma

D. Oncocytoma

E. Renal medullary carcinoma

F. MiT family translocation RCC

G. FH-deficient RCC (HLRCC syndrome)

H. SDH-deficient RCC

I. Wilms tumour (favourable histology)

J. Angiomyolipoma

(1) A 4-year-old child has a 9 cm renal mass. Histology shows triphasic architecture with blastemal small round blue cells, epithelial tubular structures, and mesenchymal stromal component. Nuclei are uniform without anaplasia. **Answer: I**

(2) A 60-year-old man has a 6 cm renal mass. Histology shows nests of polygonal cells with abundant clear cytoplasm and chicken-wire vasculature. PAX8 and CA9 are positive; CK7 is negative. **Answer: A**

(3) A 55-year-old patient has a 4 cm renal mass. Histology shows large polygonal cells with pale eosinophilic granular cytoplasm, perinuclear halos, raisinoid nuclei, and prominent cell membranes ('plant cell' appearance). Hale colloidal iron shows diffuse cytoplasmic positivity. CK7 is diffusely positive. **Answer: C**

(4) A 25-year-old patient has a 3 cm renal mass. Histology shows papillary architecture with clear cytoplasm. TFE3 nuclear immunohistochemistry is positive. **Answer: F**

(5) A 35-year-old woman with TSC1 mutation has bilateral renal masses. Histology of the dominant lesion shows abnormal thick-walled vessels, epithelioid smooth muscle, and adipose tissue. HMB45 and melan-A are positive. **Answer: J**

Chapter 23 — Skin (medical dermatopathology)

Medical dermatopathology covers the inflammatory dermatoses, bullous disorders, infectious conditions, drug eruptions, and connective tissue diseases as they present on skin biopsy. The discipline is built on pattern recognition — interface, spongiotic, psoriasiform, granulomatous, vasculitic, and other classical patterns are the diagnostic framework, with direct immunofluorescence (DIF) the principal ancillary for autoimmune bullous and connective tissue diseases. The FRCPath Part 1 candidate is expected to recognise the principal entities within each pattern, interpret the DIF findings, and integrate clinical and histological information for a structured report. Cutaneous tumour pathology is covered in Volume 2 — surgical dermatopathology.

23.1 Normal skin histology

Skin comprises three layers — epidermis (stratified squamous epithelium with keratinisation), dermis (fibrocollagenous tissue with vessels, nerves, and adnexal structures), and subcutaneous tissue (subcutis, predominantly adipose). The epidermis has four layers in non-acral sites (stratum basale, spinosum, granulosum, corneum) and an additional stratum lucidum in acral sites. The basal layer contains keratinocyte progenitor cells, melanocytes (one per ten basal keratinocytes, providing pigmentation), and occasional Merkel cells (mechanoreceptors). The spinous layer shows characteristic intercellular bridges (desmosomes — disrupted in pemphigus). The granular layer contains keratohyalin granules (precursors of soft keratin). The cornified layer is anucleate keratinised material.

The dermis is divided into papillary dermis (thin layer immediately beneath the epidermis, with finer collagen, small vessels, and prominent inflammatory and lymphatic content) and reticular dermis (thicker collagen bundles, vessels, nerves, and adnexal structures). Adnexal structures include hair follicles, sebaceous glands, eccrine and apocrine sweat glands. The subcutis comprises fat lobules separated by fibrous septa containing larger vessels and nerves. The dermoepidermal junction (DEJ) is the basement membrane zone — a complex laminar structure with hemidesmosomes, lamina lucida, lamina densa, and anchoring fibrils — and is the principal site for many autoimmune blistering disorders.

23.2 Pattern recognition in inflammatory dermatoses

Inflammatory skin disease is approached by recognising the dominant histological pattern, which narrows the differential diagnosis markedly. The principal patterns are interface (dermoepidermal junction inflammation with basal keratinocyte damage), spongiotic (intraepidermal oedema with intercellular fluid accumulation), psoriasiform (regular epidermal acanthosis with thinned suprapapillary plates), granulomatous (organised collections of histiocytes), vasculitic (vessel wall inflammation with fibrinoid necrosis), and a small number of additional patterns. Each pattern has a discrete differential informed by clinical context, immunofluorescence, and ancillary findings.

Inflammatory dermatosis patterns at a glance

Interface: DEJ inflammation, basal vacuolar change, apoptotic keratinocytes. Lupus, lichen planus, GVHD, EM, TEN, drug eruption.

Spongiotic: intraepidermal oedema, perivascular lymphocytic infiltrate. Eczema, contact dermatitis, atopic, nummular.

Psoriasiform: regular acanthosis, parakeratosis, thinned suprapapillary plates, neutrophilic microabscesses. Psoriasis, pityriasis rubra pilaris, secondary syphilis.

Granulomatous: histiocyte aggregates. Sarcoid (naked), granuloma annulare (palisading), necrobiosis lipoidica, foreign body, TB, leprosy.

Vasculitic: vessel inflammation with fibrinoid necrosis. LCV, urticarial, ANCA-associated, immune complex.

Bullous: intraepidermal (pemphigus) or subepidermal (BP, DH, LABD) with DIF patterns.

23.3 Interface dermatitis

Discoid lupus erythematosus (DLE) shows classical interface dermatitis with hyperkeratosis, follicular plugging, atrophy of the epidermis, vacuolar change at the basal layer, apoptotic (necrotic) keratinocytes, basement membrane thickening on PAS staining, perivascular and periadnexal lymphocytic infiltrate, and dermal mucin (demonstrable on Alcian blue staining). DIF shows a granular IgG and C3 deposition along the dermoepidermal junction — the 'lupus band' — present in affected skin and (in systemic lupus) in unaffected sun-protected skin. Subacute cutaneous LE shows interface dermatitis with less follicular plugging and is associated with anti-Ro/SSA antibodies.

Lichen planus shows a lichenoid interface infiltrate (dense band-like lymphocytic infiltrate at the DEJ) with sawtooth rete ridges, hypergranulosis, hyperkeratosis, basal vacuolar change, apoptotic keratinocytes (Civatte bodies — eosinophilic globules in the lower epidermis), and pigment incontinence (melanin in dermal macrophages). DIF may show fibrin and IgM in Civatte bodies. Erythema multiforme shows interface dermatitis with subepidermal cleavage and apoptotic keratinocytes; the spectrum extends to Stevens-Johnson syndrome and toxic epidermal necrolysis (TEN) — both characterised by full-thickness epidermal necrosis with subepidermal cleavage. Graft-versus-host disease (GVHD, cutaneous) shows interface dermatitis with apoptotic keratinocytes, basal vacuolar change, satellite cell necrosis (lymphocyte adjacent to apoptotic keratinocyte), and lichenoid or sclerodermoid changes in chronic disease.

23.4 Bullous diseases and direct immunofluorescence

Autoimmune bullous diseases are classified by the level of cleavage and the underlying antibody target. Pemphigus vulgaris shows intraepidermal cleavage just above the basal layer (suprabasal acantholysis) with characteristic loss of intercellular adhesion (acantholytic cells). DIF shows intercellular IgG and C3 in the epidermis ('chicken-wire pattern' or 'fishnet'). The autoantibody targets are desmoglein 3 (mucosal-dominant) and desmoglein 1 (mucocutaneous). Pemphigus foliaceus shows superficial intraepidermal cleavage (within the granular layer) with anti-desmoglein 1 alone.

Bullous pemphigoid (BP) shows subepidermal cleavage with a brisk eosinophilic infiltrate in the dermis and within the blister cavity. DIF shows linear IgG and C3 along the basement membrane zone. The autoantibody targets are BP180 (collagen XVII, the hemidesmosomal transmembrane protein) and BP230 (intracellular hemidesmosomal protein). The serum BP180 NC16A ELISA correlates with disease activity. Pemphigoid gestationis is a related entity in pregnancy with the same target antigens. Mucous membrane pemphigoid (cicatricial pemphigoid) shows similar features with scarring outcomes affecting mucosae predominantly.

Dermatitis herpetiformis (DH) shows subepidermal cleavage with neutrophilic microabscesses at the tips of dermal papillae. DIF shows granular IgA deposition at the tips of dermal papillae. The disease is the cutaneous manifestation of coeliac disease (gluten enteropathy), and the underlying antibody is anti-epidermal transglutaminase (TG3) and anti-tissue transglutaminase (TG2). Gluten-free diet is curative. Linear IgA bullous dermatosis (LABD) shows similar morphology with linear (not granular) IgA along the BMZ on DIF; the disease may be idiopathic or drug-induced (vancomycin is the classical association).

Bullous disease DIF patterns at a glance

Pemphigus vulgaris: intercellular IgG + C3 in epidermis ('chicken-wire'); anti-desmoglein 3 (and 1 in mucocutaneous).

Pemphigus foliaceus: intercellular IgG + C3 in upper epidermis; anti-desmoglein 1.

Bullous pemphigoid: linear IgG + C3 along BMZ; anti-BP180 (NC16A) and BP230.

Pemphigoid gestationis: linear C3 along BMZ in pregnancy; same antigens as BP.

Dermatitis herpetiformis: granular IgA at tips of dermal papillae; gluten enteropathy.

Linear IgA bullous dermatosis: linear IgA along BMZ; vancomycin-induced common.

Epidermolysis bullosa acquisita: linear IgG along BMZ with sublamina densa pattern; anti-collagen VII.

23.5 Granulomatous, vasculitic, and other entities

Sarcoidosis shows non-caseating granulomas with relatively scant lymphocytic infiltrate ('naked granulomas'), often with multinucleated giant cells and Schaumann or asteroid bodies. The granulomas are typically dermal and may involve the subcutis (subcutaneous sarcoid — Darier-Roussy). Granuloma annulare shows characteristic palisading granulomas around foci of degenerated collagen and mucin in the mid-to-deep dermis. Necrobiosis lipoidica (associated with diabetes) shows broad zones of altered collagen ('necrobiosis') with palisading granulomas and prominent plasma cells, often with vascular involvement. Cutaneous tuberculosis (lupus vulgaris, erythema induratum) and leprosy (tuberculoid versus lepromatous spectrum) are infectious granulomatous diseases with specific morphological features.

Leukocytoclastic vasculitis (LCV) is the principal small vessel cutaneous vasculitis, characterised by neutrophilic infiltration of small dermal vessels with fibrinoid necrosis of vessel walls and karyorrhectic debris ('leukocytoclasia' — nuclear dust). DIF may show IgA in dermal vessels (supporting IgA vasculitis, formerly Henoch-Schonlein purpura) or IgG/C3 in immune complex disease. Urticarial vasculitis shows similar features with overlying urticaria. The cutaneous vasculitides are sub-classified per Chapel Hill principles (see Chapter 18). Drug eruptions can produce a wide range of morphological patterns — morbilliform (the commonest), urticarial, vasculitic, lichenoid, fixed drug eruption, DRESS syndrome, TEN/SJS. The clinical history of recent drug exposure is the principal diagnostic tool.

Cutaneous connective tissue disease produces characteristic patterns. Discoid lupus is interface as discussed. Systemic sclerosis (scleroderma) shows progressive dermal fibrosis with thickened collagen bundles, loss of adnexal structures, and atrophy of the epidermis. Morphea (localised scleroderma) shows similar fibrosis without systemic features. Dermatomyositis shows interface dermatitis with prominent dermal mucin and a clinical context (heliotrope rash, Gottron papules, proximal muscle weakness). The candidate should integrate clinical and histological features for the connective tissue diseases.

23.6 Reporting and key points

Chapter 23 — key points

Reaction patterns: Psoriasiform, spongiotic, lichenoid, vesiculobullous, granulomatous, vasculitic, panniculitic, perivascular dermatitis.

Psoriasis: Regular acanthosis, parakeratosis, Munro microabscesses, Kogoj pustules, suprapapillary plate thinning, dilated dermal capillaries.

Lichen planus: Wedge-shaped hypergranulosis, sawtooth rete, lichenoid band, Civatte (apoptotic) bodies, pigment incontinence.

Bullous diseases — DIF: Pemphigus vulgaris (intercellular IgG/C3, suprabasal split); bullous pemphigoid (linear BMZ IgG/C3, subepidermal split with eosinophils); dermatitis herpetiformis (granular IgA at papillary tips); linear IgA disease (linear IgA at BMZ); pemphigoid gestationis (linear C3 at BMZ).

Granulomatous dermatoses: Sarcoid (naked granulomas), TB (caseation), leprosy (perineural granulomas, AFB on Fite stain), granuloma annulare (palisaded with central mucin), necrobiosis lipoidica (palisaded with central degenerated collagen).

Cutaneous vasculitis: Leukocytoclastic small vessel (palpable purpura, IgA in HSP); medium vessel (PAN, livedo, ulcers); ANCA-associated (GPA, MPA, EGPA); recognise mimics — pigmented purpuric dermatoses, Schamberg disease.

Panniculitis: Septal (erythema nodosum, scleroderma morphea-related) vs lobular (lupus profundus, pancreatic, alpha-1 antitrypsin, infective, cytophagic histiocytic).

23.7 Chapter SBAs

Q23.1. Recognition of pemphigus vulgaris versus bullous pemphigoid is the central diagnostic question in autoimmune bullous disease. A 60-year-old woman with widespread blistering has a skin biopsy showing intraepidermal cleavage just above the basal layer with characteristic acantholytic cells in the blister cavity. Direct immunofluorescence shows intercellular IgG and C3 in the epidermis with the classical 'chicken-wire' pattern. Which single statement best describes the diagnosis and the underlying autoantibody target?

A. Bullous pemphigoid — anti-BP180.

B. Pemphigus vulgaris — anti-desmoglein 3 (with anti-desmoglein 1 in mucocutaneous disease).

C. Dermatitis herpetiformis — anti-epidermal transglutaminase.

D. Linear IgA bullous dermatosis — anti-LAD-1.

E. Epidermolysis bullosa acquisita — anti-collagen VII.

Answer: B

Pemphigus vulgaris is characterised by intraepidermal cleavage just above the basal layer (suprabasal acantholysis) with loss of intercellular adhesion producing acantholytic cells. The DIF pattern of intercellular IgG and C3 in the epidermis ('chicken-wire' or 'fishnet') is diagnostic. The autoantibody target is desmoglein 3 (the principal target in mucosal-dominant pemphigus vulgaris) with additional anti-desmoglein 1 antibody in mucocutaneous disease (explaining the spread to the skin in addition to mucosae). Pemphigus foliaceus by contrast shows superficial intraepidermal cleavage in the granular layer with anti-desmoglein 1 alone — explaining the typical sparing of mucous membranes which express predominantly desmoglein 3.

Option A (BP) shows subepidermal cleavage with linear BMZ deposition and anti-BP180. Option C (DH) shows granular IgA at tips of dermal papillae and gluten enteropathy. Option D (LABD) shows linear IgA along the BMZ. Option E (EBA) shows linear IgG along the BMZ with sublamina densa pattern and is anti-collagen VII.

Q23.2. Direct immunofluorescence patterns are highly specific for individual bullous diseases. A 45-year-old man with intensely pruritic vesicles on the elbows, knees, and buttocks has a skin biopsy. Light microscopy shows subepidermal cleavage with neutrophilic microabscesses at the tips of dermal papillae. DIF shows granular IgA deposition at the tips of dermal papillae. Anti-tissue transglutaminase serology is positive. Which single statement best describes the diagnosis and the associated systemic disease?

A. Bullous pemphigoid — no systemic association.

B. Pemphigus vulgaris — paraneoplastic association.

C. Dermatitis herpetiformis — gluten enteropathy (coeliac disease) is the underlying systemic disease.

D. Linear IgA bullous dermatosis — drug-induced.

E. Epidermolysis bullosa acquisita — anti-collagen VII.

Answer: C

Dermatitis herpetiformis (DH) is the cutaneous manifestation of coeliac disease (gluten enteropathy), characterised by intensely pruritic grouped vesicles on extensor surfaces (elbows, knees, buttocks).

The histology shows subepidermal cleavage with neutrophilic microabscesses at the tips of dermal papillae. DIF shows granular IgA at the tips of dermal papillae — the defining diagnostic feature. The autoantibody targets are epidermal transglutaminase (TG3) and tissue transglutaminase (TG2), both involved in the cross-reactivity between cutaneous and intestinal autoimmunity. Anti-tissue transglutaminase serology supports the diagnosis. The systemic implications include nutritional consequences of coeliac disease, increased risk of small bowel lymphoma, and need for gluten-free diet (which usually controls both the skin and intestinal disease).

Option A would show linear IgG/C3 along the BMZ. Option B shows intercellular IgG+C3 in the epidermis. Option D shows linear IgA. Option E shows linear IgG with sublamina densa pattern.

Q23.3. Granulomatous dermatitis differential is structured by the type and pattern of granulomas. A 45-year-old woman with type 1 diabetes has bilateral pretibial plaques. Biopsy shows broad zones of altered ('necrobiotic') collagen in the mid-to-deep dermis with palisading histiocytes at the periphery, scattered multinucleated giant cells, prominent plasma cells, and characteristic vascular involvement. Mucin is not particularly prominent. Which single diagnosis is most appropriate?

A. Sarcoidosis.

B. Granuloma annulare.

C. Necrobiosis lipoidica.

D. Foreign body granuloma.

E. Lupus vulgaris (cutaneous tuberculosis).

Answer: C

Necrobiosis lipoidica is the granulomatous dermatosis classically associated with diabetes mellitus (around 60 per cent of cases occur in diabetic patients, though the entity may occur in non-diabetic patients). The clinical presentation is typically bilateral pretibial plaques with characteristic yellow-brown atrophic centres and telangiectasias. The histology shows broad zones of altered ('necrobiotic') collagen in the mid-to-deep dermis with palisading histiocytes at the periphery, multinucleated giant cells, prominent plasma cells (in contrast to most other granulomatous dermatoses), and characteristic vascular involvement (sometimes with frank vasculitis). Mucin is typically minimal — distinguishing necrobiosis lipoidica from granuloma annulare, which shows prominent mucin in the centres of granulomas.

Option A (sarcoid) shows naked granulomas without prominent plasma cells or necrobiosis. Option B (granuloma annulare) shows palisading granulomas with prominent central mucin and no plasma cells. Option D (foreign body) shows polarisable material or birefringent fragments. Option E (cutaneous TB) requires demonstration of acid-fast bacilli or positive PCR.

23.8 Chapter EMQ

EMQ 23.1. Medical dermatopathology. For each scenario, select the single most appropriate diagnosis from the option list. Each option may be used once, more than once, or not at all.

A. Pemphigus vulgaris

B. Pemphigus foliaceus

C. Bullous pemphigoid

D. Dermatitis herpetiformis

E. Linear IgA bullous dermatosis

F. Discoid lupus erythematosus

G. Lichen planus

H. Sarcoidosis

I. Granuloma annulare

J. Necrobiosis lipoidica

(1) A 60-year-old man with mucosal and skin blisters has a biopsy showing suprabasal acantholysis. DIF shows intercellular IgG and C3 in the epidermis. Anti-desmoglein 3 antibodies are detected. **Answer: A**

(2) A 35-year-old man with intensely pruritic vesicles on elbows and knees has a biopsy showing subepidermal blister with neutrophilic microabscesses at dermal papillary tips. DIF shows granular IgA at dermal papillae tips. **Answer: D**

(3) A 40-year-old woman with a malar rash has a facial biopsy showing hyperkeratosis, follicular plugging, basal vacuolar change, periadnexal lymphocytic infiltrate, and dermal mucin. DIF shows granular IgG and C3 along the dermoepidermal junction ('lupus band'). **Answer: F**

(4) A 50-year-old patient has annular plaques on the dorsum of the hands. Biopsy shows palisading histiocytes around foci of degenerated collagen and prominent mucin in the mid-dermis. **Answer: I**

(5) A 55-year-old patient on vancomycin therapy develops tense subepidermal vesiculobullous lesions. Biopsy shows subepidermal blister with neutrophilic infiltrate. DIF shows linear IgA along the basement membrane zone. **Answer: E**

Abbreviations

The list below collates abbreviations used across both volumes of this companion series. Abbreviations not included here are spelled out at first use in the relevant chapter. Where an abbreviation is contested or has shifted with classification revision — for instance the replacement of bronchioloalveolar carcinoma terminology in current WHO usage — the legacy term is annotated.

AAH	atypical adenomatous hyperplasia (lung)	**HPV**	human papillomavirus
ABMR	antibody-mediated rejection	**IBD**	inflammatory bowel disease
AIN	acute interstitial nephritis; anal intraepithelial neoplasia	**ICCR**	International Collaboration on Cancer Reporting
AJCC	American Joint Committee on Cancer	**IF**	immunofluorescence
AMR	antibody-mediated rejection	**IgA**	immunoglobulin A
ANCA	antineutrophil cytoplasmic antibody	**IHC**	immunohistochemistry
ARDS	acute respiratory distress syndrome	**IPMN**	intraductal papillary mucinous neoplasm
BAC	bronchioloalveolar carcinoma (legacy term)	**IPF**	idiopathic pulmonary fibrosis
BSH	British Society for Haematology	**ISH**	in situ hybridisation
CD	cluster of differentiation	**KRAS**	Kirsten rat sarcoma viral oncogene
CIN	cervical intraepithelial neoplasia	**LCNEC**	large cell neuroendocrine carcinoma
CK	cytokeratin	**MEN**	multiple endocrine neoplasia
CKD	chronic kidney disease	**MMR**	mismatch repair
CRC	colorectal carcinoma	**MPN**	myeloproliferative neoplasm
DAB	3,3′-diaminobenzidine	**MSI**	microsatellite instability
DCD	donation after circulatory death	**NAFLD**	non-alcoholic fatty liver disease
DLBCL	diffuse large B-cell lymphoma	**NASH**	non-alcoholic steatohepatitis
EGFR	epidermal growth factor receptor	**NICE**	National Institute for Health and Care Excellence
EMQ	extended matching question	**NSCLC**	non-small cell lung carcinoma
FFPE	formalin-fixed, paraffin-embedded	**NSIP**	non-specific interstitial pneumonia
FISH	fluorescence in situ hybridisation	**pCR**	pathological complete response
FNA	fine-needle aspiration	**PTC**	papillary thyroid carcinoma
FNAC	fine-needle aspiration cytology	**PTLD**	post-transplant lymphoproliferative disorder
FRCPath	Fellowship of the Royal College of Pathologists	**RCPath**	Royal College of Pathologists
FSGS	focal segmental glomerulosclerosis	**SBA**	single best answer
FTC	follicular thyroid carcinoma	**SCC**	squamous cell carcinoma
FNH	focal nodular hyperplasia	**SCLC**	small cell lung carcinoma
GBM	glomerular basement membrane	**TBM**	tubular basement membrane

GIST	gastrointestinal stromal tumour	**TCC**	transitional cell carcinoma (legacy term)
GIT	gastrointestinal tract	**TCMR**	T-cell-mediated rejection
H&E	haematoxylin and eosin	**TMA**	thrombotic microangiopathy
HCC	hepatocellular carcinoma	**TNM**	tumour, node, metastasis
HER2	human epidermal growth factor receptor 2	**UC**	ulcerative colitis
HIV	human immunodeficiency virus	**UIP**	usual interstitial pneumonia
HSV	herpes simplex virus	**WHO**	World Health Organization

Key Sources and Further Reading

Citation across both volumes is restricted to the following authoritative source set. Secondary textbooks and uncurated online compendia are not cited. Readers are directed to the most recent versions of each document; revision dates change frequently, and the version current at the time of manuscript completion (May 2026) is annotated where ambiguity may arise.

WHO Classification of Tumours, Fifth Edition (Blue Books)

The fifth edition of the WHO Classification of Tumours — the canonical reference for tumour nomenclature, grading, and biological behaviour across this volume — supersedes the fourth edition site by site as each new fascicle is published. The relevant individual volumes for Volume 1 are listed below; further volumes covering the systems addressed in Volume 2 of this companion are listed in the corresponding back matter of that volume.

WHO Classification of Tumours Editorial Board. Digestive System Tumours. 5th ed. Lyon: International Agency for Research on Cancer; 2019.

WHO Classification of Tumours Editorial Board. Thoracic Tumours. 5th ed. Lyon: International Agency for Research on Cancer; 2021.

WHO Classification of Tumours Editorial Board. Endocrine and Neuroendocrine Tumours. 5th ed. Lyon: International Agency for Research on Cancer; 2022.

WHO Classification of Tumours Editorial Board. Urinary and Male Genital Tumours. 5th ed. Lyon: International Agency for Research on Cancer; 2022.

WHO Classification of Tumours Editorial Board. Skin Tumours. 5th ed. Lyon: International Agency for Research on Cancer; 2024.

AJCC Cancer Staging Manual

Amin MB, Edge SB, Greene FL, et al., editors. AJCC Cancer Staging Manual. 8th ed. New York: Springer; 2017 (corrected printing, 2018).

Royal College of Pathologists — Cancer Datasets

The RCPath dataset library — covering all major site-specific cancers and updated on a rolling basis — is the canonical reporting reference for United Kingdom practice. The datasets listed below are those most directly relevant to the chapters of Volume 1. Readers should download the current version of each dataset directly from the RCPath website at the time of examination preparation; revisions occur on a rolling basis.

Royal College of Pathologists. Dataset for histopathological reporting of oesophageal carcinoma. London: RCPath; current edition at time of preparation.

Royal College of Pathologists. Dataset for histopathological reporting of gastric carcinoma. London: RCPath.

Royal College of Pathologists. Dataset for histopathological reporting of colorectal cancer. London: RCPath.

Royal College of Pathologists. Dataset for histopathological reporting of hepatocellular carcinoma. London: RCPath.

Royal College of Pathologists. Dataset for histopathological reporting of pancreatic carcinoma. London: RCPath.

Royal College of Pathologists. Dataset for histopathological reporting of lung cancer. London: RCPath.

Royal College of Pathologists. Dataset for histopathological reporting of thyroid carcinoma. London: RCPath.

Royal College of Pathologists. Tissue pathways for medical renal biopsies. London: RCPath.

Royal College of Pathologists. Tissue pathways for medical liver biopsies. London: RCPath.

International Collaboration on Cancer Reporting (ICCR) Datasets

ICCR datasets harmonise reporting elements across participating jurisdictions — and frequently inform the structure of national datasets, including the RCPath datasets listed above. The site-specific ICCR documents most relevant to this volume are listed.

International Collaboration on Cancer Reporting. Histopathology reporting datasets — Digestive System; Thoracic; Endocrine; Urinary; Skin. Sydney: ICCR; current editions.

BSH Guidelines (Haematology Overlap with Histopathology)

British Society for Haematology. Guidelines for the diagnosis and investigation of trephine biopsy in chronic myeloproliferative neoplasms. Br J Haematol; current edition.

British Society for Haematology. Guidelines for the investigation and management of lymph node enlargement. Br J Haematol; current edition.

NICE Clinical Guidance

National Institute for Health and Care Excellence. Colorectal cancer — diagnosis and management. NG151. London: NICE; latest revision.

National Institute for Health and Care Excellence. Lung cancer — diagnosis and management. NG122. London: NICE; latest revision.

National Institute for Health and Care Excellence. Suspected cancer — recognition and referral. NG12. London: NICE; latest revision.

National Institute for Health and Care Excellence. Chronic kidney disease — assessment and management. NG203. London: NICE; latest revision.

Examination Preparation Notes

The notes below summarise the practical structure of the FRCPath Part 1 Histopathology written examination as it stood at the time of manuscript completion. Candidates should verify the current specification on the Royal College of Pathologists' website before any sitting, since paper structure, marking weight, and topic distribution are revised at intervals.

Paper structure

The Part 1 written paper combines two question formats — single best answer (SBA) items, each with five options of which one is the strongest fit, and extended matching questions (EMQs) with an option list of ten items shared across five stems. The paper is delivered electronically over a fixed sitting — and candidates are expected to manage time across both formats. Per-item time discipline is more important than item-by-item perfection.

Topic distribution

Coverage spans the full histopathology syllabus, with explicit reference to the WHO Classification of Tumours, the RCPath cancer datasets, the ICCR datasets, and current NICE pathways. The medical organ systems addressed in Volume 1 (gastrointestinal, hepatobiliary, pulmonary, cardiovascular, endocrine, renal, and medical dermatopathology) and the foundational laboratory sciences (fixation, processing, immunohistochemistry, frozen sections, autopsy, molecular techniques, quality assurance) together account for a large proportion of the typical paper. Volume 2 covers the remaining systems.

Approach to SBAs

Each SBA stem in this volume is constructed mechanism-first — that is, the clinical or histological detail necessary to discriminate between the five options is foregrounded rather than buried. Candidates are advised to read each stem twice, identify the discriminating feature before scanning the option list, and only then evaluate options. A practical pace of sixty to ninety seconds per item approximates the examination tempo — with longer items balanced against shorter items across the paper.

Approach to EMQs

EMQs invite a different cognitive habit — the option list of ten items is shared across five stems, and the examiners construct option lists to discriminate near-miss diagnoses. The disciplined approach is to read the entire option list first, group the options mentally by category (entity, immunohistochemical signature, syndromic association, classification term), and only then read the first stem. Hasty stem-first reading commonly costs candidates one or two marks per EMQ block.

Use of the recommended sources

The citation policy of this companion is intentionally narrow. Candidates are urged to consult — in current form, downloaded at the time of preparation — the relevant RCPath cancer datasets and the relevant WHO 5 chapters; ICCR datasets where the RCPath version is silent or outdated; AJCC TNM 8 for staging conventions; and NICE pathways for clinical context. Time spent on uncurated online compendia is poorly correlated with examination performance — and is not recommended.

Sittings and registration

FRCPath Part 1 sittings occur on a published schedule, with separate Spring and Autumn diets. Registration, eligibility criteria, fee structures, and venue allocations are administered directly by the Royal College of Pathologists. Candidates outside the United Kingdom should verify centre availability and visa or travel requirements well in advance of the registration deadline.

Index

References are to chapter and section numbers (e.g. 2.7 = Chapter 2, section 7), not page numbers. This convention survives layout revisions and supports cross-reference between the print and digital editions. Volume 2 cross-references are flagged where the principal coverage lies in that volume.

A

AJCC TNM 8 5.1, 8.4, 9.3, 11.2, 14.1, 15.2, 16.4, 22.5
Aldosteronoma 20.2
ALK fusion 2.6, 3.6, 15.4
Amyloid (Congo red) 1.7, 17.4, 18.6, 21.3
Amyloidosis, cardiac (AL, ATTR) 17.4
Anaplastic thyroid carcinoma 19.4
Anal pathology 11.7
ANCA-associated vasculitis 18.3, 21.3, 23.6
Antibody-mediated rejection (cardiac) 17.2
Antibody-mediated rejection (renal) 21.5
Antigen retrieval 2.2
Appendiceal mucinous neoplasia (LAMN, HAMN, PMP) 10.4
Artefacts (crush, cautery, drying, pigment, floater) 1.9
Atherosclerosis 18.4
Autoimmune hepatitis 12.4
Autopsy (hospital, coroner, forensic, Scotland) 6.1, 6.2, 6.3, 6.4

B

Banff schema (liver) 12.7
Banff schema (renal) 21.5
BAP1 (mesothelioma, uveal) 16.3
Barrett's oesophagus 8.3
Basal cell carcinoma (BCC) 23.6
Bethesda system (cervical, TBSRTC) 7.5, 7.6
Bethesda TBSRTC (thyroid) 7.6, 19.6
BRAF V600E (CRC, melanoma, PTC) 2.7, 3.7, 11.5, 19.2
Bullous pemphigoid 23.4

C

Calcium oxalate 21.4
Carcinoid (lung) 15.7
Cases of Note (RCPath) 5.5
Chapel Hill vasculitis classification 18.1
Cholangiocarcinoma 12.6, 13.4

M

MASH (NAFLD/NASH) 12.3
MCN (pancreas) 14.5
Medullary thyroid carcinoma (MEN 2) 19.4
Membranous nephropathy (PLA2R) 21.2
MEN 2 (RET) 19.4, 20.4
Mesothelioma 16.1, 16.2, 16.3
Minimal change disease 21.2
Mismatch repair (MMR IHC) 2.7, 3.10, 11.4
MSI testing 3.10
MTAP (mesothelioma) 16.3
Myocarditis 17.3

N

Never events 5.5
NICE clinical guidance Back matter
NIFTP 19.5
NSIP (non-specific interstitial pneumonia) 15.6

O

Oncocytoma (renal) 22.7
Organising pneumonia (OP) 15.6

P

p16 (cervix, oropharynx, vulva) (see Vol 2)
p53 (mutant pattern interpretation) 2.6
Pancreatic ductal adenocarcinoma (PDAC) 14.1, 14.2
Pancreatic neuroendocrine tumours (PanNETs) 14.6
PanIN 14.3
Pap stain 7.2
Papillary RCC 22.3
Papillary thyroid carcinoma (PTC) 19.4
Paragangliomas 20.4
Parathyroid pathology 19.7
PD-L1 (clones, scoring) 2.6, 15.5
Pemphigus vulgaris 23.4
Perls stain (iron) 1.7, 12.1

Cholecystitis (xanthogranulomatous) 13.1
Chromophobe RCC 22.3
Chronic hepatitis (staging) 12.2
CIDP 18.6
Clear cell RCC 22.2
Coeliac disease (Marsh) 10.1, 10.2
Cone biopsy interpretation (see Vol 2)
Controls (positive, negative, internal) 1.7, 2.3
Coroner's autopsy 6.2
CRC reporting 11.2
Crohn's disease 10.3, 11.3
Cytology (Pap, Romanowsky, cell block, ROSE) 7.2, 7.3, 7.4

D

DCIS (see Vol 2)
Decalcification (EDTA, formic acid) 1.3
Diffuse alveolar damage (DAD) 15.6
Digital pathology (WSI, RCPath validation) 1.8
Direct immunofluorescence (DIF) 21.1, 23.4
Disseminated intravascular pathology (see Vol 2)
Duct of Luschka 13.3

E

EBV (Helicobacter, gastric, lymphoma) 9.5
Eosinophilic oesophagitis 8.7
EQA (UK NEQAS) 1.10, 5.3
ER, PR (breast — see Vol 2) 2.5
Errors (classification, RCA, never events) 1.10, 5.3, 5.5
Examination preparation Back matter
Extended Matching Questions (EMQ) Back matter

F

FH-deficient RCC (HLRCC) 22.4
FIGO staging 5.1
FISH (break-apart, dual-probe) 2.4, 3.6
Fixation (NBF, Bouin, B5, glutaraldehyde) 1.2
FNCLCC grading (see Vol 2)
Follicular thyroid carcinoma 19.4
Frozen section (indications, contraindications) 4.1, 4.2

G

Gallbladder carcinoma 13.2
Gastric adenocarcinoma (Lauren, WHO 5, TCGA) 9.3, 9.4, 9.5
Giant cell arteritis 18.2

Phaeochromocytoma (PASS, GAPP, SDHB) 20.3
PitNETs (pituitary) 20.1
Placenta (see Vol 2)
Polymerase chain reaction (PCR, ddPCR) 3.3
Post-infectious glomerulonephritis 21.3
PRAS, MASS, BWH staging (see Vol 2 dermatopathology)
Primary biliary cholangitis (PBC) 12.4
Primary sclerosing cholangitis (PSC) 12.4, 13.4
Procurator Fiscal (Scotland) 6.4
Psoriasis 23.2

Q

Quality management (IQC, IQA, EQA) 1.10, 5.2

R

RCPath datasets 5.1, Back matter
Reaction patterns (skin) 23.1
Renal cell carcinoma (WHO 2022) Chapter 22
Renal transplant pathology (Banff) 21.5
Reporting standards (synoptic, ICCR, RCPath) 5.1
RET (MTC, MEN 2) 19.4
Reticulin (Gomori) 1.7, 12.5
Romanowsky stains (Diff-Quik, MGG) 7.2
Root cause analysis (RCA) 5.5
ROSE (rapid on-site evaluation) 7.4

S

Salivary gland tumours (see Vol 2)
Sarcoidosis 10.6, 23.5
SCC (oesophageal, anal) 8.4, 11.7
SDH-deficient tumours 2.6, 20.3
Sentinel lymph node (breast, melanoma) 4.3, (see Vol 2)
Serrated polyps (SSL, TSA) 11.1
Single Best Answer (SBA) Back matter
Skin tumours (BCC, SCC, melanoma) 23.6, (see Vol 2)
Solitary fibrous tumour 16.6
Special stains (panels and controls) 1.7
Squamous cell carcinoma (lung) 15.2
Steatohepatitis (MASH) 12.3
Sudden cardiac death 17.7
Sydney biopsy protocol (gastric) 9.1
Synoptic reporting 5.1

T

GIST (see Vol 2 — Soft Tissue)
Goblet cell adenocarcinoma 10.5

H

H&E staining 1.6
Hans algorithm (see Vol 2)
HDGC (CDH1) 9.6
Helicobacter pylori 9.1, 9.2
Hepatocellular carcinoma (HCC) 12.5
HER2 (gastric, breast) 2.5, 9.3
HSV oesophagitis 8.2
Human Tissue Act 2004 1.11
Hypertrophic cardiomyopathy 17.5

I

IBD-associated dysplasia 11.6
IgA nephropathy 21.3
IgG4-related disease 12.4, 13.5, 18.7
Immunohistochemistry (IHC) Chapter 2
Indications for frozen section 4.1
INPC/Shimada 20.6
INRG staging (neuroblastoma) 20.7
Intraoperative communication (closed-loop) 4.4
IPMN 14.4
ISH (EBER, HPV mRNA, FISH) 2.4
ISHLT cardiac rejection grading 17.1
ISO 15189 1.10, 5.2

K

Klatskin tumour 12.6
KRAS, NRAS (CRC, lung) 11.5, 15.4

L

Lichen planus 23.3
Liquid biopsy (ctDNA) 3.11
Liver transplant biopsy (Banff) 12.7
Lung adenocarcinoma patterns (IASLC 2020) 15.1, 15.3
Lupus nephritis (ISN/RPS) 21.3
Lynch syndrome (MMR IHC) 2.7, 3.10, 11.4

Takayasu arteritis 18.1
Thrombotic microangiopathy 21.4
Thyroid carcinoma — WHO 5 19.4
Tissue banking 1.11
TNM staging 5.1
Tubular adenoma 11.1
Tubulointerstitial nephritis 21.4
Turnaround time (TAT) 5.5

U

UIP (usual interstitial pneumonia) 15.6
UK NEQAS 1.10, 5.3
Ulcerative colitis 11.3

V

Validation of WSI 1.8
Variant interpretation (ACMG, AMP, ESCAT) 3.5
Vasculitis (Chapel Hill) 18.1
VHL 20.4, 22.2

W

Whipple disease 10.2
WHO Classification of Tumours, 5e Back matter
WHO/ISUP grading (RCC) 22.2, 22.3
Wilms tumour 22.6

X

Xanthogranulomatous cholecystitis 13.1

Z

Ziehl-Neelsen (acid-fast) 1.7

Made in the USA
Monee, IL
13 September 2026

62973774R00142